ESSENTIAL CLINICAL SKILLS IN NURSING

Sara Miller McCune founded SAGE Publishing in 1965 to support the dissemination of usable knowledge and educate a global community. SAGE publishes more than 1000 journals and over 800 new books each year, spanning a wide range of subject areas. Our growing selection of library products includes archives, data, case studies and video. SAGE remains majority owned by our founder and after her lifetime will become owned by a charitable trust that secures the company's continued independence.

Los Angeles | London | New Delhi | Singapore | Washington DC | Melbourne

ESSENTIAL CLINICAL SKILLS IN NURSING

EDITED BY
DEBORAH ROWBERRY,
LEE GAUNTLETT AND
LIBOR HURT

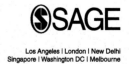

Los Angeles | London | New Delhi
Singapore | Washington DC | Melbourne

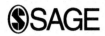

Los Angeles | London | New Delhi
Singapore | Washington DC | Melbourne

SAGE Publications Ltd
1 Oliver's Yard
55 City Road
London EC1Y 1SP

SAGE Publications Inc.
2455 Teller Road
Thousand Oaks, California 91320

SAGE Publications India Pvt Ltd
Unit No. 323–333, Third Floor, F-Block
International Trade Tower, Nehru Place
New Delhi 110 019

SAGE Publications Asia-Pacific Pte Ltd
3 Church Street
#10-04 Samsung Hub
Singapore 049483

Editor: Laura Walmsley
Development editor: Jessica Moran
Editorial assistant: Sahar Jamfar
Production editor: Martin Fox
Marketing manager: Ruslana Khatagova
Cover design: Sheila Tong
Typeset by: C&M Digitals (P) Ltd, Chennai, India
Printed in the UK

Library of Congress Control Number: 2022944854

British Library Cataloguing in Publication data

A catalogue record for this book is available from the British Library

ISBN 978-1-5297-7103-9
ISBN 978-1-5297-7102-2 (pbk)

At SAGE we take sustainability seriously. Most of our products are printed in the UK using responsibly sourced papers and boards. When we print overseas we ensure sustainable papers are used as measured by the PREPS grading system. We undertake an annual audit to monitor our sustainability.

This book is dedicated to everyone that has helped along the way. In particular to colleagues that did not get to finish it with us, Brian Mfula and Gerwyn Panes. Always missed.

CONTENTS

Guide to Using Your Book ix

Online Resources xiii

About the Editors xv

About the Contributors xvii

Acknowledgements xxi

Publisher's Acknowledgements xxiii

Introduction xxv

Part I Essential Knowledge for Clinical Skills **1**

1 Evidence-Based Practice and Clinical Skills 3
   Libor Hurt

2 The Importance of Assessment 29
   Deborah Rowberry, Peter Sewell and Wendy Churchouse

3 The Importance of Communication 51
   Deborah Rowberry

Part II Clinical Skills for Nursing Care **69**

4 History Taking and Examinations 71
   Lee Gauntlett and Peter Sewell

5 Dignity, Comfort, Rest and Sleep 119
   Sarah Tait and Louise Giles, with Sarah Kingdom-Mills (learning disabilities contribution)

6 Hygiene and Skin Integrity 135
   Nicola Tingle and Nerys Williams, with Sarah Kingdom-Mills (learning disabilities contribution)

7 Nutrition and Hydration 171
   Helen Beckett and Lovely Sajan

8 Bladder and Bowel Health 209
   Jemma Gustafson and Trudi Petersen

9 Mobility and Safety 251
   Jamie Wheeler and Lovely Sajan, with Sarah Kingdom-Mills (learning disabilities contribution)

10 Respiratory Care 283
    Gabby Wilcox

11 Preventing and Managing Infection 313
    Lisa Duffy and Lee Gauntlett

12   End of Life Care   349
     Hywel Thomas, Deb McNee, Alison Young, Wendy Mashlan, Julie Hayes and Nicola Dawkins

13   Medication Administration   375
     Nicola Henwood

Index   429

GUIDE TO USING YOUR BOOK

Essential Clinical Skills in Nursing includes a variety of learning features that have been specially designed to help you succeed in your studies.

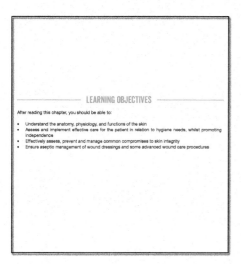

LEARNING OBJECTIVES

An overview of the knowledge and skills you should acquire from reading each chapter.

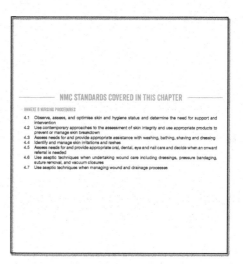

NMC STANDARDS

A list of the key *Annexe B – The Future Nurse Standards (NMC 2018)* covered in Chapters 4–13.

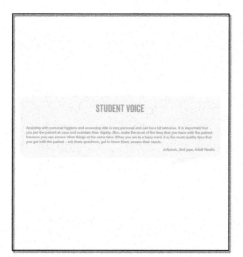

STUDENT VOICE

Short quotes from real Nursing students, offering advice, reassurance, and first-hand insights.

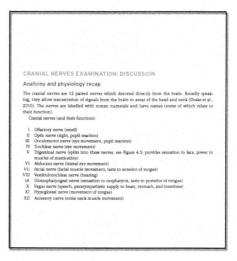

ANATOMY AND PHYSIOLOGY RECAP

High-level overviews of the key anatomy and physiology.

CARDIOVASCULAR AUSCULTATION: DISCUSSION

Cardiovascular auscultation (listening of sounds) is a routine examination performed by a range of health professionals in a variety of settings. It is suitable to be conducted alongside the respiratory examination.

The examination is performed with the heart anatomy in mind; we have four heart chambers and four valves which are located beneath the rib cage. The valves are auscultated beneath specific rib spaces whilst the examiner also palpates the carotid pulse. This allows the relationship between the pulse and the cardiac sounds to be correlated.

— CARDIOVASCULAR AUSCULTATION: STEP BY STEP —

- Ideally the patient's chest should be fully exposed, so the examination should be conducted in a closed room or behind curtains to maintain dignity. Furthermore, a blanket could be used to protect the patient's modesty to loosely cover the chest wall, and lifted for placement of the stethoscope.
- Palpate (feel) the radial pulse, assess rate and rhythm (for one minute).
- Compare radial pulses by palpating each pulse simultaneously, looking for any sign of radial-radial delay between them.
- Ask patient to open mouth and look at tongue/oral mucosa (it may be suitable to use a pen torch and tongue depressor for this step; you may need to action the movement required for some patients to understand what is required here).
- Hold the diaphragm of the stethoscope between the index and middle finger of your dominant hand and place the stethoscope onto the patient's chest, using gentle pressure. While palpating the carotid pulse with your non-dominant hand, auscultate the anterior chest wall in four different positions:
  o 2nd intercostal space, right sternal edge (aortic valve)
  o 2nd intercostal space, left sternal edge (pulmonary valve)
  o 5th intercostal space, right sternal edge (tricuspid valve)
  o 5th intercostal space, mid clavicular line (mitral valve)
- Check lower limbs for signs of peripheral oedema; press on the ankles and lower legs. See if your finger marks remain in the skin.
- Once the examination is complete, ask the patient to cover themselves or redress.
- Document your examination findings.

CLINICAL SKILLS: DISCUSSION

Brief discussions on the relevant theory, rationale and person-centred considerations behind each skill.

CLINICAL SKILLS: STEP BY STEP

Step-by-step instructions for performing each skill.

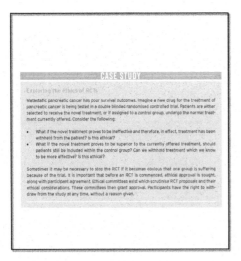

CASE STUDY

Exploring the ethics of RCTs

Metastatic pancreatic cancer has poor survival outcomes. Imagine a new drug for the treatment of pancreatic cancer is being tested in a double blinded randomised controlled trial. Patients are either selected to receive the novel treatment, or if assigned to a control group, undergo the normal treatment currently offered. Consider the following:

- What if the novel treatment proves to be ineffective and therefore, in effect, treatment has been withheld from the patient? Is this ethical?
- What if the novel treatment proves to be superior to the currently offered treatment, should patients still be included within the control group? Can we withhold treatment which we know to be more effective? Is this ethical?

Sometimes it may be necessary to stop the RCT if it becomes obvious that one group is suffering because of the trial. It is important that before an RCT is commenced, ethical approval is sought, along with participant agreement. Ethical committees exist which scrutinise RCT proposals and their ethical considerations. These committees then grant approval. Participants have the right to withdraw from the study at any time, without a reason given.

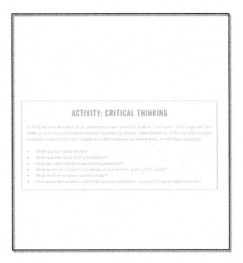

ACTIVITY: CRITICAL THINKING

In 1998 Andrew Wakefield et al. published a (now retracted) study in The Lancet which suggested the MMR vaccine may lead to developmental disorders in children (Wakefield et al., 1998). Considering what has been covered within this chapter and after reviewing the above study, answer these questions:

- What was the study design?
- What was the study trying to achieve?
- How was information analysed and presented?
- What would be a good study design to achieve the goals of this study?
- What level of evidence was the study?
- How would the evidence affect the general population, including those in deprived areas?

CASE STUDY

Real-world examples of clinical skills in practice, showcasing the experiences and requirements of a range of patients.

ACTIVITY

Practical activities that help you to hone your skills and reflect on what you have learnt so far.

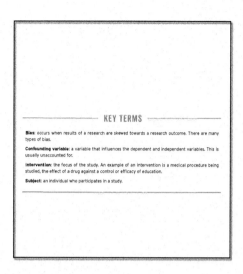

GO FURTHER

A selection of relevant resources, including journal articles, websites and videos, that enable you to go one step further in your studies.

KEY TERMS

Technical terms or key concepts highlighted within the text and accompanied by short explanations.

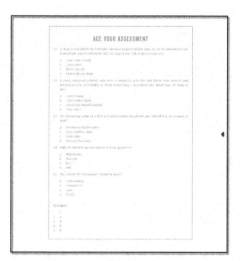

ACE YOUR ASSESSMENT

A selection of multiple-choice questions at the end of each chapter allowing you to test your understanding of the content.

ONLINE RESOURCES

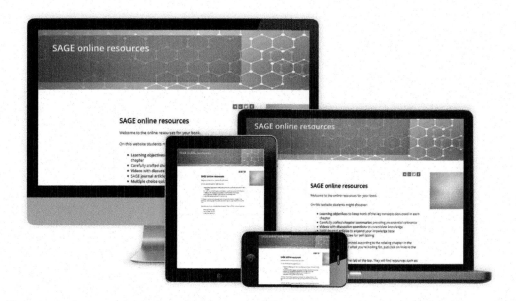

Students and instructors can visit https://study.sagepub.com/rowberry to access over **25 videos** demonstrating clinical skills in practice, from oxygen administration to venepuncture, cannulation and more.

A **video teaching guide** is also available to instructors and features chapter overviews and questions relating to each video.

USING THE QR CODES IN THE BOOK

QR codes have been placed throughout the book to direct you straight to relevant video content.

Got an iPhone?

- Open the camera app on your phone
- Hold the camera over the QR code of the video you want to watch
- Tap the notification when it appears

Got an Android?

- Open the camera app on your phone or download a QR scanner app
- Hold the camera or open the app over the QR code of the video you want to watch
- Tap the notification when it appears

ABOUT THE EDITORS

EDITOR

Deborah Rowberry is a Senior Lecturer at Swansea University working in the Department of Nursing. She has over 20 years clinical experience in a variety of settings including, neurology, acute medicine, cardiac ITU and nephrology and moved into education almost 15 years ago. Deborah is a Fellow of the Higher Education Academy and a double recipient of the University's Excellence in Learning and Teaching Award. Deborah has previous experience as a Clinical Skills Educator for postgraduate medicine and undergraduate Medical Students. Deborah's specialist and research interest areas include Simulation Based Education and Interprofessional Education.

CO-EDITORS

Dr Lee Gauntlett is a trainee anaesthetist working in South Wales with experience in intensive care medicine. His career began working as a healthcare support worker in several hospitals in the Midlands and volunteering within the British Red Cross, starting medical training in 2013. He came to the medical profession as a mature student from a marketing background and recognises the value in diversity. He is keen to teach nurses, medical students, and allied health professionals, strongly believing that a multidisciplinary approach to learning can lead to beneficial patient outcomes.

Dr Libor Hurt was born in the Czech Republic and moved to the UK aged 11. He began working as a hospital porter in the summer holidays and evenings after college and carried on doing this whilst reading Medical Sciences at De Montfort University. Following this, he pursued a further MSc by Research in Learning Technology there, before eventually going on to study medicine at Swansea University. He rotated through several medical and surgical specialities and ultimately began working as a general surgery speciality trainee. Dr Hurt enjoys teaching and mentoring, actively participating whenever given the opportunity to do so. He has presented his research at both a national and international level on a wide variety of topics, such as antibiotic treatment of appendicitis during the Covid-19 pandemic and outcomes of hepatic metastasectomy in patients with anal squamous cell carcinoma. In his spare time, Dr Hurt enjoys exploring the diverse Welsh landscape.

ABOUT THE CONTRIBUTORS

Helen Beckett is a Senior Lecturer in Children's Nursing at Swansea University working in the Department of Nursing. Helen is a Registered Children's Nurse and has over 18 years clinical experience in a variety of paediatric settings including burns, medicine, surgical and High Dependency Care (HDU). Helen holds a Master's degree in Education for Health Professions and is a Fellow of the Higher Education Academy. Helen is field lead for Children's Nursing Pre-registration Nursing at Swansea University, and has specialist interest in Acute care, clinical skills, and Simulation Based Education.

Wendy Churchouse (BEM – MSc Cardiology, RGN, ENG, DipN, Cert Ed, FETC, NNEB) is a Senior Lecturer in Non-Medical Prescribing, Swansea University. Her extensive clinical background encompasses haematology, diabetes and vascular surgery. However, for over 30 years, she has focused on cardiac care working in primary, secondary and tertiary care. Wendy has been fortunate to work with highly motivated teams and has pioneered various service developments and innovations. She was involved in the development of the Welsh NSF for CHD and acted as clinical expert on NICE heart failure and ICD/CRT guidelines. In 2016, she was awarded the Queens British Empire Medal for developing patient focused services and patient support groups. She regularly speaks at national conferences and has numerous publications related to the above specialties.

Lisa Duffy has advanced experience and knowledge of the practical and theoretical issues relating to Infection Prevention and Control practice and education. Lisa's clinical experience spans several roles, from Senior Clinical Nurse working as a member of the IP&C Team capturing all aspects of prevention, investigation, surveillance and control of infection. She has also promoted the provision of safe environments of care for service users, the public and staff in terms of Infection Prevention and Control. Lisa has been a Senior Lecturer at Swansea University for six years and as well as Programme Director for Undergraduate Nursing. She has also worked with Health Education and Improvement Wales (HEIW) focusing on IP&C education and workforce transformation. Lisa made a substantive contribution to the assessment and supervision of pre-registration nursing within the fields of adult, child and mental health. Additionally, Lisa is the regional education officer for the Infection Prevention Society which provides the opportunity to collaborate with other IP&C professionals both nationally and internationally.

Louise Giles (MAEd, PGDip, BSc (Hons), RGN, SFHEA, FNF Scholar) has been a practising registered nurse for the past 35 years with experience in several care environments, clinical roles, managerial roles, leadership roles, practice development and education roles. This has provided Louise with a great depth of knowledge and skills that offer a solid foundation to current and future professional practice along with writing for journals and books.

Jemma Gustafson (RGN, BAc, BSc, PgCertHE) is a clinical skills Lecturer in the Faculty of Medicine, Health and Life Science at Swansea University, teaching a range of modules on pre-registration courses, a healthcare certificate course and return to practice. Jemma currently leads on the first module for the BSC

Pre-registration Adult Nursing course, working collaboratively and informing teaching within local health boards. Previously an educator in practice as a clinical skills trainer with a speciality in vascular access, Jemma is a registered adult nurse with a background in acute care, clinical decision. Jemma has expertise in teaching nursing skills and simulation at all levels of the pre-registration programme with a particular interest in developing contemporary support mechanisms for students to gain quick access and information.

Nicola Henwood is an Adult Registered Nurse. She qualified from Swansea University in 2009 and has since worked in a variety of inpatient and community areas in the UK and Australia. She has gained additional qualifications in teaching, as well as a master's in Public Health and Health Promotion. For a short time, she returned to Swansea University as a lecturer, before moving to Children's Mental Health Services.

Sarah Kingdom-Mills is a Learning Disability Nurse, working as a Care Home Education Facilitator at Health Education Improvement Wales. Her clinical experiences vary from acute inpatient assessment and treatment, specialist learning disability and autism services to complex behavioural challenges and continuing healthcare needs. Sarah had two decades of clinical experience within the learning disability field of nursing within health and social care settings prior to working in practice education. Sarah is an alumnus with the RCN and has been a finalist in the Nurse of the Year Awards for the category of 'Supporting Education and Learning in Practice'; she also chairs the All-Wales Practice Educator Forum and is a Bevan Commission Exemplar for her work in creating student nurse placements within care homes. Key interest areas are effective communication, advocacy and best interest; she has been involved in these areas for many years. She feels that the profile of learning disabilities is being positively raised through several forums, and this is work that she continues to champion within her professional career.

Deb McNee is a Child Nursing Lecturer at Swansea University predominantly teaching undergraduate nursing students. She has held this position for four years and teaches across many other disciplines including public health, paramedics and osteopathy. Her background is in child health with over 30+ years' experience. Most of this experience was within primary care, first as a children's nurse and then as a Health Visitor. She holds an MSc in Specialist Community Public Health Nursing and has a specialist interest in vulnerable groups, health promotion, paediatric palliative care and end of life care.

Trudi Petersen (RMN, BSc, PgDip, MSc.Econ) trained as a psychiatric nurse between 1987 and 1990. She has worked in substance misuse and dual diagnosis, health promotion and both acute and longer term mental health settings. She has worked as a clinician, a manager, a lecturer and a research practitioner. She has worked in NHS, third sector and private settings. She currently works as the Projects and Innovations lead for Welsh care provider Fieldbay Ltd. Her interests include behaviour and behaviour change, psychological aspects of physical health conditions, brain injury, effective engagement and knowledge transfer and innovations in nursing. Trudi holds an honorary lecturer's position with Swansea University.

Lovely Sajan is a highly motivated and enthusiastic educator with great passion for clinical skills teaching. She gained her clinical expertise from her experience in the NHS in medical and cardiac areas, continuing healthcare and haemoglobinopathy settings for 16 years. She also has six years of background in teaching in higher education and is currently working as a lecturer at Swansea University. She holds an MSc in Nursing Science, with additional teaching qualifications and accreditations. She is devoted to her career and loves to support and develop students in gaining knowledge, skills and expertise required in their profession as a qualified nurse.

Peter Sewell (MSc Advanced Practice, BSc Critical Care, Dip Nurs. RGN. FICM Assoc.) is an Advanced Critical Care Practitioner and part-time Senior Lecturer in Advanced Practice and Non-medical Prescribing at Swansea School of Health and Social Care. He qualified as a RGN in 2003 and has worked in Acute and Critical Care services since. He was an Intensive Care and Critical Care Outreach charge nurse until 2013, when he trained to become an Advanced Critical Care Practitioner in Morriston Hospital, Swansea.

Sarah Tait is a Senior Nurse Lecturer in the Mental Health Department of the School of Health and Social Care at Swansea University. She began her nursing career in 1991 and qualified as a Registered General Nurse (RGN) in 1995 and a Registered Mental Health Nurse (RNMH) in 2001. In 2014, Sarah became recognised as a Fellow of the Higher Education Academy (FHEA). Sarah completed a MA in Education for Health Professionals in 2016. Sarah predominantly teaches within the pre-registration nursing curriculum and is an academic mentor to pre-registration nursing students on a variety of full-time and part-time programmes. Sarah also teaches and leads a module on the postgraduate, Advanced Practice and Education – MSc in Advanced Practice. Sarah is the Mental Health Field Lead for the BSC Mental Health Nursing Programme.

Hywel Thomas has been qualified as a mental health nurse since 1997. A 25-year mental health nursing career has been a mixture of clinical practitioner working in several inpatient and community settings notably within the older persons mental health speciality and pre-registration education delivering on the current Nursing and Midwifery Council (NMC, 2018). Hywel has been employed at Swansea University initially as a Lecturer and now Senior Lecturer from January 2012 to the present date. His responsibilities as a senior lecturer involve delivering teaching on the current pre-registration, part time and masters nursing programmes and curriculum development as module and field lead. He is currently the Mental Health Undergraduate Admissions Tutor within the Faculty of Medicine, Health & Life Science, Swansea University.

Gabby Wilcox is a sister in a busy emergency department in Swansea with responsibility for teaching and assessing. She registered in 2005 and began her career in respiratory nursing. Since then, she has worked in burns, critical care and emergency nursing, spanning several UK hospitals as well as spending time working in France and the Middle East. Gabby has a Masters in Critical Care from Cardiff University and a PGCE from Swansea University. She is incredibly passionate about clinical skills teaching and patient assessment; her special areas of interest lie in major incident response, trauma care and resuscitation.

Nerys Williams is an Adult Nursing Senior Lecturer in the pre-registration and the master's level nursing programmes at Swansea University. Nerys has a clinical background in burns and reconstructive surgery, working in burns intensive care, burns theatre, plastics trauma and as a Plastics Trauma Nurse Practitioner and Burns Outreach Clinical Nurse Specialist.

Jamie Wheeler is a Lecturer in Mental Health Nursing. He has worked in several clinical settings and has a wealth of experience. Jamie is Lead for Manual Handling training for the faculty as well as responsible for Violence and Aggression education.

ACKNOWLEDGEMENTS

Writing this book has been fun (no, not a typo). The process has been made so much more enjoyable and easy because of the constant and invaluable help from a very special set of people, Laura (we do not know what we would have done without you), Jess, Charlotte and Sunita – thank you all sincerely.

PUBLISHER'S ACKNOWLEDGEMENTS

The publishers would like to thank all of the academic reviewers who contributed thoughtful and helpful feedback on various parts of the book throughout the development stages, as well as those who contributed video content.

Hannah Ames, University of Plymouth

Sean Baker, University of Chester

Patience Bamisaye, Anglia Ruskin University

Lesley Butcher, Cardiff University

Katrina Emerson, University of East Anglia

Deborah Fallon, University of Manchester

Gary Francis, London South Bank University

Barbara Howard Hunt, Birmingham City University

Calvin Moorley, London South Bank University

Fiona Knights, University of Huddersfield

Michelle O'Reilly, Edinburgh Napier University

Suhaylah Patel, University of Central Lancashire

Debbie Rainey, Queens University Belfast

Boikhutso Shianyana, University of Plymouth

Pamela Young, University of the West of Scotland

INTRODUCTION

The aim of this book was always to provide a supportive resource for clinical skills in the nursing curriculum. Annexe B of the NMC's *The Future Nurse* standards (https://www.nmc.org.uk/globalassets/sitedocuments/standards-of-proficiency/nurses/future-nurse-proficiencies.pdf) was the rationale and drive for developing the book. The overall focus was to have a resource that both learners and faculty could use when teaching the additional clinical skills.

Using the book – The chapters follow *The Future Nurse* platforms and skills covered are outlined in each chapter as step by step instructions. Chapters include an anatomy and physiology recap where appropriate as a starting point for learners. This does not seek to replace a deeper understanding of the relevant anatomy knowledge. The skills are supported by a series of video guides; users can use the QR codes to access the links.

We value and have ensured equality, diversity and inclusivity are addressed where reasonably practicable but do recognise limitations to this. Learners should also recognise the importance of this area when practicing. The editors and contributors come from a diverse background, some with experience outside of nursing. We hope this brings several different perspectives to the chapters. We have also included field specific aspects of care where able to do so and had contributors from all four fields of nursing.

Learners – as student nurses you will learn many new topics including an array of clinical skills. We hope you use this book and video guides to support your clinical practice and university learning. Chapters and clinical skills have been written from a generic aspect, it is important for your learning that you consider any specific policies that are applicable to the Health Boards or Trusts you work with, they can vary and there will be differences in different clinical/practice areas. Remember to try the multiple-choice questions at the end of each chapter to enhance your learning.

Faculty – As with any book, there are limitations and this one is no different. The aim was always to outline the pure skill, with additional care and treatment aspects included where possible. It does not include everything; we hope it is a starting point for supporting your teaching or clinical skills labs.

We hope you enjoy using it as much as we all enjoyed contributing to it.

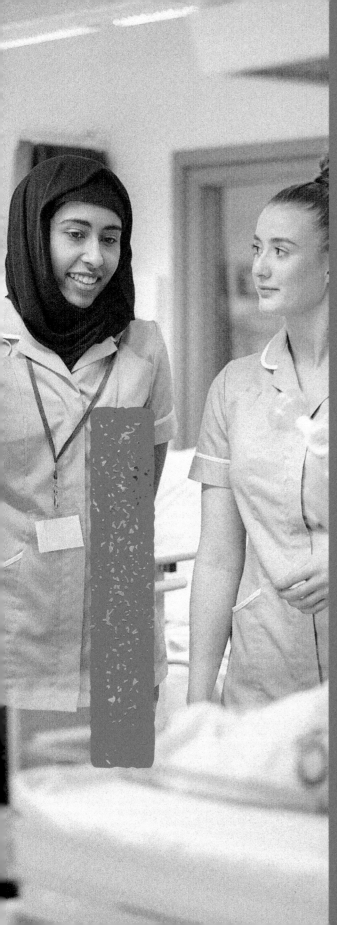

ESSENTIAL KNOWLEDGE FOR CLINICAL SKILLS

1   EVIDENCE-BASED PRACTICE
    AND CLINICAL SKILLS   3

2   THE IMPORTANCE OF
    ASSESSMENT   29

3   THE IMPORTANCE OF
    COMMUNICATION   51

EVIDENCE-BASED PRACTICE AND CLINICAL SKILLS

1

LIBOR HURT

LEARNING OBJECTIVES

After reading this chapter, you should be able to:

- Identify the importance of evidence-based nursing practice
- Describe different levels of evidence hierarchy
- Describe different study designs
- Design a search strategy
- Assess the quality of a source
- Know how to begin appraising research
- Recognise the utility of various clinical skills in practice

STUDENT VOICE

I remember the humbling honesty of my mentor when she told the patient on the colorectal ward that she didn't know much about the hormonal treatment for breast cancer. It was then that I realised that I didn't necessarily need to know everything, but I definitely needed to know how to find the information that I need!

Jenni, 2nd year, Adult Nursing

INTRODUCTION

With the advent of the internet, information has become more available than ever before. Patients will search the internet for answers to their ailments; medical professionals can utilise the same network to access information. However, just because information is available, it does not always mean that it is reliable, that it has been researched, scrutinised and peer reviewed or is accepted by a professional body via consensus.

Now more than ever nurses are within the public eye. Often their choices for treatments are scrutinised and must be justified. This means that nurses should be able to use evidence to justify their practice. NMC standards state that the role of the registered nurse within the 21st century is to 'play a vital role in providing, leading and coordinating care that is compassionate, **evidence-based** and person–centred' (NMC, 2018a: 3).

What does this mean? How do you analyse information to ensure that it is safe for your patients? This chapter will outline the hierarchy of scientific evidence and its application to evidence-based nursing care. It will discuss how evidence-based practice is the process of attaining, analysing, and applying research to improve clinical practice and patient outcomes. Evidence-based practice allows us to deliver the highest quality care which is cost-efficient and responsible. It must be noted that nurses should be able to piece together various sources of evidence to provide care for patients and this will not always include the highest levels of evidence. A nurse should however be equipped with the skills to determine the value of the evidence that they are appraising. To understand the value of research evidence, we will explore the hierarchy of evidence and discuss levels of strength next.

HIERARCHY OF EVIDENCE

For us to be able to assess evidence in the form of research, we must first appreciate that not all research is equally reliable. Therefore, not all evidence is equal and some pieces of evidence have greater validity than others. There exists a hierarchy of evidence. To illustrate this, Figure 1.1 orders different types of research by the relative strength of the evidence they produce. Level 1 produces the highest quality evidence with each subsequent level being thought of as less rigorous. Each level is defined below and subsequently discussed further. Figure 1.1 demonstrates the different levels of evidence, with pale blue representing the weakest levels and dark blue the strongest levels.

--- KEY TERMS ---

Validity: results representing true findings among individuals with similar characteristics outside of the study as within the study.

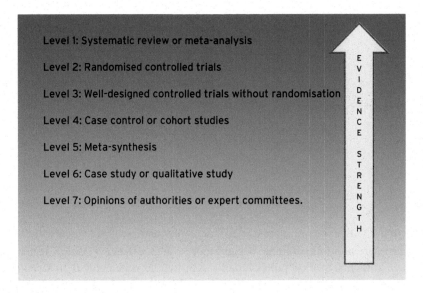

Figure 1.1 Hierarchy of evidence

STUDY DESIGN

The framework or methods and procedures utilised to collect and analyse data are called the study design. A particular study design is dependent upon the research question, resources available to the researcher and ultimately the aims of the study. Study design can be descriptive or analytical (Ranganathan, 2018). An example of a descriptive study is a case study or case report. Analytical studies can further be observational such as cohort studies or experimental such as randomised controlled trials. These types of study design are discussed in more detail below in their respective hierarchical order.

Level 1: Systematic review and meta analysis

Systematic review and meta-analysis combine, analyse and present data from high quality studies, typically randomised controlled trials, and form the highest level of evidence. These comprehensive studies essentially provide a summary of the research available pertaining to a particular question (Averis and Pearson, 2003). To conduct a systematic review, the study design will contain a protocol of key steps. Firstly, the research question must be defined, and this is often done using the PICO model discussed within the research question portion of this chapter. Then the inclusion and exclusion criteria are listed to ensure consistency and relevance to the research question. A search is performed, usually via a journal database, and the identified studies are scrutinised against the inclusion and exclusion criteria. Data is then extracted and analysed (Egger et al., 2022). It can often be combined and is typically presented in a table format.

A systematic review will often carry out statistical analyses of combined data from the various studies included to form new statistical conclusions. This is called a meta-analysis. It is important to note that not all systematic reviews will contain a meta-analysis. A meta-analysis is only ever available in a systematic review and not in other levels of evidence.

Meta-analyses provide stronger statistical evidence due to an increased number of subjects or accumulated results, when compared to results from a single study. Nonetheless, even meta-analyses are susceptible to bias, for example, if they contain data from disparate studies. This can produce unreliable results and we must always aim to scrutinise the research method, before accepting the outcomes provided (Greco et al., 2013).

In summary, a systematic review is the process through which studies are selected, analysed and their evidence is synthesised. A Meta-analysis is the statistical process of combining data obtained in a systematic review.

Level 2: Randomised controlled trials

--- **KEY TERMS** ---

Bias: occurs when results of a research are skewed towards a research outcome. There are many types of bias.

Confounding variable: a variable that influences the dependent and independent variables. This is usually unaccounted for.

Intervention: the focus of the study. An example of an intervention is a medical procedure being studied, the effect of a drug against a control or efficacy of education.

Subject: an individual who participates in a study.

Randomised controlled trials (RCTs) are the most rigourous method of testing a hypothesis and are therefore regarded as a gold standard when testing an intervention. They are an example of an experimental study design where an intervention is compared to a control.

A subject is usually randomly assigned to one of two groups. The group which has the intervention that is being tested, such as a new vaccine, or a group which acts as a comparison or control. Participants are randomly assigned a group, which is thought to reduce selection bias. This randomisation further allows us to minimise confounding variables and arguably produces more accurate data (Suresh, 2011).

RCTs can further be improved by designing the study as a double-blind RCT. In this study design, neither the researcher nor the subject knows which intervention they are giving or getting. Again, this is an attempt to reduce bias, including that of the placebo effect. A placebo is usually inert and used as the control; the placebo effect occurs when a change can be attributed to the treatment expectations of a subject rather than the action of the intervention (Colloca and Benedetti, 2005).

Although an RCT is arguably the best method of investigating an intervention, it too has its own drawbacks. It is important to be aware of this. Results from an RCT may not always mimic real life. This is because such studies can be designed with stringent inclusion and exclusion criteria, for example a novel treatment for asthma may exclude smokers or those with existing pulmonary disease. In real life asthma often forms a part of a list of comorbidities which may preclude the treatment from working. Thus, study criteria may not always translate to real patients whose medical needs are complex.

Interventions can also be carried out in highly controlled settings which may not always be replicated within the clinical setting, whether this is on the wards, clinic or out in the community.

Finally, it may not be appropriate to carry out an RCT due to ethical considerations. For example, consider a RCT which aims to establish the efficacy of immune therapy treatment for haematological malignancy. There may be treatment and control arms. It would be unethical to carry on the study if it became apparent that the treatment arm is superior in terms of improving overall survival.

CASE STUDY

Exploring the ethics of RCTs

Metastatic pancreatic cancer has poor survival outcomes. Imagine a new drug for the treatment of pancreatic cancer is being tested in a double blinded randomised controlled trial. Patients are either selected to receive the novel treatment, or if assigned to a control group, undergo the normal treatment currently offered. Consider the following:

- What if the novel treatment proves to be ineffective and therefore, in effect, treatment has been withheld from the patient? Is this ethical?
- What if the novel treatment proves to be superior to the currently offered treatment, should patients still be included within the control group? Can we withhold treatment which we know to be more effective? Is this ethical?

Sometimes it may be necessary to stop the RCT if it becomes obvious that one group is suffering because of the trial. It is important that before an RCT is commenced, ethical approval is sought, along with participant agreement. Ethical committees exist which scrutinise RCT proposals and their ethical considerations. These committees then grant approval. Participants have the right to withdraw from the study at any time, without a reason given.

Level 3: Well-designed controlled trials without randomisation

──────────────────── **KEY TERMS** ────────────────────

Quasi-Experimental study design: in this study design there is no random assignment to a particular group. Typically, a researcher will assign a participant to an intervention using another predefined criterion. This type of study design aims to establish a cause-and-effect relationship. The lack of randomisation influences validity as it does not minimise confounding variables.

There are many other ways in which studies assess the efficacy of an intervention. Studies can still contain an intervention without randomisation. Remember that randomisation attempts to reduce bias and therefore studies which do not randomise as part of the design are thought to be less rigourous.

The subtypes of these types of studies include:

- **Non-randomised controlled trials**, where participants are allocated to either intervention or control without randomisation.
- **Controlled before and after studies**, where outcomes are measured before introducing an intervention and after the intervention. Any outcomes are then attributed to the intervention. These types of studies can still include a control arm, and data would also be collected before the control and after. This can be used when RCTs are not possible and can often be less expensive to run. An example would be measuring cholesterol in a subject, then giving them medication to lower cholesterol and measuring it again after. The control arm would have no intervention.
- **Interrupted time series studies**, which utilise different time points in relation to the intervention. Data collection would occur at different time points prior to the intervention and after the intervention. This is a type of a quasi-experimental study design which tries to determine a cause-and-effect relationship. Different time points are utilised to establish whether the reported outcomes are due to the intervention, or mere trends over time. An example would be measuring monthly admissions to a respiratory ward and then banning smoking. This would be the interruption or intervention, then rates of admission would be measured again.

Level 4: Case control and cohort studies

Case control studies

──────────────────── **KEY TERMS** ────────────────────

Confidence interval: a range of values likely to include the population value. For example, a 95% confidence interval means that there is 95% certainty the population mean will lie between the upper and lower limit of the confidence interval.

Incidence: the proportion of an outcome developing within a defined time-period. For example, the number of new cases of a disease per year.

Odds ratio: the ratio of the odds of an exposure in the outcome group vs the odds of an exposure in the control group.

Prevalence: the likelihood of an outcome being present within a population. For example, the number of cases of a disease within a population.

Case control studies attempt to determine whether an intervention or exposure has association with an outcome. They are an example of observational study design where participants are selected based on the outcome or indeed lack of it, termed cases and controls respectively. Two groups of subjects are analysed, those with the outcome being studied (such as a particular illness or condition) and those without. Researchers would then deduce whether those in either group were subject to the intervention or exposure being studied. An example of this would be bladder cancer and the exposure or lack thereof to aniline dyes.

Because data is collected from the past in case control studies, the researcher already knows what the outcome is for each participant. In the example above, the researcher will already know if the participant had bladder cancer. Furthermore, because data is collected from the past, this would make this study design a retrospective study.

The advantages of this study design are that it can be relatively quicker than an RCT for example. Because the outcome is already known, rarer effects can be studied. For example, it allows for the study of rare diseases based on a particular exposure and allows the researchers to include all known subjects with the rare disease. This is faster than providing the exposure as an intervention and waiting for the rare outcomes to occur. Case control studies can also be useful when evaluating disease outbreaks. This is because a particular exposure may lead to a disease. The outcomes of a case control study may then be used to justify more rigourous study designs looking at the exposure effect relationship in more detail.

Case control studies produce an odds ratio. This is a measure of the association between an exposure or intervention and the studied outcome.

Figure 1.2 demonstrates the formula for calculating the odds ratio.

	Outcome/Case	No Outcome/Control
Exposed or Intervention	a	b
Not Exposed/No Intervention	c	d

$$\text{Odds Ratio} = \frac{(a \times d)}{(b \times c)}$$

Figure 1.2   Formula for calculating the odds ratio

Case control studies then go on to give us the confidence interval.

Studies that are case controlled do not collect prevalence or incidence data about the outcome because these data are not relevant to the conditions of this type of study.

Cohort studies

KEY TERMS

Attributable risk: proportion of the outcome occurring that can be attributed to the exposure or intervention.

Populations: people with a predefined characteristic.

Relative risk: the probability of an outcome in an exposed group vs probability of an outcome in an unexposed group. For example, the probability of developing bladder cancer in dye workers (exposed) vs those not working with dyes (unexposed).

Whilst case control studies look at different subject groups retrospectively and try to determine a relationship between exposure and outcome, cohort studies are a type of a longitudinal study which collect data about participants over a certain period. They too are an example of observational study design and can either be investigating outcomes forward in time (prospective outcomes), or backward in time (retrospective outcomes).

Cohort studies do not contain control groups, nor do they offer an intervention or exposure. Subjects can often share a common characteristic such as location, gender or ethnicity. Populations may be identified by the presence of an exposure and can be followed until an outcome occurs. An example of this would be a population being studied in a city area with heavy pollution (exposure) until they develop lung disease (outcome).

The disadvantages of such a study design are that they can often have a long duration, which can be costly. A large sample size is required for this type of study, and because participants are actively selected, they are subject to selection bias. Cohort studies are useful because they can assess causality, multiple outcomes at once, they are excellent at studying rare exposures and can calculate both incidence and relative risk. Relative risk is the chance of an outcome, not an absolute.

Figure 1.3 shows a formula for calculating the relative risk and Figure 1.4 demonstrates the formula for attributable risk. Please note that you are unlikely going to be calculating these and the formulas are provided for information only.

	Outcome/Case	No Outcome/Control
Exposed/Intervention	a	b
Not Exposed/No Intervention	c	d

$$\text{Relative Risk} = \frac{(a \,/\, a + b)}{(c \,/\, (c + d)}$$

Figure 1.3 Calculating relative risk

	Outcome/Case	No Outcome/Control
Exposed/Intervention	a	b
Not Exposed/No Intervention	c	d

$$\text{Attributable Risk} = \frac{(a \,/\, a + b)}{(c \,/\, (c + d)}$$

Figure 1.4 Calculating attributable risk

Let's summarise how case control studies and cohort studies differ:

Case control studies identify cohorts based on the presence or absence of an outcome and determine whether an exposure was present or absent. For example, subjects with lung cancer and whether they smoked or not and subjects without lung cancer and whether they smoked or not.

Cohort studies identify cohorts based on the presence of an exposure and determine whether an outcome develops or not. For example, whether smokers (exposed group) go on to develop lung cancer or not vs non-smokers (unexposed group) going on to develop lung cancer or not.

Case Control Study
Outcome → Was there an exposure?
Cohort Study
Exposure → Is there an outcome?

Figure 1.5   Case control vs cohort study

Level 5: Meta-synthesis

KEY TERMS

Qualitative data: data that cannot be easily expressed in numbers such as narration, pictures, videos. They are often sourced through interviews, observations or patient diaries.

Quantitative data: data that can be measured and statistically analysed. This can be numerical in nature (blood pressure, cholesterol) or data that is transformed into categories (e.g. yes/no or very satisfied/satisfied/neutral/dissatisfied/very dissatisfied).

Often studies may yield qualitative data, and this may therefore not always be conducive to statistical analysis. Meta-synthesis offers a study design in which a research question is answered through a comprehensive qualitative data search. The data is then assessed and combined.

Meta-syntheses are useful because they attempt to answer the rationale behind something. They answer the '*why*' and often relate to human experiences in relation to the question, rather than objective measures. These can include behaviours, wishes, needs, and even expectations. In fact, this is true of all qualitative studies. Meta-syntheses are useful because they identify new concepts within findings, and then attempt to interpret the new concepts to deduce and determine new understandings.

Numerous methods of analysing qualitative data have been produced. We'll discuss two next: meta-ethnography and thematic analysis.

A popular method of analysing qualitative data is called meta-ethnography. Initially developed by Noblit and Hare (1988), it is one of the earliest methods, and the most used in healthcare research (Hannes and Macaites, 2012). Ethnography is a process of qualitative data collection whereby researchers immerse themselves and interact with their environment, allowing them to gain a deeper understanding of the problem or the research question. Examples of ethnographic data collected could be interviews or photographs. Meta-ethnography therefore combines qualitative data and combines data from research, finding new interpretations rather than just combining data to present.

Thematic analysis is another common method of analysing qualitative data, developed by Holton in the 1970s. In this method, qualitative data is analysed and interpreted to deduce common patterns. These common patterns are then further interpreted to generate recurring themes (Holton, 1973).

Other methods include grounded theory, narrative synthesis, meta-summary, critical interpretive synthesis, and framework synthesis. This list is not exhaustive and serves to underpin the fact that qualitative data is analysed via a variety of methods (Mohammed et al., 2016).

In summary, meta-synthesis is important within evidence-based nursing practice because it can often provide invaluable insights into our patients' behaviours. Going further, meta synthesis may be utilised to analyse nursing values and practices. This may give further understanding into ethics and gives research and nursing care a more human approach, tending to and understanding the human needs of both patients and caregivers.

Level 6: Case study or qualitative study

Case studies

Case studies are a lower level of evidence because they only analyse one single 'case'. They are a descriptive study design because they describe a case. This can be one or a very small number of partici-pants, a ward, a department or a unit. A case study can utilise both quantitative and qualitative data. Case studies can be useful to further analyse a single phenomenon. An example would be the labour process in a transgender male who has retained his uterus, a case that is not common but requires understanding.

Qualitative studies

Qualitative studies are descriptive studies discussed above in the meta-synthesis section of this chapter. In summary, their aim is to provide further insight into the *how* and the *why*. The researcher may first begin by trying to define *what* a phenomenon being answered is. Different qualitative research methods are then utilised, dependent on what the researcher is trying to answer. For example, if there is a phenomenon of which little is known, grounded theory may be applicable. Developed by Glaser and Strauss (1967), grounded theory is a process through which a theory is generated based on data, seeking to uncover the process of the phenomenon. An example would be how patients with peripheral vascular disease, diabetes and learning disabilities develop skills to manage their condition.

Phenomenology

Phenomenology aims to understand and re-examine an experience or a phenomenon to further under-stand it. It aims to describe an experience; an example would be a researcher asking a patient 'what did it feel like to be told that you have cancer?' Data may be collected through interviews, questionnaires or observations. Phenomenology is useful in evidence-based nursing because it considers the person holistically, giving importance to their experiences.

Two different schools of phenomenology exist. Firstly, developed by Husserl in 1913 (first trans-lated in 1931), descriptive phenomenology aims to rid the researcher of their existing knowledge, and 'bracket it', so that the research is approached in a manner devoid of preconceptions.

Interpretive (hermeneutic) phenomenology, developed by Heidegger (1927), states that it may not be possible to bracket existing knowledge. This means that the researcher may not be wholly neutral and as such allows the researcher to use their existing knowledge to interpret the experience of others.

Overall, regardless of the method used to underpin evidence-based nursing practice, qualitative research allows patients' stories and experiences to form the core of nursing practice. It allows us to understand the problem through understanding the patient fully.

Level 7: Opinions of authorities or expert committees

This is widely regarded as the lowest level of evidence and is used when higher levels of evidence are not available. This evidence may be based on expert clinical experience or may consider descriptive studies. Often more than one expert combines their experience to form a committee and provide a recommendation. This level of evidence may be used to provide a rationale for further research.

IN SUMMARY

There are a multitude of challenges when considering research as evidence, and often there are limitations also. For example, it may be costly to research rare diseases. It is therefore important that the correct study design is selected to reflect the needs of the research question. Although a randomised controlled trial is a high level of evidence, it is not always the most suited. As a student nurse you should understand the various types of study design, their strengths and weaknesses, and how to apply them to real life questions.

ACTIVITY: CRITICAL THINKING

In 1998 Andrew Wakefield et al. published a (now retracted) study in *The Lancet* which suggested the MMR vaccine may lead to developmental disorders in children (Wakefield et al., 1998). Considering what has been covered within this chapter and after reviewing the above study, answer these questions:

- What was the study design?
- What was the study trying to achieve?
- How was information analysed and presented?
- What would be a good study design to achieve the goals of the study?
- What level of evidence was the study?
- How would the evidence affect the general population, including those in deprived areas?

ACTIVITY: PAUSE AND REFLECT

Consider a time when you were presented with a question from a patient which you did not know the answer to.

- How did not knowing make you feel? Consider that the patient might feel the same. They might feel anxious or helpless.
- How did you feel after you learnt more about the medication? Was there a point at which you researched the evidence and felt more confident?
- How could this be communicated to the patient to empower them?

UNDERSTANDING COMMON TEST TERMS

Patients frequently undergo diagnostic tests as part of their health journey, and the test is often the focus of a study. Research aims to define the usefulness of novel methods. An example of this would be lateral flow testing during the Covid-19 pandemic. Sensitivity and specificity are often reported. But what does this mean? How does this apply to evidence-based nursing?

In this section of the chapter, we will discuss and define sensitivity, specificity and positive and negative predictive values. These will be underpinned with pertinent examples.

True and false positives and negatives

First, we must understand what a true positive and a true negative is. Consider an individual who has undergone a diagnostic test to determine whether they have a particular illness or condition, in the example given above, comparing the results of a Covid-19 lateral flow test to the actual presence or absence of a Covid-19 infection. This is shown in Figure 1.6:

	Condition Present	Condition Not Present
Test Positive	True positive	False positive
Test Negative	False negative	True negative

Figure 1.6 Defining true and false positives and negatives

- If a patient has the condition and the test is positive, the outcome of the test is termed a **true positive**.
- If a patient does not have the condition and the test is positive, the outcome of the test is termed a **false positive**.
- If a patient has a condition, and the test is negative, the outcome of the test is termed a **false negative**.
- If a patient does not have a condition and the test is negative, the outcome of the test is termed a **true negative**.

It is therefore clear that for a test to be useful in clinical practice we would like the highest number of true positive values, where the test correctly shows the presence of a condition, and we would also like the highest number of true negative values reported, where the test correctly shows that a condition is not present.

Sensitivity

Sensitivity is the ability of a test to correctly identify the presence of a condition. In sensitivity we ask: Of those with the condition, how many were true positive? This is usefully expressed mathematically using the following calculation:

Sensitivity = True positive / (True positive + False negative)

Specificity

Specificity is the ability of a test to correctly identify the absence of a condition. In specificity we ask: Of those without the condition, how many were true negative? The mathematical calculation to determine specificity is as follows:

Specificity = True negative / (True negative + False positive)

The metrics often used within sensitivity and specificity are percentages. It is therefore clear that for a test to be absolutely accurate, it should have a 100% sensitivity and 100% specificity. In real life however, this is not always true.

We can go on to determine further useful values.

Positive predictive value

Positive predictive value is the ability of a test to correctly determine which of those testing positive have the condition. It is calculated as follows:

Positive Predictive Value = True positive / (True positive + False positive)

Negative predictive value

Negative predictive value is the ability of a test to correctly determine which of those testing negative do not have the condition. It is calculated as follows:

Negative Predictive Value = True negative / (True negative + False negative)

Similarly to the metrics used within sensitivity and specificity, positive and negative predictive values are often reported in terms of percentages. For a test to be absolutely accurate, it would have 100% positive predictive values and 100% negative predictive values.

ACTIVITY: WHAT'S THE EVIDENCE?

This activity will help you form an overview of the common test terms used. Although it is unlikely that you will ever have to calculate them in practice, it is important to know what the values represent.

A novel blood test has been developed to detect the presence of cervical cancer. Results of the test were then confirmed against existing testing techniques to establish accuracy. Out of 115 patients with cervical cancer, 95 had a positive test. Out of 243 patients without cervical cancer, 21 had a positive test.

Using these results, let us now calculate:

- Sensitivity
- Specificity
- Positive Predictive Value
- Negative Predictive Value

We will first begin by designing a table.

	Cervical Cancer	No Cervical Cancer	Total Row
Test Positive			
Test Negative			
Total Column			

Overall Total

Next, we will use the results data to fill in the blank values. This will give us the following table:

	Cervical Cancer	No Cervical Cancer	Total Row
Test Positive	95	21	116
Test Negative	20	223	243
Total Column	115	244	359

Overall Total = 359

Finally, we will use this table to make our calculations.

- Sensitivity = 95 / (95 + 20) = 0.83 = 83%
- Specificity = 223 / (223 + 21) = 0.91 = 91%
- Positive Predictive Value = 95 / (95 + 21) = 0.82 = 82%
- Negative Predictive Value = 223 / (223 + 20) = 0.92 = 92%

Questions

- What does each value tell us?
- Is this a good test? Would you recommend using this test to determine the presence of cervical cancer?

DEVELOPING AS AN EVIDENCE-BASED NURSE BEYOND SCIENTIFIC RESEARCH

It is impossible for research to have tested every possible situation and every possible variable. There is more to evidence-based practice than the hierarchy of evidence, important as it is. A nurse should be able to treat whichever situation they encounter independently. They should be able to assess and appraise it. Where do you turn to when research is limited? In the next portion of the chapter, we will discuss some other sources of evidence which can underpin nursing practice and discuss the importance of combining all sources of evidence together to underpin care.

Patterns of knowing

Barbara Carper was an influential nursing theorist and in 1978 outlined four fundamental patterns of knowing:

1   **Empirical Knowledge** is found within research and in textbooks. It has undergone the scientific research method and can be proven.

2   **Aesthetic Knowledge** refers to the Greek origin of 'aesthetic' meaning to perceive, apprehend and notice (Lidell and Scott, 1940). Unlike empirical knowledge, which is objective, aesthetic knowledge is subjective. It is the knowledge that feels right and looks correct. It requires the nurse to have knowledge of the whole situation and the patient's circumstance. It requires the nurse to interpret, understand and utilise empathy holistically.

3   **Personal Knowledge** derives itself from the nurse's experience and self-understanding. It requires empathy.

4   **Ethical Knowledge** requires awareness of moral codes and various beliefs. To some extent, it may be argued that ethical knowledge can vary between cultures and individuals.

These ways of knowing empower the nurse and provide knowledge (or evidence) through which to justify nursing practice (Carper, 1978). It is important to acknowledge that as a nurse develops through formal education such as lectures and through placement, gaining knowledge and new skills, feeding into Carper's four ways of knowing, some learning will be through a concept described as the hidden curriculum, lessons learnt via experience.

Sources of evidence

Roycroft-Malone et al. (2004) introduced a four key concept model for evidence. Knowledge from research evidence, knowledge from clinical experience, knowledge from patient experience and knowledge from local context. It is the amalgamation and overlap of these concepts that create a patient-centred evidence-based care. The authors state that research has become the main source of evidence for practice (Roycroft-Malone et al., 2004). Although research is regarded as robust, it can become superseded by new emerging research and therefore the answers it yields aren't always absolute. Research is also subject to interpretation and thus different interpretations can yield different answers. This is the case even when there are defined clinical topics amenable to the scientific method (Dopson et al., 2002). Therefore, it is important to bring together evidence from different sources and apply it to the clinical question, care or context.

Clinical experience is an ever-evolving source of evidence and is something that is accrued during the professional life. It is consistent with Carper's Personal Knowledge discussed above. Research shows that nurses not only draw on their own clinical experience but also on that of others to help their practice (Thompson et al., 2001). Despite this, some argue that clinical experience is subject to bias and personal views. It is argued that clinical knowledge, like research knowledge, should be analysed, critiqued and evaluated for it to become valid (Upshur, 1997). Observations that have been reflected on and exposed to critique and verification have been termed 'affirmed experience' (Stetler et al., 1998). When evidence from research is combined with evidence from experience, it can be very powerful, yet if there is a discrepancy between the two, then actual practice may be varied (Ferlie et al., 1999). It is important to acknowledge that clinical experience is an evolving process and that it, too, is subject to change as new evidence comes to light. Furthermore, sometimes it is necessary to evolve the clinical experience of a body of professionals. A nurse may be dissuaded from using novel research to inform their practice just because other colleagues are not doing the same. Improving clinical practice involves reasoning skills as well as skills in finding new research and evidence so that it is integrated and utilised (Benner et al., 2008).

Knowledge from patients and carers must not be undervalued, yet the documented literature on this is sparse. Farrel and Gilbert (1996) state that there are two distinctions in the concept of involvement in healthcare: collective and individual. Collective involvement in healthcare entails a group or a collective of individuals that participates in the delivery of a healthcare service and healthcare planning strategies. An example of a collective involvement is that of NICE, where there is patient representation at a national level, via the development of guidelines. Individual involvement pertains to episodes of care. A patient brings with them their previous experiences and knowledge about themselves, their mind, body and social life (Farrell and Gilbert, 1996).

The final source of evidence for evidence-based nursing is from a local context. Often local evidence is derived from the three sources discussed above as well as local quality improvement projects, audits, organisation culture and direction, local policy, services available and multisource feedback. This has been described as internal evidence (Stetler, 2003). Local sources of evidence are not as recognised as research evidence and thus their potential should be explored within the literature (Roycroft-Malone et al., 2004). Nonetheless, it forms a valuable source for evidence-based nursing when used in conjunction with all three other sources.

Pillars of critical practice

Ann Glaister discusses critical practice in health and social care and gives us three pillars of critical practice. Critical thinking and practice allow nurses to develop a holistic and inclusive model of professional practice, one which can adapt to new sources of information. This includes not just evidence but also the patients' individual circumstances.

These pillars are forging relationships, seeking to empower others and making a difference.

- **Forging relationships** means working with others so that nurses can incorporate diverse perspectives to form a view of the situation. They can then use these views to understand what the issue at heart is and try to answer it with existing evidence. Forging relationships will allow the nurse to develop clinical experience.
- **Seeking to empower** allows us to appreciate that not all people within this world are treated equally. It allows us to recognise that there are minorities who may become disadvantaged within health and social care. For example structural racism towards ethnic minorities can reinforce employment inequalities, and this can in turn affect physical and mental health. We must therefore work to minimise this power imbalance. This feeds into knowledge from patient experience as it is the patient that knows themselves the best. We can use this evidence to create a plan to help them.
- The final pillar, **making a difference**, encompasses a wide spectrum of improvement. The concept centres around the prospect that nurses and other practitioners make assessments and interventions with the aim of improving health. This may include treatment of an infection, or emotional upset. It may also include aiming to improve a patient's circumstance for the better as part of social justice and improving their access to health and opportunities. For example, an elderly patient may not be able to afford carers financially but having carers would allow them to stay in their own home. Nursing staff along with social services would be able to organise these. The patient would have this new safety net and support. For nurses it ultimately means playing a role in helping patients recover from an illness as a whole person (Glaister, 2008).

Ellis (2019) states that a nurse appraises evidence in all forms, including those above. This allows the informed action to become patient-centred care. Ellis states that there are influences and dispositions of an evidence-based nurse. Dispositions involve being questioning, reflective, critical and moral. Influences are based around research evidence, law, ethics as well as hospital policies and patient preference among others.

Evidence-based nursing encompasses lessons learnt far beyond available research, and draws on the cumulative experience of the nurse and their tutors, guided by professional standards and guidelines.

RESEARCHING EVIDENCE

Imagine you are a first-year nursing student on an orthopaedic ward. Your patient has cognitive impairment, chronic kidney disease and a fractured neck of femur. Their neck of femur fracture is because of osteoporosis. You have been asked by your nurse in charge whether you would recommend a novel monoclonal antibody treatment for the management of osteoporosis in this patient. This is because their renal function precludes them from utilising the usual first line therapy. You have never heard of a monoclonal antibody before and decide to review available research before making a recommendation. Where do you begin?

Searching for evidence within the vast amount of information available can seem like a daunting task. There are specialists available who are dedicated to finding knowledge. As an example, librarians are often an excellent source of help when attempting to find information and they can guide you through the process.

Within this section of this chapter, we will outline a method for the search process, and will go on to discuss how to critique the search output.

Search strategies

As you will be aware, information exists in different formats. For example, within books but also electronically stored, free and paid for through online publications and through journal articles. Your institution may be able to facilitate access to articles which would normally require a payment and again specialist or hospital librarians are a good source of help for this.

A search strategy entails a series of steps which will lead onto the output of evidence. These are discussed below in Figure 1.7.

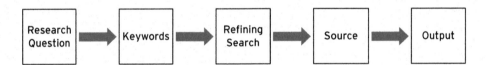

Figure 1.7   Steps in a search strategy

Research question

To find evidence you must first decide what the problem is, what you'd like to find out and what kind of evidence integrity you need. This information will often be apparent from your clinical practice, from patients or from your colleagues. A helpful aid in trying to decide what your research question is, is to utilise PICO.

PICO is a mnemonic made up of the elements of a good research question (Richardson et al., 1995):

- **P – Population**. This encompasses your group of patients. For example, post-partum patients, or geriatric patients.
- **I – Intervention**. This considers what treatment, intervention or exposure is being considered.
- **C – Comparison**. Are there any alternatives to what the intervention is? Is there a control? Placebo?
- **O – Outcome**. What is the clinical outcome? What would you like to see?

As part of the PICO process, thought should be given to the period from which evidence will be included, to ensure that evidence is as up to date as it can be.

An example of a question trying to identify the impact of different chemotherapies in non-Hodgkins lymphoma on patient survival could be:

- **P** – non-Hodgkins lymphoma
- **I** – cyclophosphamide
- **C** – cisplatin
- **O** – overall survival

When considering qualitative research, the aid becomes PEO. This isn't generally as complex as PICO because you are only considering a population, exposure and outcome.

- **P** – Population
- **E** – Exposure
- **O** – Outcome

Although PICO and PEO have been outlined above, they are not the only frameworks for designing research questions and indeed can be modified further to narrow down the question. For example, a time frame may be added or a particular setting. Other frameworks include SPICE (setting, population, intervention, comparison, evaluation) (Booth et al., 2018) or SPIDER (sample, phenomenon, design, evaluation, research type) (Cooke et al., 2012).

ACTIVITY: HAVE A GO

Using the PICO format above, formulate a research question for the above scenario on an orthopaedic ward.

Keywords

The next phase is trying to assess what words will be used in electronic databases and search engines. Care must be taken to ensure that thought is given to different names for the same thing; this is especially true in healthcare as often there are medical terms attributed to various conditions. For example, myalgia is a term used for pain in muscles. Hypertension is used for high blood pressure. Epistaxis means nosebleed.

It may be useful to generate a list of key words which try to encompass your PICO question as much as possible. A librarian may again be able to help generate this list. It's important to be aware that although useful in generating key words, a thesaurus may not be able help with medical terminology.

Refining search

Although it is possible to simply insert keywords into a database or a search engine, the outcome can be improved through trying to inform the search engine of how the key words are related to each other.

George Boole, a mathematician in the 19th century, developed a way through which concepts can either be combined or excluded. This gave advent to *Boolean operators*. These are words in between key words to link the keywords in several ways.

- **AND** – this operator links keywords together and ensures the search engine or database outputs all keywords within the result. It narrows a search. An example of this would be Pregnancy AND folic acid AND neural tube defects. Sometimes search engines automatically insert this operator within the words, and this is something to be aware off. To overcome this, you can use "quotations" so that exact wording is used. For example, "hormone therapy" AND "transgender".
- **OR** – this operator is used to connect two or more similar key words. This means that your search will be broadened. An example of this could be babies OR children OR infants OR kids AND breastfeeding AND development.
- **NOT** – this operator is used when you want to exclude a word from your search. This therefore narrows the search by instructing the search engine or the database to ignore a concept. An example would be "medical honey" NOT manuka.

Sources

There are many sources of information available, on the internet or physical. A news article or report is a source of information, as is a book or a journal article. As discussed earlier, not all sources of information are identical in the strength of their evidence. For example, an article about a product claiming to have health benefits on a website which is trying to sell it will be less robust than a journal article detailing the results of a scientific double blinded randomised controlled trial testing the active ingredient of that product.

We must therefore decide what sources of information we are seeking and consider how robust their information is likely to be. There exist many credible sources of information outside of the journal scope. Some examples include key organisations such as the Department of Health or the National Institute for Health and Care Excellence or more specific support websites such as Cancer Research UK.

Policy documents, whether hospital or national policy, are another good source of information.

With regards to journal articles, it may often be useful to search that article's reference list to identify sources which the authors found useful, and by extension you may find useful also.

A librarian will again be able to guide you through the process of source selection. To some extent the source you select may be reliant on what the search question is.

Output

It is useful to keep a record of the search and the results generated thereof. Often databases will allow you to save your search within your profile. This will allow you to access the information faster if required again. When information is found, it is important to appraise how reliable that information is, and to an extent this is carried out through deciding how reliable the source is.

A systematic process often helps in deciphering complex questions. To assess the output it may be useful to consider the following:

- Who are the authors? What makes the authors qualified to write on the subject at hand? Do they have any qualifications? Are they reputable? Do the authors make use of referencing to draw on established knowledge?
- What is the source? Is the source susceptible to any bias? Is it peer-reviewed? Is it sponsored? What is the agenda of the source? Is the source current and up to date? Is it relevant?
- Who are the audience? Is the article or information targeted at academics? Practitioners? Is it targeted at the general population?

Following the above method will provide a framework towards being able to find and appraise evidence and to decide whether it is reliable and worthwhile.

ACTIVITY: CRITICAL THINKING

Now that you've generated a research question using the PICO format for your monoclonal anti-body treatment in osteoporosis, generate a list of key words which can be used in conjunction with Boolean operators to give you the research studies that you need to make a recommendation. What level of evidence would you accept? Where would you find this evidence?

APPRAISING EVIDENCE

Evidence found through a rigourous research process should not just be taken at face value, because not all research is rigourous. Nurses should decide whether it is well designed and useful. A critique should therefore form a normal part of the research process.

To critique a research study, the person carrying out that critique is assessing the study to decide what its strengths and weaknesses are (Brink and Wood, 2001). It may be useful to follow a structured framework. This framework can follow the structure of the article that is being critiqued. There are many ways in which evidence can be appraised. The framework used will also be adapted to the type of study being appraised. Some helpful sources have been suggested at the end of this section. It is important to be aware of available tools that can be used to help appraise evidence. For example, the CASP tool is a tool which helps appraise the strengths and limitations of qualitative studies (CASP, 2022). Below we will discuss a basic framework for appraising evidence, one that you can begin to expand upon in your clinical practice.

Title

What does the title indicate about the research? Is it informative? A title which states 'Breastfeeding versus bottle feeding: A multicentre comparative study' gives more information than just 'Is breast-feeding beneficial?'

Whilst a title should be informative and give a good idea of what the article or research is about, it should also not be too long. The title should consider the variables or theories being studied.

Introduction

This section of an article will usually describe the rationale for the research being undertaken.

- Does the article provide a clear rationale and outline what the research question is?
- Do the authors carry out a literature review to outline established knowledge?
- Is the literature holistic, ensuring all available literature has been considered, but focusing on contemporary knowledge?

The introduction should set the scene, and therefore discuss the problem or gap in research.

- Why it is important enough to warrant the study?
- Does the introduction clearly outline the aims of the study?

A theoretical framework outlines theories behind the research problem. These frameworks support a study by utilising existing evidence to draw on theoretical aspects. A conceptual framework outlines and relates together variables within a study. A conceptual framework can be used to generate research questions in qualitative studies or generate hypotheses in quantitative studies (Varpio et al., 2020).

Methods

A thorough methods section should enable the reader to be able to duplicate the research process. Furthermore, it should be comprehensive so that the reader can go on to evaluate the methods used to carry out the research, deciding whether they are reliable.

It is important to decide whether the method selected is appropriate for the research question. For example, it may be more useful to collect qualitative interview data for a study analysing perceptions than it would be to use Likert scale questions. Some points to consider are:

- Do the authors of the research identify how they selected their participants?
- Do they discuss the inclusion and exclusion criteria?
- Do they discuss any controls as comparative measures?
- Do the authors outline limitations of their study or methods?
- If the research involves participants, was ethical approval sought?
- Do they outline ethical considerations?

Results

This section concerns itself with the reporting of important results. It should provide understandable information which allows the reader to see how the authors reached their conclusions. Some points to consider are:

- Does the results section contain the *relevant* data?
- Does the results section discuss data which may disprove the null hypothesis?
- Do the authors identify statistical analysis used, and provide pertinent p values and confidence intervals?
- Does the way data is presented make the analysis clear?

Discussion

Within the discussion section, the authors will generally discuss the results of the study in relation to established research. Within this section, the authors should aim to use their data to justify and argue why their theories are proved or disproved. Some points to consider are:

- Do the authors analyse their results within the context of the research question?
- Do the conclusions draw on any analysis made?
- Do the authors make the important results known?

Furthermore, the authors should go on to make suggestions for further research. They should identify any gaps in research or use the current study to establish why more research is required.

Conclusion

This section should not provide any new concepts. Rather it should provide a summary of the key points and indicate why the study is useful. Suggestions for further research may be made here rather than within the discussion section.

The authors should declare any limitations and sources of bias, including sponsorship.

GO FURTHER

Read the below sources to learn in more detail about appraising evidence:

- Cathala, X. and Moorley, C. (2018) 'How to appraise quantitative research', *Evidence-Based Nursing*, 21 (4): 99-101.
- Moorley, C. and Cathala, X. (2019) 'How to appraise qualitative research', *Evidence-Based Nursing*, 22 (1): 10-13.
- Moorley, C. and Cathala, X. (2019) 'How to appraise mixed methods research', *Evidence-Based Nursing*, 22 (2): 38-41.

ACTIVITY: WHAT'S THE EVIDENCE?

Consider the scenario posed earlier in this chapter regarding a patient requiring treatment for osteoporosis.

Now that you have a PICO research question and a list of keywords, find an article which aims to address this question.

Analyse the article for its strengths and limitations as well as the outcome. Compare the strengths and limitations to decide how useful the article is.

INTRODUCTION TO CLINICAL SKILLS AND THEIR APPLICATION TO PRACTICE

With the advent of new information, new critical thought and research, nursing continues to evolve and with it the requirements which equip nurses to be able to deliver excellent patient-centred care. No two patients or situations are the same. Evidence-based nursing and being able to correctly search for and scrutinise information is one key skill a nurse can possess.

The Nursing and Midwifery Council (NMC) publication *The Code* gives the professional standards of practice and behaviours which nurses and midwives must uphold. Statements within *The Code* portray what good practice looks like. *The Code* is split into four sections (NMC, 2018b):

- Prioritise People
- Practice Effectively
- Preserve Safety
- Promote Professionalism.

The NMC also provide standards for proficiency for registered nurses, which portray the skills, knowledge and attributes which all nurses must hold. The standards, among others, list all the individual clinical skills a nurse should possess. These are discussed within the relevant sections of this book.

Next we will discuss a theoretical scenario which is not too dissimilar from real life. It will highlight the multitude of skills, clinical, research and more, that a nurse must possess in their arsenal.

Nursing in action

Consider a hospital bay full of patients with different ailments:

- Sikshya in bed 1 has not passed urine and is complaining of abdominal pain.
- Ilona in bed 2 is frail, has dementia and is not eating.
- Morwen in bed 3 has a malodorous wound and learning difficulties, therefore keeps picking at it.
- Sonam in bed 4 is feeling overwhelmed and anxious as they are awaiting a scan for a suspected malignancy, family have rung the ward and are not happy as they haven't been updated for days.

It quickly becomes obvious that to be able to help with all those scenarios, a very wide set of skills will be required of a nurse. Critical thinking will be required. Priorities will need to be set. Careful selection of appropriate nursing assessments and interventions will need to be made. Communication, collaboration, and multidisciplinary effort are an integral part of the process.

Sikshya in bed 1: Personal experience will tell the nurse that they should carry out an abdominal examination to palpate for a distended bladder. The patient will be able to tell the nurse what symptoms they have and outline their patient evidence. Following this assessment, patient evidence, and with the aid of a bladder scanner, which has undergone research evidence for assessing urinary volumes, the nurse will determine that Sikshya has gone into urinary retention. To alleviate suffering and resolve the acute issue, the nurse will know from clinical experience and learned experience that a catheter must be inserted through the urethra, into the bladder, draining the urine. This process must be carried out in a way which minimises the risk of introducing infection and developing problems further down the line. Clearly the skills required here are abdominal examination, aseptic non-touch technique and catheter insertion. Perhaps followed by effective communication of events to the medical team, using a structured and concise approach. The nurse may then further draw on their clinical experience and recall the various causes of urinary retention, including constipation and urinary tract infections and be able to further assess these, using local evidence in the form of local policy and protocols.

Ilona in bed 2: The skills required are different again. Assessment should be made as to why the patient is not eating and what their nutritional status is. Formal tools may be used according to local policy (local evidence) or tools that have research evidence behind them. Further specialist advice can be sought from allied health specialities such as dietetics. Considerations need to be made:

- Will Ilona have the necessary energy to recuperate from her ailment?
- Will this affect her skin integrity and place her at risk of developing pressure ulcers?
- Do Ilona's family understand what is happening?

The nurse should be able to utilise nutritional assessments and skin assessments among others to decide on the best interventions to support Ilona. These will be evidence based. If nasogastric feeding is to be used, local policy can be checked to determine indications for nasogastric feeding as well as the protocol to be followed.

Morwen in bed 3: A review of the wound should be made, and consideration given as to whether the wound is infected. Again, a nurse can use personal experience, and research evidence learnt to assess the wound and perhaps knowledge from Chapter 6. They will be able to use local evidence and personal experience to determine if a swab should be sent. Knowledge of wound healing should be applied. Perhaps the nurse may wish to recommend consideration of antibiotics to the medical team. Personal experience and research evidence will guide further:

- Does Morwen need to have her observations checked?
- Is she systemically unwell from this?
- Does Morwen understand what is happening?

The nurse will then be able to look for and find evidence, tools and strategies which will help aid communication with Morwen.

Sonam in bed 4: The nurse will be able to determine that Sonam requires emotional support. Perphaps there may be qualitative evidence to help. Some things which need to be considered are:

- What are some of the strategies through which emotional support can be given?
- Is the family also feeling anxious and therefore feel like there is a lack of communication?
- Is there anything that can be done to empower Sonam?
- Can sources of information be identified and assessed for credibility and suitability so that the patient is able to understand them?

The above scenarios, although theoretical, are not too dissimilar to some real life examples. A multitude of skills will be required from a nurse, and they should have knowledge of where to seek information and evidence to support the interventions used. Carper's ways of knowing apply in the above scenarios as well as evidence frameworks posed by Roycroft-Malone et al.

The above scenario may seem daunting. Whilst colleagues will be able to help, it serves to underpin the vast array of clinical skills which will be required to intervene for each patient. The following chapters within this book will discuss the clinical skills required of a qualified nurse, and work towards empowering you and providing you with the knowledge to be able to practice them in a safe and effective manner. As you develop your experience, knowledge and skill, you will be able to deal with bays such as the one described above. What once would have been a daunting task may now be second nature.

CHAPTER SUMMARY

This chapter discussed the hierarchy of research evidence, outlining the strengths of each level. Systematic reviews form the highest level of research evidence and opinions of authorities or expert committees the lowest level. Common test terms have been discussed as often these are discussed within the literature, namely sensitivity and specificity. Evidence-based nursing has been discussed at length and different theories outlined, showing that evidence-based nursing goes far beyond scientific research. Frameworks for forming a research question have been discussed and a framework for appraising evidence demonstrated. Finally, a clinical scenario has demonstrated evidence-based nursing in action.

ACE YOUR ASSESSMENT

Q1   A study found within the Cochrane database pulled together data across 10 randomised controlled trials and presented the data as a forest plot. This is an example of a

a   Case control study
b   Case series
c   Meta analysis
d   Observational study

Q2   A study analysed patients who were exposed to asbestos and those who weren't and determined the probability of them developing a mesothelioma. What type of study is this?

a   Cohort study
b   Case control study
c   Quasi-experimental design
d   Case series

Q3   The percentage value of a HPV test being positive in patients who had HPV is an example of what?

a   Positive predictive value
b   False positive value
c   Odds ratio
d   True positive value

Q4   AND, OR and NOT are an example of what operators?

a   Nightingale
b   Boolean
c   Elis
d   NMC

Q5   The C in the PICO mnemonic stands for what?

a   Confounding
b   Comparison
c   Case
d   Clarity

Answers

1   C
2   A
3   D
4   B
5   B

GO FURTHER

Nursing and Midwifery Council (NMC) (2018a) *Future Nurse: Standards of Proficiency for Registered Nurses*, NMC, May 17. https://www.nmc.org.uk/standards/standards-for-nurses/standards-of-proficiency-for-registered-nurses/ (accessed October 5, 2022).

Nursing and Midwifery Council (2018b) *The Code*. London: NMC. https://www.nmc.org.uk/globalassets/sitedocuments/nmc-publications/nmc-code.pdf (accessed October 5, 2022).

Ellis, P. (2011) *Evidence-based Practice in Nursing*. London: Sage.

REFERENCES

Averis. A. and Pearson, A. (2003) 'Filling the gaps: Identifying nursing research priorities through the analysis of completed systematic reviews', *JBI Reports*, 1 (3): 49–126.

Benner P., Hughes R.G. and Sutphen M. (2008) 'Clinical reasoning, decisionmaking, and action: Thinking critically and clinically', in: R.G. Hughes (ed.) *Patient Safety and Quality: An Evidence-Based Handbook for Nurses*. Rockville, MD: Agency for Healthcare Research and Quality (US), pp. 87–109.

Booth. A., Noyes. J., Flemming, K., Moore, G., Tunçalp, Ö. and Shakibazadeh, E. (2018) 'Formulating questions to explore complex interventions within qualitative evidence synthesis', *BMJ*, 4 (1): 1–7.

Brink. P. J. and Wood. M. (2001) *Basic Steps in Planning Nursing Research: From Question to Proposal* (5th edition). London: Jones and Barlett.

Carper, B. (1978) 'Fundamental patterns of knowing in nursing', *Advances in Nursing Science*, 1 (1): 13–24.

Colloca L. and Benedetti, F. (2005) 'Placebos and painkillers: Is mind as real as matter?', *Neuroscience*, 6 (7), 545–52.

Cooke. A., Smith, D. and Booth, A. (2012) 'Beyond PICO: The SPIDER Tool for qualitative evidence synthesis', *Qualitative Health Research*, 22 (10): 1435–43.

Critical Appraisal Skills Programme (CASP) (2022) *Qualitative Studies Checklist*. https://casp-uk.net/casp-tools-checklists/ (accessed October 7, 2022).

Dopson. S., FitzGerald, L., Ferlie, E., Gabbay, J. and Locock, L. (2002) 'No magic targets! Changing clinical practice to become more evidence based', *Health Care Management Review*, 27 (3): 35–47.

Egger, M., Higgins, J. P. T. and Smith, G.D. (eds) (2022) *Systematic Reviews in Healthcare: Meta-analysis in Context* (3rd edition). Oxford: John Wiley & Sons.

Ellis, P. (2011) *Evidence-based Practice in Nursing*. London: Sage.

Farrell, C. and Gilbert, H. (1996) *Health Care Partnerships*. London: Kings Fund.

Ferlie E., Wood, M. and Fitzgerald, L. (1999) 'Some limits to evidence-based medicine: A case study from elective orthopaedics', *Quality in Health Care*, 8 (2): 99–107.

Glaister, A. (2008) 'Introducing Critical Practice', in: S. Fraser and S. Matthews (Eds.) *The Critical Practitioner in Social Work and Healthcare*. London: Sage, pp. 17–23.

Glaser, B.G. and Strauss, A.L. (1967) *The Discovery of Grounded Theory: Strategies for Qualitative Research*. New York, NY: Aldine de Gruyter.

Greco, T., Zangrillo, A., Biondi-Zoccai, G. and Landoni, G. (2013) 'Meta-analysis: Pitfalls and hints', *Heart Lung and Vessels*, 5 (4): 219–25.

Hannes, K. and Macaitis, K. (2012) 'A move to more systematic and transparent approaches in qualitative evidence synthesis: Update on a review of published papers', *Qualitative Research*, 12: 402–42.

Heidegger, M. (1996) *Being and Time*. Albany, NY: State University of New York Press.

Holton. G.J. (1973) *Thematic Origins of Scientific Thought: Kepler to Einstein*. Cambridge, MA: Harvard University Press .

Husserl, E. (1931 [1913]) *Ideas: General Introduction to Pure Phenomenology* (trans. W.R.B. Gibson). London: Routledge.

Karimi, H. A. (2015) 'Florence Nightingale: The mother of nursing', *Nursing and Midwifery Studies*, 4 (2): e29475.

Liddell, S. and Scott, R. (1940) *A Greek–English Lexicon* (9th edition). Oxford: Clarendon.

Mohammed, M., Moles, R.J. and Chen, T.G. (2016) 'Meta-synthesis of qualitative research: The challenges and opportunities', *International Journal of Clinical Pharmacy*, 38 (3): 695–704.

Nightingale, F. (1979 [1852]) 'Cassandra: An essay', *American Journal of Public Health*, 100 (9): 1586–7.

Noblit, G.W. and Hare, R.D. (1988) *Meta-ethnography: Synthesizing Qualitative Studies*. Thousand Oaks, CA: Sage.

Nursing and Midwifery Council (NMC) (2018a) *Future Nurse: Standards of Proficiency for Registered Nurses*, NMC, May 17. https://www.nmc.org.uk/standards/standards-for-nurses/standards-of-proficiency-for-registered-nurses/ (accessed October 5, 2022).

Nursing and Midwifery Council. (2018b) *The Code*. London: NMC. https://www.nmc.org.uk/globalassets/sitedocuments/nmc-publications/nmc-code.pdf (accessed October 7, 2022).

Ranganathan, P. (2018) 'Study designs: Part 1 – An overview and classification', *Perspectives in Clinical Research*, 8 (6): 184–6.

Raso, A., Marchetti, A., D'Angelo, D., Albanesi, B., Garrino, L., Dimonte, V., Piredda, M. and De Marinis, M.G. (2019) 'The hidden curriculum in nursing education: A scoping study', *Medical Education*, 53 (10): 989–1002.

Richardson, W. S., Wilson, M.C., Nishikawa, J. and Hayward, R.S. (1995) 'The well-built clinical question: A key to evidence-based decisions', *ACP Journal Club*, 123 (3): A12–13.

Roycroft-Malone, J., Seers, K., Titchen, A., Harvey, G., Kitson, A. and McCormack, B. (2004) 'What counts as evidence in evidence-based practice?', *Journal of Advanced Nursing*, 47 (1): 81–90.

Stetler, C.B. (2003) 'Role of the organization in translating research into evidence based practice', *Outcomes Management for Nursing Practice*, 7 (3): 97–103.

Stetler, C. B., Brunell, M., Giuliano, K.K., Morsi, D., Prince, L. and Newell-Stokes, V. (1998) 'Evidence-based practice and the role of nursing leadership', *The Journal of Nursing Administration*, 28 (7/8): 45–53.

Suresh, K.P. (2011) 'An overview of randomization techniques: An unbiased assessment of outcome in clinical research', *Journal of Human Reproductive Sciences*, 4 (1): 8–11.

Thompson, C., McCaughan, D., Cullum, N., Sheldon, T.A., Mulhall, A. and Thompson, D.R. (2001) 'The accessibility of research-based knowledge for nurses in United Kingdom acute care settings', *Journal of Advanced Nursing*, 36 (1): 11–22.

Upshur, R. (1997) 'Certainty, probability and abduction: Why we should look to C.S. Peirce rather than Gödel for a theory of clinical reasoning', *Journal of Evaluation in Clinical Practice*, 3 (3): 201–6.

Varpio, L., Paradis. E., Uijtdehaage, S. and Young, M. (2020) 'The istinctions between theory, theoretical framework, and conceptual framework', *Academic Medicine*, 95 (7): 989–94.

Wakefield, A. J., Murch, S.H., Anthony, A., Linnell, J., Casson, D.M., Malik, M. [...] and Walker-Smith, J.A. (1998) 'Ileal-lymphoid-nodular hyperplasia, non-specific colitis, and pervasive developmental disorder in children', *Lancet*, 351: 637–41.

Zandi, A. (2014) *Concepts and Theories of Nursing with a Sound Heart Model*. Tehran: Heidari.

THE IMPORTANCE OF ASSESSMENT

2

DEBORAH ROWBERRY, PETER SEWELL AND WENDY CHURCHOUSE

LEARNING OBJECTIVES

After reading this chapter, you should be able to:

- Identify the importance of assessment in a variety of settings
- Discuss the stages of the Nursing Process
- Identify the links between clinical reasoning, decision-making and patient assessment
- Develop confidence in conducting patient assessment remotely

STUDENT VOICE

The more I learn about nursing assessment, the more I realise there is so much more to learn about nursing assessment.

Nia, 3rd year, Child Health

INTRODUCTION

We use assessment to identify patients' problems, which allows us to put interventions in place to help the patient. The assessment process should always involve the patient, have the patient at the centre and aim to understand the patient, rather than concentrating on merely their illness. The way nurses assess patients has evolved and the nurse's role has also changed over the years, most recently with the introduction of the latest NMC Standards of Proficiency in 2018. As a student nurse, recognising the complexity of assessment early in your studies is key to help understand your ongoing learning needs.

Evidence-based care underpins effective, quality patient assessment (see Chapter 1). It is important to build therapeutic relationships with patients based on mutual trust as this allows the patient to share honestly what their concerns are during the assessment process. Accurate patient assessment is also essential. Accuracy not only helps ensure patient safety and ensure we are meeting patients' needs but is also vital for our colleagues and other members of the healthcare team, in order that the assessment process provides a true picture. This ensures any subsequent treatment is appropriate and timely. However, this can be more difficult to do. Many factors can affect this process, if the patient is in pain, for instance, their concentration levels may be lessened. If patients have a communication barrier, this must be addressed early in the assessment process. The complex systems and teams that nurses work in mean there is a constant stream of distraction in the workplace, making the process of accurate, safe, quality patient assessment more difficult and complex to achieve. The chapter will look a little further into aspects of assessment.

THE NURSING PROCESS

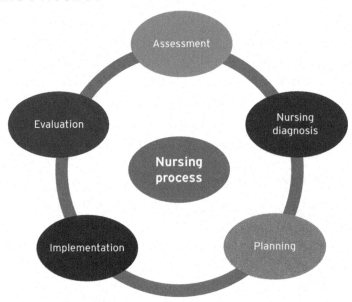

Figure 2.1   The Nursing Process

Source: Toney-Butler and Thayer, 2022

The Nursing Process helps the nurse understand the patient as a whole person. It aims to provides individual, person-centred nursing care. Originating in the US in 1958 by Ida Jean Orlando (as cited in Toney-Butler and Thayer, 2022), the Nursing Process concept was then introduced to the UK in 1977 and still guides nursing care today. The earlier version of the nursing process was a four-stage (APIE) approach and the Nursing Diagnosis element (ADPIE) was added in 1960. It is a systematic approach which relies on evidence-based practice, a patient-centred approach and critical thinking. As illustrated in Figure 2.1, the Nursing Process comprises five sequential stages, beginning with assessment. This chapter will focus mostly on that first stage; however, further resources are provided at the end of the chapter which you can read to help deepen your understanding of the Nursing Process.

CLINICAL REASONING AND DECISION MAKING

KEY TERMS

Clinical reasoning: describes the process by which nurses (and other healthcare professionals) gather information and cues, process this information, come to an understanding of a patient problem or situation, plan and implement interventions, evaluate outcomes, and reflect on and learn from the process (Levett-Jones et al., 2010).

Central to the Nursing Process is *clinical reasoning* (see Go Further section for more information). The terms *clinical reasoning, clinical judgment, problem solving, decision-making,* and *critical thinking* are often used interchangeably in the literature on this topic. The clinical reasoning process is not a linear one. It is more often conceptualised as a spiral or cycle of linked experiences. The clinical reasoning process takes skill to learn and master and is dependent upon a 'critical thinking approach and attitude'. It can be influenced by a person's philosophical perspective and preconceived values and beliefs.

Levett-Jones (2010) outline the five rights of clinical reasoning, relating to the ability to:

1   Collect the RIGHT information
2   Take the RIGHT action
3   For the RIGHT patient
4   At the RIGHT time
5   And for the RIGHT reason

Whilst clinical reasoning is a complex theory to take on board, particularly early in your chosen programme, many of the underpinning skills are somewhat easier to understand.

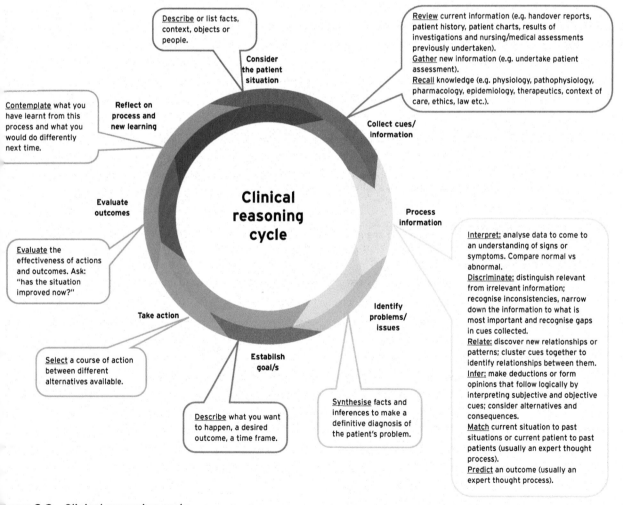

Figure 2.2   Clinical reasoning cycle

Source: Levett-Jones et al. (2010: 517)

Fundamental communication skills, team working in healthcare, the process of reflective practice and understanding evidence-based practice are some of the grounding aspects involved in clinical reasoning.

Figure 2.2 may be useful as a revision point.

ACTIVITY: PAUSE AND REFLECT

Take a few minutes to watch the following videos, to help your understanding of the clinical reasoning cycle:

- DID-ACT (2016) 'What is Clinical Reasoning?' (YouTube video), December 5. https://www.youtube.com/watch?v=gud5xeHmvXw (accessed October 7, 2022).
- NorthTec | Te Pūkenga (2019) 'Clinical Reasoning Scenario', (YouTube video), April 10. https://www.youtube.com/watch?v=OxKILfnHM1k (accessed October 7, 2022).

What examples have you seen in practice? Where have you witnessed clinical reasoning?

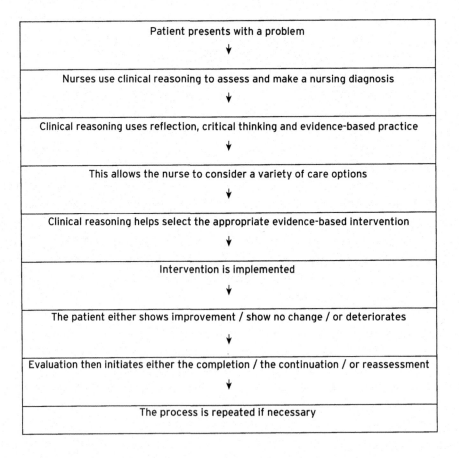

Figure 2.3 Clinical reasoning and decision-making in the Nursing Process

Critical thinking and clinical reasoning involve differentiating the facts gathered through patient assessment. This, then helps the clinical practitioner make decisions about the patient's treatment and care. Let us consider what this might look like in relation to the Nursing Process of assessment, diagnosis, planning, implementation and evaluation. The flow chart in Figure 2.3 helps process how and where clinical reasoning is used in the Nursing Process.

GATHERING PATIENT INFORMATION FOR ASSESSMENT

Having introduced the wider themes of the Nursing Process and clinical reasoning, this next section will focus more closely on assessment itself. The process of assessment is structured, and this structure will differ depending on your field of study and area of work. It uses various methods of gathering patient information and often involves the use of assessment tools, many of which will be introduced over the course of the book.

To begin, three main methods of gathering patient information are listed below. Depending on the situation, you may find that you use more than one method to build a complete picture of the patient. Methods of gathering patient information for assessment include:

- **Hardcopy documentation** – many clinical practice areas use this format; it can be perceived as flexible as it can be completed anywhere with little technology. However, many areas are moving away from this method as it can be time consuming and difficult for other healthcare team members to access when needed.
- **Digital systems** – this is a more modern way of recording and documenting information; it is perceived as a safer alternative to paper and pen systems. This method also allows records to be centralised, completed in real time and more accessible by those needing the information. There is also less repetition of documentation when using digital systems.
- **Virtual assessments** – reviewing patients virtually using virtual platforms (for example Zoom or Microsoft Teams) has been used because of the pandemic. However, it has benefits for long-term use (further information on this method can be found in this chapter).

Regardless of the method, you will often be looking for the same kind of information about the patient. This patient information is often subcategorised as Subjective and Objective data. The following table helps explain this.

Table 2.1   Subjective – Objective data

Subjective Data	Subjective/Objective	Objective Data
Demographic patient information: name, address etc. Gather from the patient or their family/friend.	Past medical history: chronological order, this can be Subjective or Objective dependent on the situation, or a mix of both.	Test results, diagnostics, vital signs.
Social information: again, gathered directly from the patient or their family/friend.	Referral information: passed to our colleagues, team members. Relies on previous stages and can sit in both subcategories.	
Presenting complaint: the patients' symptoms as explained by the patient.	GP medication history, prescriptions. Until a more detailed approach has been taken, this can sit in both subcategories.	

Important note: Visual observations taken by the nurse or other colleagues, not to be confused with Vital Signs, is subjective data.

Often the subjective and objective data gathered by nurses needs to be communicated to other healthcare professionals and team members – the challenges of this are discussed in more depth in Chapter 3.

Assessment tools

Assessment tools look to gather information that may not have been directly observed, they often using a numbering or scoring system to give an overall score which is used to help calculate risk. The overall scoring number may then help direct us to what care is needed. When completed accurately and effectively, assessment tools assist the assessment process and enhance patient safety and quality care. In your background reading throughout your studies, you will encounter many literature pieces that critically discuss the barriers and challenges in this area. Poorly or inadequately completed assessment tools can cause harm or potential risks to patients in our care. Education and understanding of these tools are vital to their thorough and safe completion. You will work with your practice supervisors and assessors when in placement and have opportunities to use assessment tools. You may also be introduced to these in your skills labs or simulation-based education opportunities.

Some of the assessment tools you will use on a regular basis are (this is not an exhaustive list):

- Nutritional Assessments
- Falls Risk Assessment
- Manual Handling Assessment
- Skin Integrity Assessment
- SEPSIS Risk Assessment
- Cognitive Assessment

ACTIVITY: PAUSE AND REFLECT

Ms Chandros is a 59-year-old Greek woman who speaks little English. She is accompanied by her granddaughter and husband. Her granddaughter is 15 years old and acts as the interpreter for the family. Ms Chandros is presenting with abdominal pain; she has not opened her bowels for five days and cannot eat or drink due to the pain.

Make a list of the assessment tools you have encountered in placement and identify which may be applicable to assessing Ms Chandros.

- What is their purpose?
- Did you encounter any problems using or understanding them? If so, what were they?
- How was the patient involved in their completion?

Incorrect or inaccurate assessment tools can cause harm to patients. Problems occur when the nurse over- or underestimates the risk involved. If we lack the knowledge to complete them, we may make errors, and this would not be acceptable. Take your time to understand these tools, ask questions and make sure to practise, as completing an assessment tool once (or twice) does not make us expert in this. Nurses have multiple documents to complete in any given shift, which can cause some complacency towards these tools – 'another box to tick'. Many of the reports into care inequalities or failings will cover this area of nursing. Whilst there are many documents to complete, we need to still have respect for each one. As a student nurse, take time to understand what happens with the assessment tool after it has been completed, who then uses this to plan care or treatment for instance, as this helps give an understanding of their importance and enormity. Practice supervisors and assessors will work with you to increase your knowledge and proficiency in this area. However, you also need to remember your responsibility to complete your own reading and study in this area. Read extensively on the assessment tools commonly used in your chosen field of nursing and remember to draw on the topics we covered in Chapter 1: what and where is the evidence base for this tool?

ETHICAL DILEMMAS IN ASSESSMENT AND DECISION MAKING

Ethics is a set of principles that guides a person's behaviours or specific activities. It is grounded in the rights and wrongs of what a person should do. You will have teaching in more detail on ethics during your programme. It is important to include ethics in this chapter to understand and heighten our awareness of how they impact our work. When assessing patients, we have a number of points to consider; for instance gaining consent, does the patient have capacity, patients' freedom of choice as well as our ability to impart information to the patients so that they understand the information being given or the request being made. Ethics can influence all these areas.

When you encounter these early in your studies, they can be overwhelming and put you in a difficult or uncomfortable situation. It is important you seek support from your academic mentor and assessor as well as practice staff. Your wellbeing is extremely important, so please make yourself familiar with your institution's support networks. If you prefer to use external sources for support, here are some that can be useful:

- https://www.nhs.uk/nhs-services/mental-health-services/
- https://www.mind.org.uk/get-involved/active-monitoring-sign-up
- https://www.kooth.com/

Further reading on ethical principles is needed to broaden your knowledge (please see links in the Go Further section at the end of the chapter). It is likely to be a core component of your programme of study.

CASE STUDY

Cody

Cody is working as a student nurse and is assessing a patient, Biji. During the assessment process Biji discloses to Cody that she believes her daughter is stealing money from her home. Her daughter is the only other person with a key and Biji has noticed money missing on several occasions over the last 12 weeks, often when she has been out of the house to do shopping or visit friends. Biji asks Cody not to say anything as her daughter is one of the Senior Nurses in the hospital.

Questions

1   What should Cody consider in this situation?
2   What should Cody's immediate action be?
3   What are your own concerns in relation to this case study if you were in Cody's position?

It can be difficult to truly know if we are always working in the patients' best interests. This can be because of daily challenges such as lack of time, resources, or knowledge and understanding. Ethics in theory and ethics in practice can give rise to conflicting and challenging situations. Inequity can occur between ethical behaviour and ethical thinking. It is key to add here that ethical situations can arise for several reasons, for example:

- lack of resources
- patient/client/family expectations of service
- cultural considerations.

These areas can be difficult to navigate as a student as they are multifactorial situations. Nurses are morally accountable for their practices and have a responsibility to work within legal and proficiency frameworks. As a student you may not always feel competent or proficient to do what is asked of you. Seeking support when this happens is paramount to your wellbeing and psychological safety, as well as that of the patient.

Using ethical principles in our everyday practice can help with decision-making and other processes, including the assessment process, but they can cause conflict, resulting in ethical and moral dilemmas. Understanding and using clinical reasoning will help problem-solve when faced with these dilemmas. As a student it is important for you to recognise this area of practice, reflect on events you observe or are involved in, seek help for the patient in the first instance and seek support for yourself when you become overwhelmed.

REMOTE CONSULTATIONS AND PATIENT ASSESSMENT

During your nurse education, you will work in a variety of service or care settings with a large component in hospital care. Most inpatient hospital nursing care is provided face-to-face and requires physical contact. However, sometimes, particularly in an outpatient or community setting, patients are reviewed, assessed and managed without any physical contact. This method of patient care can be conducted by telephone or electronic forms of communication such as email, phone video or computer video. In these situations, the terms remote, virtual or telehealth care are used.

In 2020, the Covid-19 pandemic had a global impact on healthcare as all sectors tried to reduce the transmission of the virus by avoiding physical contact, and this led to the increased use of remote consultations (Gilbert et al., 2020; Jiménez-Rodriguez et al., 2020; Portnoy et al., 2020; Churchouse et al., 2021). The National Health Service (NHS) was at an early stage of digitalised healthcare, but the pandemic triggered a digital revolution throughout the UK (Churchouse et al., 2021). Prior to the pandemic, there had been a measured transition to remote care across a broad range of services, for example cardiac device care such as implantable defibrillators or pacemakers follow up, or chronic conditions such as heart failure care (Fauchier et al., 2005; Crossley et al., 2011; Flodgren et al., 2015). In the community, some General Practitioner (GP) surgeries introduced various types of remote care (Atherton et al., 2018) and reviews, including telephone consultations or telehealth care ('digital packages'). These forms of healthcare were favoured by some (Downes et al., 2017; Atherton et al., 2018) but many patients preferred face-to-face consultations (Thiyagarajan et al., 2020). However, during the pandemic, remote consultations removed the need to travel or enter healthcare settings (Thiyagarajan et al., 2020; Churchouse et al., 2021), as this was considered beneficial in reducing the risk of transmission of the virus between clinician and patient. Because of this, patients were more accepting of remote consultations (Locke et al., 2020; Churchouse et al., 2021).

Following the pandemic, remote consultations and assessments have become permanent features and nursing students need to be confident and competent in this new form of healthcare. Most of the knowledge, skills and expertise used for conventional face-to-face care is transferrable to remote care but some key principles of good practice need to be considered.

Key principles for safe remote practice

The principles of remote care are not dissimilar to conventional face-to-face practice, as the needs of the patients continue to be central and supported by good communication skills, astute assessment skills, evidence-based care, safeguarding and governance. However, both nursing students and qualified staff should consider the following principles.

Confidentiality

During the pandemic, either due to 'shielding' or 'self-isolating', many healthcare professionals provided remote consultations from non-traditional locations such as their office or home. Whilst this practice has reduced from its peak during the pandemic, it is good practice that regardless of the 'location' of the video consultation, efforts are made to ensure the 'office' environment is professional and conducive to the consultation. This includes ensuring that any identifiable information such as other patients' medical records, x-rays etc. are not visible to the camera and that the consultation cannot be easily heard by other people.

In the unlikely event of working from home, safeguarding your own personal information is also important (GMC et al., 2019). Equally important is ensuring that your family members or neighbours do not overhear the patient's consultation (GMC et al., 2019; Chua et al., 2020). Furthermore, the use of a Virtual Private Network (VPN) system should be provided by healthcare providers (Trust or health board) as this provides a private and secure online system (Shacklock, 2020).

Confirming the patients identify at the start of the remote consultation is important. Also ensuring that the patients' confidentiality is maintained in their home is necessary. This involves asking the patient to check that the consultation cannot be seen, heard or recorded by others. If another person is present in the patient's home or room, their relationship to the patient should be checked and that their presence is consensual (GMC et al., 2019). This should be documented.

Depending on the nature of the remote consultation, it is sensible to confirm the patient's actual location, in case they are conducting the remote consultation from a relative's or friend's address rather than their own home. This information would be important if their health status/condition deteriorated suddenly and an emergency '999' response crew needed to be arranged; as sending the '999' response to their home address would be futile if they were at a different address (Royal College of General Practitioners, 2020a).

Medical records and documentation

As with any face-to-face consultations, it is necessary to have access to the patient's health records and documentation (Nursing and Midwifery Council, 2019). In the UK, many care providers have access to patients' electronic records. When accessing the electronic records, either the patients must provide verbal consent (GMC et al., 2019) or the healthcare professional must provide a reasonable explanation for why they are accessing the records without the patient's permission. Without this, the health professional could be in breach of the Data Protection Laws.

Record keeping is essential for any form of care. Any difficulties or limiting factors that affected the consultation, such as the patient having hearing difficulties or any technical issues occurring during the consultation ('buffering' or loss of sound), should be clearly documented. In addition, if the consultation mode changed from a telephone to video or vice versa, this should also be documented. Finally, the outcome of the remote consultation, including the management plan, safety-netting and follow up must be documented (Abbs et al., 2020; Royal College of General Practitioners, 2020b).

New experiences

For most nursing students, some qualified staff, patients and their relatives or carers, a remote consultation would be a new experience. There may be concerns associated with this, fears around technical issues occurring. Many health boards and departments have detailed guidance on remote consultations including information leaflets explaining what to do if technical issues occur and outlining what is going to happen during the assessment. Allaying the patients concerns and possible anxiety is paramount. Being empathetic, patient and providing clear communication are essential.

Patient assessment

The reason or nature of the remote consultation will vary depending on the type of the service and/or the patient's needs. A telephone call can be used to triage and risk assess the patients' needs (Al Hasani et al., 2020) or used to follow up a patient after an admission or some form of treatment. A web-based video conferencing tool such as 'Attend-anywhere' provides a way of visually assessing the patient. Regardless of the format of the remote consultation, when assessing and reviewing the patient it is important that a combination of open and closed questions is used to obtain a full history and holistic picture. Similarly, avoid 'leading' questions, for example instead of asking the patient if their 'toenail is red and swollen', ask them to *tell you* what their toe looks and feels like. Equally important is actively listening to the patient's answer along with the associated non-verbal communication. Here, the use of video consultations outweighs the use of telephone consultations.

Physical assessment/examination

One of the main challenges when conducting remote consultations is the inability to perform a physical examination. This is also a cause of concern for some patients, who feel they are not receiving a complete and accurate assessment (Powell et al., 2017). For a conventional face-to-face assessment, a detailed clinical history combined with a 'top to toe' visual check of the patient helps form the clinical picture (Churchouse et al., 2021). With creativity, detailed instruction and patient participation remote consultations offer a limited but sound medium to assess a patient. For example, reviewing the patients' physical appearance (unkempt), their manner (relaxed, distressed) and significant clinical signs such as cyanosis and pallor are achievable via a well-lit computer screen and camera.

Also, some vital signs can be assessed remotely. These include asking the patient to place their hand on their chest to allow an assessment of the respiratory rate and chest movements. It may be possible to show the patient how to take their own pulse or to get them to tap out its approximate speed and rhythm. Some patients may have a home thermometer, blood pressure or glucose monitor or self-monitoring devices such as a smart device mobile phone or watch. Whilst these may not be accepted strictly as medical equipment, they may be useful in the first instance to provide some limited data.

It may be extremely challenging for both the patient and the health professional to undertake intimate examinations via a remote consultation. If this is required, it must be dealt with cautiously and in a sensitive and professional manner (Abbs et al., 2020; Royal College of General Practitioners, 2020).

In line with face-to-face consultations, a chaperone should be used/offered and documented even if declined by the patient. It is important to note that family members acting as a chaperone is not recommended in such clinical situations, and another member of the clinical team could be used as an online chaperone. However, an intimate examination may not be appropriate within the scope of a remote consultation. The Royal College of General Practitioners (2020a) provide fundamental principles for undertaking intimate clinical assessments remotely which are transferrable to all disciplines.

On a general note, it is important to consider in every case whether it is appropriate clinically, or from the patient's perspective, to undertake physical examinations remotely or whether this needs to be done in person. There needs to be a risk versus benefit assessment by the clinician, in partnership with the patient. As a nursing student, it essential that you follow the service or teams agreed practice/policy in regards to any patient assessment via a remote consultation. This is because each clinical area would have undertaken a risk assessment and/or agreed criteria outlining the limitations of a remote consultation. This would maintain patient safety and standards of care.

However, one of many lessons learnt from the Covid-19 pandemic was the innovative way some health professionals led in the production of validated alternatives to face-to-face consultations (see guidance in the Go Further section).

Safety-netting and aftercare plan

For the majority of remote consultations, there will need to be a clear plan for aftercare (follow-up) and/or guidance on what the patient must do if their symptoms do not improve within a specified period, or the treatment plan is not implemented.

Table 2.2 **Safety-netting post remote consultation**

WHAT should prompt them to act?	'If your temperature is still above 38 degrees'
WHEN does your advice apply?	'In 48 hours from now'
WHERE should they go?	'Go to the emergency department'
HOW should they get there?	'Via an ambulance'
CHECK understanding	'Can you repeat that plan back to me'

Source: Abbs et al. (2020: 19)

It is good practice to check the patient's understanding of the instructions/guidance, and ideally ask the patient to write the instructions down, for example, 'do shoulder rotations 5 times a day... Hannah, the community nurse, will phone back on Tuesday 3rd June @ 10am'.

Whilst you may be familiar with remote consultations, the patient may have been under considerable stress during the consultation and will only remember a fraction of what has been said. Therefore, it is important to prompt them to write down the information. This is particularly important if there are language or communication issues, the patient is elderly or has specific learning needs. If the patient is unable to do this, ask a relative to write the instructions.

Similarly, the assessment and the safety-netting guidance and management plan must be documented clearly and concisely in the patient health records in line with NMC guidance.

Limitations of remote consultations

The Covid-19 pandemic necessitated that health professionals and managers rapidly evaluate their practice and services. This facilitated creativity and practice innovation which triggered a change in approach towards remote consultations (Churchouse et al., 2021). There is no doubt that the introduction of remote consultations contributed greatly to the delivery of healthcare in the UK during the peaks of the pandemic and afterwards. However, remote consultations are not a panacea and have limitations.

Firstly, inequity in access is an issue. Not all patients have access to computer and mobile technology, and this includes access to the internet. During the pandemic, this was illustrated by school pupils from less affluent areas of the UK struggling to access computers and/or the internet. Therefore, it is reasonable to hypothesise that this issue also applies to adults living in deprived areas. In addition, it has been extensively documented that those from deprived areas have higher levels of ill health, comorbidity and mortality rates (Marmot et al., 2010; 2020; 2021). Therefore, a proportion of the patient groups with the greatest healthcare needs (those from deprived areas) could be disadvantaged using remote consultations.

Furthermore, individuals who are homeless, regardless of the geographical location (deprived or affluent areas of the UK), are less likely to have access to a computer with internet connection or a reliable telephone for a telephone consultation.

Even when technology and access to the internet is readily available, this does not mean that remote consultations are suitable for others. For example, the elderly or individuals with learning needs, communication or language issues (Raven et al., 2013; Atherton et al., 2018) may also have practical problems using a remote consultation. It is acknowledged that many senior adults confidently and competently use computers, commonly known as the 'silver surfers.' However, for many, especially those with dementia or other conditions affecting cognition, and/or communication issues such as hearing or vision impairment, the use of the computer or telephone can be extremely challenging. Such issues are not restricted to the elderly as they can affect all age groups.

Individuals with learning needs, mental health or capacity issues, language barriers or individuals experiencing physical or emotional abuse (Raven et al., 2013; Greenhalgh et al., 2016; Atherton et al., 2018; GMC, 2020) may be left vulnerable with the use of remote consultations. Remote consultation may create a barrier to the ability of individuals to speak without coercion or prevent them speaking freely about abuse or without fear of retribution. As stated previously, clarifying and documenting the consensual presence of another person during the remote consultation and their relationship with the patient is vital (GMC et al., 2019).

Another limitation of remote consultations is the sometimes-complex nature of the consultation. Patients with complex needs such as Attention Deficit Hyperactivity Disorder (ADHD), multiple co-morbidity or palliative care are examples (Greenhalgh et al., 2016; GMC, 2020). In addition, there may be practical issues such as a need for the patient to check their heart rate or expose a part of their body, i.e., show their swollen knee to the camera, and this interaction requires assistance from a family member or another person. If the patient has no social or family support, then a remote consultation is inappropriate.

In conclusion, remote consultations have become a core component of healthcare and student nurse interaction with patients. Working with patients via a remote consultation requires the same rigour and attention to detail as conventional face-to-face care. However, it is important that the limitations of remote consultations are acknowledged and considered within the context of the clinical situation and the individual patient's needs (GMC et al., 2019; Abbs et al., 2020; Royal College of General Practitioners, 2020).

ASSESSMENT OF PATIENTS IN ICU SETTINGS

Critical illness is the failure of one or more of the body's vital organs or systems, because of a disease or injury. This causes physiological instability and will usually lead to death within minutes or hours if left untreated. Intensive care aims to support these body systems using a range of therapeutic interventions using machinery and medication; in Intensive Care this is often referred to as simply 'support'. During admission to the Intensive Care Unit (ICU), patients will go through stages of physiological deterioration and recovery, often many times, before they will reach a level of stability where they can be discharged from ICU, or instead where they continue to deteriorate, and they unfortunately die.

Because of this precarious physiological state, any changes to the patient's condition must be detected as early as is possible for appropriate measures to be taken in response, often immediately. Intensivists (medical professionals specially trained in critical care) aim to avoid anything happening to a patient in an uncontrolled way – because of this, cardiac arrests in Intensive Care are relatively rare. Detecting changes to the patient's physiological state early requires intense vigilance through continuous assessment and monitoring of all body systems – therefore it is called Intensive Care. Intensivists use a range of medical devices and clinical assessments to monitor for any changes to the patient's physiological, psychological and emotional state, providing a continuous cycle of assessment and intervention.

As well as monitoring for signs of deterioration, it is important that any *improvements* in the patient's condition are noticed early, as this will allow 'support' to be reduced. Much of the 'support' in ICU comes with significant side effects and so much of the care that takes place in Intensive Care is directed at reducing the risk of harm to the patient. A good example of this is with the use of ventilators; we know that if we give the patients artificial breaths that are too large, it can cause serious short- and long-term damage to the lungs. Therefore, Intensive Care clinicians will carefully try to adjust ventilation, to ensure the patient is given adequate respiratory support, without giving them too much. It is the ICU nurse's responsibility to continuously monitor and assess a range of measurements in relation to ventilation, which can then be used as the basis for assessing whether changes to the ventilator are indicated.

Assessment in ICU is a team effort, with patient reviews undertaken at different times by multiple members of the ICU multidisciplinary team (medical staff, physiotherapist, dieticians, speech and language therapists, psychologists), but the continuous monitoring and assessment is the role of the ICU nurse. The role and responsibilities of the ICU nurse is characterised by an attention to detail through careful assessment. This requires the nurse to collect and document a huge range of information, with continuous collation of objective data such as heart rate, blood pressure and oxygen saturations alongside information that is perhaps more subjective, such as levels of sedation or the amount of sleep a patient is having – all this information will then be used by the ICU nurse and other members of the MDT to establish the patients' immediate and future needs.

The systematic approach to problem solving encompassed in the nursing process – assess, diagnose, plan, implement and evaluate – should be applied to all care settings, although the way it is applied will depend on an individual patients' needs and the environment in which the care is provided. Within an Intensive Care environment, this process is applied constantly, and often numerous issues will be addressed simultaneously. Assessment and intervention will often occur at the same time, with treatments being adjusted with immediate effect.

ICU nursing assessment involves not only physiological assessment, but as with all nursing care, it requires a holistic assessment which considers emotional, social and spiritual needs, to identify the patient's specific individual needs. The ICU nurse applies a continuous cycle of assessment, intervention and reassessment which involves visual, auditory and even olfactory observation; this involves analysis and interpretation of a wide range of information from various sources: clinical monitors and equipment, blood tests, assessment tools as well as communication with the patient and their significant others.

Assessment by the ICU nurse will begin even before the patient is admitted, with some assessments taking place at defined points during admission, whilst others are continuous and ongoing. Some of the different types of assessment used by ICU nurses are outlined next.

Environmental assessment and safety checks

Even before a new patient arrives in Intensive Care, assessment of the patient's bed area and the surrounding environment must be undertaken by the ICU nurse. This is not specific to this setting, this happens in all inpatient facilities but is very important as the patient may rapidly deteriorate, requiring immediate intervention without delay. The nurse must prepare the patient's bed area, ensuring that all equipment (such as ventilators, drug pumps and equipment for emergency procedures) are ready and checked and that drugs that will be required are ready for when the patient arrives.

Alarms settings on monitors need to be assessed. Whilst these are prevalent in the ICU setting, all areas will have these, specific to the patients being cared for in any given area. These must be set at levels that provide early identification of changes in the patient's condition, but at the same time, they must not be allowed to continuously sound as this may be distressing to the patients and irritating to staff! Throughout the patient's admission, the ICU nurse must be able to effectively assess what are acceptable parameters for these alarms, taking into consideration the physiological state of the patient and the circumstances at the time. There may be times, such as the end of life, when alarms will be silenced altogether.

Other important environmental factors that any ward or area must assess before and throughout admission include cleanliness, light and noise. Environmental cleanliness is particularly important in ICU as the patients are very vulnerable to infections. Both excessive light and noise have been implicated as having a significant impact on the patient's mental health during ICU admission and on the quality and quantity of sleep.

Systems-based assessment

As Critical Care is primarily engaged in the support of body systems, patients are often assessed using a systems-based approach (an approach based on bodily systems, see table below – these can vary from area to area). This approach would normally be utilised on admission and on a daily

Table 2.3 Systems Approach Assessment

What is being assessed	How you would assess it
Neurological	Glasgow coma score Sedation score Peripheral neurological observations Pupils
Respiratory	Airway: whether can maintain own airway, type of airway adjunct used, endotracheal cuff pressures, security of endotracheal tube Respiratory signs (sputum production, auscultation, arterial blood gas analysis, oxygen saturations, respiratory rate) Suction: need for oral or deep tracheal secretion suctioning Humidification: need for humidification and appropriate type Ventilation: mode of ventilation and ventilator parameters Efficacy of paralysing agents Monitoring for signs of pressure damage due to ventilation devices on face (masks etc.) Appropriate positioning in bed (dependent on underlying disease, whether ventilated)

What is being assessed	How you would assess it
Cardiovascular	Heart rate / rhythm Blood pressure Fluid balance (hourly) Electrolyte imbalance DVT prophylaxis methods Intra-aortic balloon pump Full blood count Blood transfusion reaction Lactate levels Peripheral perfusion Tissue oedema Invasive intravenous and monitoring lines (patency, infection, security)
Gastrointestinal	Potential/actual nutritional deficit Nasogastric feed absorption - gastric residual volumes Bowel movements Blood sugars Stoma health
Renal	Urine output (hourly) Arterial blood gas analysis (bicarbonate levels, base excess) Dialysis - dialysis parameters and fluid loss
Microbiology/ infection	Temperature Full blood count Actual infection sites - changes indicative of infection (exudate from wounds, purulent sputum etc.)
Muscular skeletal/ skin	Wounds and dressings Wound drains Pressure damage and other skin integrity issues Personal hygiene needs Loss of muscle tone
Psychological/pain	Basic comfort Pain - type of pain, source, response to analgesia Risk of sensory deprivation Sleep (quality, quantity) Low mood/anxiety Delirium Patient knowledge on condition/progress
Sociocultural	Family updates - by medical and nursing team (need to provide update) Specific family needs (complex social structure), young children, pets, vulnerable adults Spiritual needs Protection of vulnerable adult risk (where appropriate)

or shift basis and will be used as the basis for identifying specific goals in relation to patient care. The initial period after the emergency admission of an Intensive Care patient is often a very busy period, when life supporting procedures and treatments are commenced. The Intensive Care nurse as part of the MDT will be continuing assessing the patient's physiological state, their blood pressure, heart rate and rhythm, urine output, consciousness levels, blood tests, pain etc. Skills that underpin this assessment include a knowledge of normal and abnormal physiology and the ability to apply this to different patients who may have quite different levels of what normal is, depending on their disease process or injuries

An approach to systems-based assessment used in Intensive Care (as well as other areas) is outlined in Table 2.3, with examples of what and how the Intensive Care nurse may assess these. Further in-depth information on the following topics can be found in other chapters in this book.

Soon after admission, more formal aspects of assessment will begin, when the Intensive Care nurse will complete admission documentation. This will include a holistic medical, social, cultural and spiritual assessment, which may involve receiving information from the patient if they are well enough to answer questions, or family/friends who accompany them if they are not.

ACTIVITY: PAUSE AND REFLECT

Consider how you may begin a patient assessment if neither the patient nor a family member/friend is able to supply reliable information at this time.

Using a holistic, individualised approach to assessment

Whilst there is a great deal of emphasis on the management of physiological problems in Intensive Care, it is essential that assessment of the patient's needs is focused on the individual, rather than applying a one-size-fits-all approach. Without this approach, assessment will inevitably result in sub-optimal goals that are not patient-centred. This principle should be applied to physiological care, as well as psychological, social and emotional support.

Individuals will have very different 'normal' physiology, for example one patient's blood pressure may be normally much lower than another in health, or a patient with COPD may normally have low oxygen saturations. It is important for an ICU to understand what is normal for a patient, to ensure that the care they provide for that individual is tailored to their individual needs.

Information about an individual patient's needs such as their likes and dislikes, their perspective on whether they would want certain interventions or treatments, and their spiritual beliefs need to be established early, to provide holistic patient-centred care that is appropriate for the individual patient.

Because of the constant contact with the patient and detailed understanding of the patient as a person, the ICU nurse is in the ideal position to act as continuous advocate for the patient, when they are unable to represent their own needs. This is a vital part of the role of ICU nurse and typifies the importance of detailed and accurate assessment, which provides the basis for the role of advocate and for the caring patient–nurse relationship that underpins this.

Care bundles and assessment tools

Care bundles are sets of evidence-based interventions that when used together have been proven to improve clinical outcomes in Critical Care patients. The bundle is designed to ensure consistent delivery of these interventions. An example of these is the ventilator care bundle (see below) which is designed to reduce the incidence of ventilator-associated pneumonia (this is a pneumonia caused as a result on intubation and ventilation removing the body's normal protective mechanisms against chest infection, such as cough). Care bundles are evident in all clinical areas as they ensure the delivery of standardised care (Lavallée et al., 2017).

An important part of the routine daily assessment of an Intensive Care nurse is to check that all elements of these bundles have been achieved or that consideration (usually by the medical team) has occurred if an intervention is not to be delivered. A significant amount of the assessment that an ICU nurse undertakes daily may be considered routine, but it is important that the suitability of even routine elements of care are appropriate for the individual patient.

Table 2.4 Ventilator care bundle

Intervention	Rationale
Head of bed raised above 30–45 degrees	To reduce risk of micro-aspiration and ventilator-associated pneumonia
Daily sedation interruption & assessment of readiness to extubate	Reduced time spent ventilated and length of stay in ICU
Use of subglottic suction	Reduce risk of micro-aspiration and ventilator-associated pneumonia
DVT prophylaxis	Minimises complication and length of stay
Use of chlorhexidine for oral care	Reduce risk of ventilator-associated pneumonia
Peptic ulcer prophylaxis	Minimises complication and length of stay

Assessment of risk

The critically unwell patient is at significant risk of harm because of the treatments and interventions initiated to support and save life. Procedures that are required to care for the patient, even seemingly simple ones, such as rolling the patient on their side to wash, carry risk such as the accidental removal of indwelling devices such as endotracheal tubes. One of the reasons a critically ill patient will have a 1:1 nurse/patient ratio is to simply allow a nurse to be able to continuously observe the patient. This helps to ensure invasive apparatus such as central and arterial lines or endotracheal tubes are not accidentally removed by the patient, which could have disastrous consequences.

Research in Intensive Care has highlighted several very specific areas of critical care intervention, that carry with them a significant risk of harm to the patient, and which may have a direct impact on the chances of the patient surviving their critical illness. One example of this is the use of sedation in ICU, which involves the use of powerful opioids and anaesthetic drugs. Most patients will require some level of sedation to ensure comfort and tolerance of Intensive Care interventions and to reduce the risk of accidental removal of indwelling devices.

Studies have shown that high levels of sedation come with significant risk: they increase the time spent on a ventilator (which has significant risk) increase time spent in ITU and reduce the ability for clinicians to properly examine the patient, particularly neurologically (Kress et al., 2017).

Only a minority of critically ill patients will have a clinical indication for continuous high levels of sedation. By minimising sedation levels and pausing sedation daily, the ICU nurse can assess whether the patient needs sedation at all, or whether they can tolerate lower levels. The nurse therefore provides continuous assessment of sedation levels, often using one of several sedation assessment tools, and will assess suitability to pause sedation daily, in order to help reduce the risk of using these drugs.

Family/Friends

Approximately 25% of patients who are admitted to Critical Care units die or will survive with significant life changing disability. The critical illness of a loved one is obviously an extremely difficult time for the family and friends of the patient, who will need regular updates of the progress and deterioration of the patient and breaking of bad news when treatment is failing.

ICU nurses will usually be the first contact for enquiries from relatives, they will accompany the relatives when they visit the patient, they will often contact them to warn them that their loved one's condition is deteriorating and will be with the family at the time of the patient's death.

Each patient's family will have specific support needs, which it is important for the ICU nurse to identify early in admission and continue to assess throughout the patient's stay. This assessment might include whether the family have been suitably updated about the patient's condition by the ICU team, whether they need support with accommodation during the admission or simply that they need some emotional support.

CASE STUDY

Dion

Dion is a 27-year-old male who is a Jehovah's Witness. He has been in the department for five days and his condition is deteriorating. His haemoglobin levels have dropped since yesterday.

Questions

What considerations are needed in relation to Dion's Care? And to updating his family?

Colleagues

Intensive Care can be a physically and emotionally challenging place to work for all members of the Intensive Care team. Examples of stressors include competing urgent demands, interpersonal conflict, complex decision-making, moral distress, rapid patient turnover, night and weekend work and patient mortality. The Covid-19 pandemic brought into sharp relief the need for staff to be aware of their own and colleagues' mental and emotional wellbeing at work. The term 'burnout' syndrome is used to describe when clinician wellbeing is compromised and can cause a range of physical and mental symptoms such as tiredness, emotional lability, frustration, anxiety and insomnia (Moss et al., 2016).

CHAPTER SUMMARY

Assessment is a key skill that all nurses will learn and use daily. There is a lot to consider when learning assessment, and it can be a lengthy process. Clinical reasoning helps in the assessment process and aids decision-making. Ethical principles also have a significant part to play when assessing patients. Intensive Care patients are often so unwell and so close to death that any small deterioration in condition can be significant. It is therefore vital that the patient is continuously monitored, and every aspect of their physical, mental and emotional state is assessed in order to identify early any required change to their care and treatment. Continuous and careful assessment allows for early detection of physiological and psychological deterioration, allowing pre-emptive and timely remedial action to be taken.

— GO FURTHER —

Ellis, P., Standing, M. and Roberts, S. (2020) *Patient Assessment and Care Planning in Nursing* (3rd edition). London: Sage.

Lecturio Nursing (2021) 'How to perform a nursing assessment' (YouTube video), August 12. https://www.youtube.com/watch?v=CiO_UD5F-GQ (accessed October 10, 2022).

Toney-Butler, T. J. and Thayer, J. M. (2022) 'Nursing Process', StatPearls, April 14. https://www.ncbi.nlm.nih.gov/books/NBK499937/ (accessed October 10, 2022).

Ellis, P. (2020) *Understanding Ethics for Nursing Students* (3rd edition). London: Sage.

Royal College of General Practitioners (2020a) *Key Principles for Intimate Clinical Assessments Undertaken Remotely in Response to COVID-19*. rcgp.org.uk, July. https://elearning.rcgp.org.uk/pluginfile.php/154305/mod_page/content/15/Key%20principles%20for%20intimate%20clinical%20assessments_July%202020.pdf (accessed October 10, 2022).

Royal College of General Practitioners (2020b) *Principles for Supporting High Quality Consultations by Video in General Practice During COVID-19*. www.england.nhs.uk, August 20. https://www.england.nhs.uk/coronavirus/wp-content/uploads/sites/52/2020/03/C0479-principles-of-safe-video-consulting-in-general-practice-updated-29-may.pdf (accessed October 10, 2022).

Cortese, S., Coghill, D., Santosk, P., Hollis, C. and Simonoff, E. (2020) 'Starting ADHD medications during the COVID-19 pandemic: Recommendations for the European ADHD Guidelines Group', *The Lancet Child & Adolescent Health*, 4 (6): E15.

Ford, G., Hargroves, D., Lowe, D., Harston, G., Rooney, G., Oatley, H. and Lough, J. (2020) *Adapting Stroke Services during the COVID-19 Pandemic: An Implementation Guide*. Oxford Academic Health Science Network. https://www.gettingitrightfirsttime.co.uk/wp-content/uploads/2022/06/Adapting-stroke-services-in-the-COVID-19-pandemic-May-2020.pdf (accessed October 10, 2022).

REFERENCES

Abbs, D.A., Hyams, A. and Ahmed, Z. (2020) *Remote Consultations Handbook – Strategies to Ensure a Safe and Effective Consultation via Video or Telephone* (2nd edition). https://gpexcellencegm.org.uk/wp-content/uploads/Remote-consultations-handbook.pdf (accessed October 7, 2022).

Al Hasani, S., Al Ghafri, T., Al Lawati, H., Mohammed, J., Al Mukhainai, A., Al Ajmi, F. and Anwar, H. (2020) 'The use of telephone consultation in primary care during Covid-19 pandemic, Oman: Perceptions from physicians', *Journal of Primary Care & Community Health*, 11: 1–8.

Atherton, H., Brant, H., Ziebland, S., Bikker, A., Campbell, J., Gibson, A. and Salisbury, C. (2018) 'Alternatives to the face-to-face consultation in general practice: Focused ethnographic case study', *British Journal of General Practice*, 68 (669): e293–e300.

Chua, I., Jackson, V. and Kamdar, M. (2020) 'Webside manner during the COVID-19 pandemic: Maintaining human connection during virtual visits', *Journal of Palliative Medicine*, 23 (11): 1507–9. https://doi.org/10.1089/jpm.2020.0298

Churchouse, W., Griffiths, B., Thomas, J., Sewell, P. and Harries, R. (2021) 'Remote consultations, prescribing and virtual teaching during the Covid-19 pandemic', *Journal of Prescribing Practice*, 3 (7): 264–72.

Cortese, S., Coghill, D., Santosk, P., Hollis, C. and Simonoff, E. (2020) 'Starting ADHD medications during the COVID-19 pandemic: Recommendations for the European ADHD Guidelines Group',

The Lancet Child & Adolescent Health, 4 (6): E15. https://www.sciencedirect.com/science/article/abs/pii/S2352464220301449?via%3Dihub (accessed October 7, 2022).

Crossley, G.H., Boyle, A., Vitense, H., Chang, Y., Mead, R.H. and CONNECT Investigators (2011) 'The CONNECT (Clinical Evaluation of Remote Notification to Reduce Time to Clinical Decision) Trial: The value of wireless remote monitoring with automatic clinician alerts', *Journal of the American College of Cardiology*, 57 (10): 1181–9. https://doi.org/10.1016/j.jacc.2010.12.012

Downes, M.J., Mervin, M.C., Byrnes, J.M. and Scuffham, P.A. (2016) 'Telephone consultations for general practice: A systematic review', *Systematic Reviews*, 6 (1): 128.

Fauchier, L., Sadoul, N. and Kouakam, C. (2005) 'Potential cost savings by telemedicine-assisted long-term care of implantable cardioverter defibrillator recipients', *Pacing and Clinical Electrophysiology: PACE*, 28 (Suppl 1): S255–S259. https://doi.org/10.1111/j.1540-8159.2005.00071.x

Flodgren, G., Rachas, A., Farmer, A.J, Inzitari, M. and Shepperd, S. (2015) 'Interactive elemedicine: Effects on professional practice and health care outcomes', cochrane.org, September 7. https://www.cochrane.org/CD002098/EPOC_interactive-telemedicine-effects-professional-practice-and-healthcare-outcomes (accessed October 7, 2022).

Ford, G., Hargroves, D., Lowe, D., Harston, G., Rooney, G., Oatley, H. and Lough, J. (2020) 'Adapting stroke services during the COVID-19 pandemic: An implementation guide'. Oxford Academic Health Science Network. https://www.gettingitrightfirsttime.co.uk/wp-content/uploads/2022/06/Adapting-stroke-services-in-the-COVID-19-pandemic-May-2020.pdf (accessed October 7, 2022).

General Medical Council (2020) 'Remote prescribing via telephone, video link or online', gmc-uk.org. https://www.gmc-uk.org/ethical-guidance/ethical-hub/remote-consultations (accessed October 7, 2022).

General Medical Council, Academy of Medical Royal Colleges, Care Quality Commission, Faculty of Pain Medicine, GDC, GOC, GPC, HeIS, HeIW, NMC, PSNI, RPS, RQIA. (2019) *High Level Principles for Good Practice in Remote Consultations and Prescribing for all Healthcare Professionals*. nmc.org.uk. https://www.nmc.org.uk/globalassets/sitedocuments/other-publications/high-level-principles-for-remote-prescribing-.pdf (accessed October 7, 2022).

Gilbert, A.W., Billany, J., Adam, R., Martin, L., Tobin, R., Bagdai, S. [...] and Bateson, J. (2020) 'Rapid implementation of virtual clinics due to COVID-19: Report and early evaluation of a quality improvement initiative', *BMJ Open Quality*, 9 (2): e000985. https://doi.org/10.1136/bmjoq-2020-000985

Greenhalgh, T., Vijayaraghavan, S., Wherton, J., Shaw, S., Byrne, E., Campbell-Richards, D., Bhattacharya, S., Hanson, P., Ramoutar, S., Gutteridge, C., Hodkinson, I., Collard A., and Morris, J. (2016) 'Virtual online consultations: Advantages and limitations (VOCAL) study', *BMJ Open*, 6 (1). https://bmjopen.bmj.com/content/6/1/e00938 (accessed October 7, 2022).

Jiménez-Rodríguez, D., Ruiz-Salvador, D., Rodríguez Salvador, M., Pérez-Heredia, M., Muñoz Ronda, F.J. and Arrogante, O. (2020) 'Consensus on criteria for good practices in video consultation: A Delphi Study', *International Journal of Environmental Research and Public Health*, 17 (15): Article #5396. https://doi.org/10.3390/ijerph17155396

Lavallée, J.F., Gray, T.A., Dumville, J., Russell, W. and Cullum, N. (2017) 'The effects of care bundles on patient outcomes: A systematic review and meta-analysis', *Implementation Science*, 12 (1): Article #142.

Levett-Jones, T., Hoffman, K., Dempsey, J., Jeong, S.Y., Noble, D., Norton, C.A., Roche, J. and Hickey, N. (2010) 'The "five rights" of clinical reasoning: An educational model to enhance nursing students' ability to identify and manage clinically "at risk" patients', *Nurse Education Today*, 30 (6): 515–20. doi: 10.1016/j.nedt.2009.10.020

Locke, J., Herschorn, S., Neu, S., Klotz, L., Kodama, R. and Carr, L. (2020) 'Patients' perspective of telephone visits during the COVID-19 pandemic', *Canadian Urological Association Journal*, 14 (9): E402–E406. https://doi.org/10.5489/cuaj.6758

Marmot, M., Allen, J., Goldblatt, P., Boyce, T., McNeish, D., Grady, M. and Geddes, I. (2010) *Fair Society, Healthy Lives*. London: Institute of Health Equity. https://www.instituteofhealthequity.org/resources-reports/fair-society-healthy-lives-the-marmot-review (accessed October 7, 2022).

Marmot, M., Allen, J., Boyce, T., Goldblatt, P. and Morrison, J. (2020) *Health Inequality in England: The Marmot Review 10 Years On*. London: Institute of Health Equity. https://www.health.org.uk/publications/reports/the-marmot-review-10-years-on (accessed October 7, 2022).

Marmot, M., Allen, J., Goldblatt, P., Herd, E. and Morrison J. (2021) *Build Back Fairer: The COVID-19 Marmot Review. The Pandemic, Socioeconomic and Health Inequalities in England*. London: Institute of Health Equality. https://www.health.org.uk/publications/build-back-fairer-the-covid-19-marmot-review (accessed October 7, 2022).

Moss, M., Good, V.S., Gozal, D., Kleinpell, R. and Sessler, C.N. (2016) 'A critical care societies collaborative statement: Burnout syndrome in critical care health-care professionals. A call for action', *American Journal of Respiratory and Critical Care Medicine*, 194 (1): 106–13

Nursing and Midwifery Council (NMC) (2019) *Standards for Prescribers*. nmc.org.uk, May 17. https://www.nmc.org.uk/globalassets/sitedocuments/education-standards/programme-standards-prescribing.pdf (accessed October 7, 2022).

Portnoy, J., Waller, M. and Elliott, T. (2020) 'Telemedicine in the era of COVID-19', *The Journal of Allergy and Clinical Immunology in Practice*, 8 (5): 1489–91. https://doi.org/10.1016/j.jaip.2020.03.008

Powell, R.E., Henstenburg, J.M., Cooper, G., Hollander, J.E. and Rising, K.L. (2017) 'Patient perceptions of telehealth primary care video visits', *The Annals of Family Medicine*, 15 (3): 225–9. https://doi.org/10.1370/afm.2095

Raven, M., Butler, C. and Bywood, P. (2013) 'Video-based telehealth in Australian primary health care: Current use and future potential', *Australian Journal of Primary Health*, 19 (4): 283–6. https://doi.org/10.1071/PY13032

Royal College of General Practitioners (2020a) *Key Principles for Intimate Clinical Assessments Undertaken Remotely in Response to COVID-19*. rcgp.org.uk, July 2020. https://elearning.rcgp.org.uk/pluginfile.php/154305/mod_page/content/15/Key%20principles%20for%20intimate%20clinical%20assessments_July%202020.pdf (accessed October 7, 2022).

Royal College of General Practitioners (2020b) *Principles for Supporting High Quality Consultations by Video in General Practice During COVID-19*. www.england.nhs.uk, August 20. https://www.england.nhs.uk/coronavirus/wp-content/uploads/sites/52/2020/03/C0479-principles-of-safe-video-consulting-in-general-practice-updated-29-may.pdf (accessed October 7, 2022).

Shacklock, J. (2020) *Covid-19 and Safeguarding*. rcgp.org.uk. https://elearning.rcgp.org.uk/pluginfile.php/148868/mod_page/content/25/COVID-19%20and%20Safeguarding%20%286%29.pdf (accessed October 7, 2022).

Thiyagarajan, A., Grant, C., Griffiths, F. and Atherton, H. (2020) 'Exploring patients' and clinicians' experiences of video consultations in primary care: A systematic scoping review', *BJGP Open*, 4 (1). doi.org/10.3399/bjgpopen20X101020

THE IMPORTANCE OF COMMUNICATION

3

DEBORAH ROWBERRY

INTRODUCTION

What is communication?

Day to day, we rarely give much thought to the way we communicate and are often unaware of how we come across to others. This is in part because communication is not always a conscious activity. Our ability to communicate with others begins as an early infant, though there is considerable debate on whether these skills are innate or learnt as we develop and grow. Communication is a two-way process and enables us to form long- and short-term relationships with those around us.

Communication can be both simple and complex and occurs simultaneously. During the process, information is transmitted by the 'sender' and a 'message' is created. The 'message' is then imparted to the 'receiver' (Bach and Grant, 2011). On the surface, the process appears to be simplistic, though this is rarely the case.

Barriers to communication in healthcare

Several barriers and potential barriers can occur. For instance, if a patient is in a lot of pain, their ability to send or receive communication effectively could be impaired as their focus is on their pain. Working in or being a patient in a busy environment will also have an impact on effective communication.

Effective, quality communication does not always come easily to patients. For example, some people find talking about difficult or emotional issues an uncomfortable experience and for this reason may consciously or subconsciously avoid them.

Societal attitudes also have a significant impact. For example, conversations around urine and faeces or genitalia embed notions of disgust and concealment, in addition, the sight, smells and sounds of our most private bodily functions are traditional fodder for comedy, from stand up to sitcom. It is perhaps no surprise that some patients and staff may perceive a degree of stigma in relation to public attitudes towards such issues. Individuals seen as having little control, for example, due to age (the very young and the very old), may generate a more sympathetic response. The language of healthcare of course differs to that of public discourses: vernacular (everyday) words and double-entendres are replaced with biologically correct terminology. Yet many people still find communication about such private bodily functions or emotive topics embarrassing and difficult.

Facts, feelings, thoughts, fears, hopes and anxieties are expressed and transferred via communication. For nurses to be successful in their profession an openness to study and improve these skills is imperative. Health professionals who are not educated in or open to furthering their communication skills can encounter significant additional challenges; for example, the inability to separate work and personal life, which can have negative effects on an individual and can potentially lead to emotional burnout if not addressed.

The physical environment, cultural considerations, unconscious bias, psychological safety as well as other key points can affect the communication process. These will be explored further in this chapter as well as referred to in other chapters.

ACTIVITY: PAUSE AND REFLECT

As a student nurse, consider a time you have worked in a busy, noisy environment, maybe a ward, department, or clinic. Perhaps the environment was 'chaotic' and there was a lot going on.

- How did the environment make you feel the very first time you entered it? Now consider how every patient feels every time they enter this environment.
- How did the environment make you feel after you had been there a few weeks? Was there a point you noticed you had become desensitised to the 'chaos', and you no longer felt the same?
- Perhaps after a while you were able to 'tune out' some of the 'chaos'.
- How might desensitisation to our environment (as staff) affect communication within the team?
- Patients are not able to 'tune out the chaos', how must this impact their communication?
- What considerations are needed for student nurses/nurses who have hearing impairments?

Understanding and being actively aware of your environment can play an important part in effective communication. When you are actively aware of the issues and understand the challenges patients face, you can factor it into your communication processes. Waiting for quieter, less busy periods to communicate complex or sensitive topics might be considered. Moving the patient to another room or space (where available) may also be an option in some areas. There are times when communication interaction is needed but no alternatives or other spaces can be located. At these times it is important to recognise the anxieties of the patients and take time to clarify what has been communicated. The patient requires and deserves the full attention of the nurse during the communication process. This can be difficult to achieve at times. The health professional should make every effort to ensure this is the case.

Developing rapport and relationships

Try to establish a professional relationship with the patients you work with, which is based on two-way communication and trust from first contact. A polite, professional, and approachable manner helps to establish the relationship. When you start the conversation:

- Introduce yourself and explain your role.
- Ask the person's name and how they would like to be addressed.
- Orientate them to their surroundings and inform them of what to expect.

However, do not dismiss the importance of a little small talk, this can help oil the wheels for future, more in depth, communication. Remember the person's name and use it; this helps to build a personal connection and is very important to patients. Often general surveys indicate the positive impact on patients when the nurse(s) caring for them remember their name.

The patient should feel valued, respected, and listened to and this cannot be achieved when we take communication for granted. Being as actively aware of our communication skills as we are of our practical skills is a good place to start. Conversations with patients should not invoke any doubts or misunderstandings on either side; for example, if, whilst in a conversation with a patient, we are distracted by another task or person, or we have our head down making notes, the patient may feel vulnerable and not listened to. Interactions like these are likely to cause ambiguity around what was said or heard and can damage our relationship with the person. Someone who perceives they are not listened to may not be forthcoming in future encounters or may become angry or frustrated that they have not been properly heard. The patient may already feel vulnerable or stressed because of what they are experiencing: the responsibility to ensure the communication interaction is as effective as possible is on the nurse or health professional.

Listening is a core skill. Individuals may not always communicate clearly for a range of reasons. Allow people plenty of time to express themselves and reassure them that you understand that what you are discussing may be a sensitive or emotive topic. Ensure that you understand the meaning of what the person is saying. Terminology can vary between areas and cultures. Vague terminology in conversations and personal interpretations can lead to a lack of clarity. This can be further complicated by the use of local slang terms or colloquialisms. Ask the person to clarify meaning. Good listening skills encourage the person to express themselves in depth. It is important to be aware of what is not said as much as what is said. These may give clues to issues that the person finds difficult to talk about.

Empathy in communication

--- **KEY TERMS** ---

Empathy: an attempt to put oneself 'in the shoes' of another person to try and understand their experiences from their point of view.

It is all too easy to assume meaning based on one's own views or expectations, but it must be remembered that what motivates one person will not necessarily be the same for another. You might have a clear vision of what your main concern is, but the patient may have very different priorities and concerns. It is important to express what these are, listen to the patient and clarify these.

Empathy differs from sympathy – feeling sorry for another person. The latter does little to help the person. Expressed sympathy may be perceived as pity and when done poorly can appear to be condescending. At worst, the patient may end up feeling unable to engage therapeutically with the nurse when discussing difficult or embarrassing topics. Empathy, on the other hand, is essential in order to maintain an emotional connection. This is not to say that the nurse should not feel compassion, indeed it would be a heartless individual who did not feel for another person and wish to help alleviate their distress (and one for whom nursing may not be the most appropriate career choice).

Empathy is expressed through careful phrasing, reflective language, and paraphrasing, for example 'You find talking about such things difficult'. 'You have said that you have been unable to be intimate with your partner, that is something you've been distressed by'. Empathy needs to be both accurate and appropriately expressed. Avoid phrases such as 'I know how you are feeling'. You cannot experience *exactly* what the person is experiencing, even if you have gone through a similar situation. Every person and situation are unique. You should strive to try and understand the individual's personal beliefs, perceptions, and emotions as much as you can with an open mind and a non-judgmental attitude, even if these do not sit comfortably with your own. This can sometimes be challenging and requires self-awareness. Reflective practice and clinical supervision can help you to develop your skill in this area. A willingness to listen to the lived experiences of patients may help the nurse to develop a broader understanding. We learn from patients in a way that we cannot learn from courses, books, or articles.

ACTIVITY: PAUSE AND REFLECT

Think about a time you personally had a positive experience communicating with a health professional as a service user or a relative. What was it about the experience that made it positive? What did they say? How did they say it? How did they listen?

Now think about a time you had a less than positive experience. What was different about this?

Communicating health information

The health information and knowledge you possess is likely to be greater than that of the patient (a generic statement of course). Be careful not to fall into the trap of using language which is too technical or involves jargon (jargon refers to language or terms used by a specific group, which is difficult for others outside that group to understand). You may spend much of your day talking to people about health-related issues. You can become used to the language of your field and profession but the person receiving care may not understand, and neither is it their responsibility to. This can even be the case with what you may consider to be non-technical terms. For example, asking a patient if they have a hard stool may conjure up an image of a particularly uncomfortable seat! Check understanding and re-word, as necessary.

Information should be provided in small, manageable 'bite-size chunks.' Too much all in one go can be confusing. Prioritise and provide options for further information. Where possible, and when appropriate, back up information with written and/or visual material. The latter should be provided in a suitable format, considering the level of literacy of the individual, their age, mental capacity, language, and cultural needs.

Verbal and non-verbal communication

Communication is often divided into two categories: verbal and non-verbal. Any interactions that contain the spoken word are referred to as verbal communications, literature sometimes includes written language in this category also.

In verbal communication equal importance is given to what and how words are spoken. However, multiple factors can influence the 'what' and 'how', for instance:

Table 3.1   What factors influence verbal communication?

Factors influencing the 'what'	Factors influencing the 'how'
Individual's age	Pace of the speech
Level of education	Clarity of the speech
Level of development	Tone of voice
Environment/distraction	Level of volume

Non-verbal communication pertains to how the individual(s) present themselves and accounts for most of all communications. Most individuals are consciously aware and make conscious decisions about the content of verbal interactions, but less so with non-verbal. Most people are significantly less aware of the messages they are sending in this manner. Non-verbal communication includes:

- Posture of body
- Eye contact (present/not present)
- Facial expressions (present? Appropriate?)
- Position of persons during interaction
- Gestures (displaying anger? Fear? Elation?)

Understanding what constitutes non-verbal communication, how it impacts others and how we can improve this aspect of ourselves can be extremely beneficial and have a positive impact on patients and others. Particularly when working with children, clients who have learning disabilities or patients for whom English is a second language, as well as those who use alternative methods to communicate, for instance, digital technology or artificial intelligence devices.

ACTIVITY: PAUSE AND REFLECT

We communicate and send messages even when we say nothing. This can be very impactful; consider the following:

1   You walk into placement on your first day, a staff member gets up from the desk and walks towards you smiling.
2   You walk into placement on your first day, there is a staff member at the desk, they remain there and do not look up when you enter.

Consider how each option might make you feel.

Non-verbal communication can enhance and reinforce verbal communication, but also contradict and impair it. Research indicates both categories affect patients' perception of nurses' levels of empathy (Montague, 2013). Health professionals who make eye contact and shake patients' hands are viewed as more approachable, kind, and empathetic. However, there are times when these interactions are not appropriate, not least when working in areas affected by Covid-19. Both verbal and non-verbal communication becomes incredible difficult to influence when touch is no longer appropriate, and masks are being worn.

Being aware of our own body language is important. Equally important is being able to interpret the body language of others.

CASE STUDY

Jackson

Jackson is a 61-year-old patient, admitted to your placement area. You approach Jackson and ask him about his day. You observe he is lying in bed on his side and his knees are bent up near his abdomen. He is usually sitting in his chair. He has his eyes closed and does not open them when you approach. You ask if he is ok. He keeps his eyes closed and responds, yes, he's fine, thank you.

Questions

1   What conflicts of verbal and non-verbal communication do you observe?
2   What questions might you ask next?

Whilst it can be useful to consider the disparities you observe with Jackson, it is important to remember not to rely solely on this method of communication. It can be open to misinterpretation. Cultural differences can influence body language and its interpretation. The acceptable proximity of individuals, whether standing or sitting, varies across cultures; this can also be personal preference. There may be times in clinical situations where you need to be in close proximity to the patient. First and foremost, assess for any safety issues when doing this. Secondly, be sensitive and address it, explain carefully to the patients, and let them know you understand their discomfort but that you will be as brief as you possibly can.

Active listening

Whilst we have briefly covered the importance of listening above, effective communication requires us to be open to learning and developing these skills. One key skill is active listening. We mentioned earlier about ensuring we clarify what is said and heard in the communication process; active listening is key here. It requires us to hear what is being said; it also requires us to repeat that back to the person with whom we are communicating by paraphrasing what was heard, thus confirming what you have heard and that both participants in the interaction share the same understanding. We may have to ask questions to further ascertain or clarify points and understanding. For this we can use open and closed questions. Examples of these are below:

Table 3.2   Examples of open and closed questions

OPEN - How? Why? What?	CLOSED - Require Yes or No response.
Why did you choose to be a nurse?	Are you a student nurse?
What does your pain feel like?	Do you have any pain?
How does the Dr think my Mum is progressing?	Did the Dr see my Mum today?

When we are rushed, distracted, or have several tasks to do at once, it can be all too easy to lose sight of how we are asking questions. Be mindful before asking the question that you are appropriately using open or closed questions. Being aware and mindful of our own behaviour, actions and communication is a vital skill needed for us to engage meaningfully in relationships with patients and others.

KEY TERMS

Self-awareness: having a conscious understanding and knowledge of our own feelings, beliefs and personality, and how they affect both our behaviour and our interactions with those around us.

STUDENT VOICE

When I started my course, I found reflection hard and did not really enjoy doing it or engaging with it, but as I have progressed and learned how to reflect on myself and be self-aware, I can say it has been hugely beneficial. Understanding how I come across to others has helped me improve. On my last placement when I was nervous, I would put my hands in my pockets so no-one could see that they were shaking. My Practice Assessor explained this made me look bored and disinterested and I was horrified to hear this, as this was not the case at all. Now when I feel anxious or nervous and worry that my hands might be shaking, I take myself away and wash my hands. This helps and gives me a few seconds to calm myself and gives a very different, more positive impression.

Luke, 2nd year, Mental Health

Communication, safety, and patient satisfaction

Working with people when they are vulnerable is a complex process, particularly in relation to communication that happens during this time. Effective communication is important to ensure shared decision-making and maintenance of person-centred care. Unfortunately, there are times when the communications are not effective, or are missed altogether, which can result in an opportunity for harm to those we care for. For instance, when patients do not fully understand their diagnosis; how or why they are taking medications; what they need to do when they return home or what to do if their symptoms worsen as harmful consequences may occur.

Patients report communication problems and poor communication as their most important concern (NIHR, 2021). Although the 2019 report indicated no serious harm to patients because of poor communication events, they did identify the events as avoidable or preventable. 22% of patients surveyed in the report indicated communication issues were the biggest cause for concern. Examples given were:

- No reliable information given about when the patients were going for surgery – resulting in unnecessary nil by mouth status and missed meals for patients as well as increased anxiety about the upcoming operation. This report shows, as do many others, that communication is seen as key to patients feeling valued and listened to.
- There are several examples in the literature that show poor communication has a financial impact on healthcare systems. Avoidable admissions or re-admissions have adverse effects on the individual, but also have cost implications for individual health boards and healthcare overall. Whilst it can appear unempathetic to discuss the impacts communications have on finances, it is a real and current problem that becomes everyone's responsibility. Understanding the full ramifications of our communication skills helps us understand how complex this area is, as well as how important it is to work to improve these skills.

How do we communicate and who do we communicate with?

When you first begin your programme of study you will be overwhelmed by the amount of communication you receive and send. We will start by looking at some areas you will experience:

Table 3.3   Where and with whom will you communicate?

	Who you will communicate with	How you will communicate with them
University	University Academic Mentor (AM)	Emails to and from your AM.
	Peer group	WhatsApp messages and groups
	University departments	Formal documents and emails
	Assessment department	Essays, assignments both formative and summative
Placement	PS/PA	Emails, Progress Achievement Documentation (PAD), In Point Assessment
	Colleagues	Formal and processional conversations, handover, social interactions, Multi-Disciplinary Team (MDT)
	Patients	Information, emotional discussions, digital interactions, British Sign Language (BSL), translations, communication appropriate for different client groups (children, clients with learning difficulties)

Emails

We need to learn early on in our studies how to send professional emails. Constructing an email is very different to constructing a text or a group message to our peers, but the lines can become a little blurred when our relationships develop. You may come to develop a frequent relationship with your AM for instance but that does not necessarily mean we should communicate with them in the same way as our peers or friends. Emails should remain professional and respectful in nature and at times may need to be shared with others. Never write anything you would not want shared with other staff in your institution. You will also send emails to other departments in university or even to your placement areas, respect and professionalism remain paramount.

Documentation

Completing documentation, for nurses (and student nurses) can feel endless. Some of this will be hard copy paper format, if this is the case it is important to take our time to complete ensuring accuracy and legibility. For some people this can take extra time or may need to be done with support. Students or staff members who have an SpLD (dyslexia for instance) may need support in this area. Disclosing this to practice staff outlining what support is needed to help you can aid both you and them. If you have any concerns in this area speak with your AM or university support, they can help you navigate the resources and systems available.

Many health boards are choosing to replace paper documentation with digital alternatives. These have proven benefits but can take a little time to get used to if these are new to you (Huxley, 2015).

Some of those benefits include sending large pieces of data more easily, avoiding repetition of paperwork, improved access to medical and other health records, improvements in co-ordination of care, improved accessibility and greater patient involvement.

Multiple points of communication sit in the verbal category. For example, formal conversations with colleagues or other healthcare professionals, emotional conversations with patients and families, handovers and transfer of care and social interactions at break times. Many of these can be difficult to navigate for some people, especially those new to healthcare. Using and learning new ways of communication, for example BSL, Finger BSL or Makaton (https://makaton.org), may be something you encounter. Indeed, in some BSc and MSc programmes, these are factored in. If these are not included in your programme you may want to do your own research to explore learning in these areas by using the Go Further resources at the end of the chapter (p. 67).

CASE STUDY

Ken

We sometimes recognise gaps in our knowledge or opportunities for new knowledge when our communication skills are challenged. Take time to read the following case study.

Ken Francis was admitted to the emergency admissions unit at 13.00. Ken had experienced an episode of severe headache prior to admission and a brief loss of consciousness at home. At the time his neighbour had called to visit, witnessed the episode, and called an ambulance.

The early shift on the unit were just handing over to the late shift, now 13.30, and reported Ken had just arrived on the unit but had not yet been admitted, no nursing documentation or assessment had yet been completed.

(Continued)

The medical differential diagnosis at this point was that Ken may have suffered a CVA (Cerebral Vascular Accident) or TIA (Transient Ischaemic Attack), the medical team were awaiting results from diagnostic tests performed.

On completion of the handover, the nurse on the late shift had the responsibility for completing the admission and assessment process for Ken.

The final part of the handover for him outlined that he had a hearing impairment, a visual impairment and was non-verbal.

Questions

1   Before considering actions, take time to find definitions for patients who are:

Blind – what variations does this include?
Deaf – what variations exist here?
Mute – what does this mean?

2   Considering the communication points discussed so far in the chapter, what does the admitting nurse need to consider in their approach to communicating with Ken?
3   How might the nurse complete the outstanding admission and assessment tasks given these communication challenges?
4   How do you think the nurse might have felt in this situation?
5   How do you think the patient might have felt?

What do nurses communicate?

The answer to this question may be another question – 'How long is a piece of string?'. For the purpose of this chapter, we will look at handover/transfer of care and breaking bad news.

Handover/transfer of care

Handoff; report; transfer of care; handover – all terms that have been used historically. You may even have heard alternatives not included in this list. The most used term is 'handover', so this is the term we will use in the rest of the chapter. This communication interaction is happening in all healthcare settings and in all nursing fields multiple times a day. It could be shift to shift handover – all the patients in one area, unit or case load are handed over to the next shift or team. It could be a patient is transferred from one area or department to another as they move through health services. A patient may become acutely unwell, or their symptoms deteriorate, and there is a handover to medical staff or escalated care. For whatever the reason, the communication process of handover happens regularly.

For student nurses it can be an area that causes anxiety. Information must be transferred accurately, succinctly and in a structured manner. Our colleagues may ask questions or clarify points, so we must be prepared to respond. If this is an area that causes you some anxiety, work with your PS/PA in placement areas to practice this skill. Maybe start small, handover one or two patients just to your PS/PA in a private area and work up from that. Whatever method you prefer to practice, the key is that you do practice. It is an important registrant skill and it takes time to become proficient. When done well handover ensures safety is maintained for patient(s); unfortunately, like all communication interactions, if it is not done well if can increase the risk of harm to patients in our care.

Your experience of handover may happen in several ways.

Table 3.4 Various ways handover occurs

Verbal Handover	Allowing receiving participants the opportunity to ask questions and clarify points about information being given.
Digital Handover	A variety of platforms or systems exist and are tailored to individual services or Health Boards.
Recorded (Audio) Handover	Completed using a portable recording device which is securely locked away. This option means both parties do not have to be present at the same time, giving time back to patient care.
Private Handover	Conducted in a private space behind closed doors, an office perhaps, or an area away from patients.
Bedside Handover	The teams visit each patient and conduct handover at each patient's bedside and in front of the patient. Usually in secondary care settings, like Medics/Surgical Ward Round.

Literature has debated handover interactions for many years (Entwistle, 2019) and whilst there is no one ideal way or method, authors do agree on several key aspects that should be considered.

Poor or miscommunication during the handover process can lead to several negative effects:

- Patient delays and prolonged stay in hospital
- Ineffective treatment or management; medication and/or treatment errors
- Unnecessary, subjective information communicated

Despite these points, handover is a key opportunity to professionally discuss the patient's care and treatment, as well as any concerns raised. When done well, safety can be maintained, tasks are not unnecessarily repeated and quality care is effective (Merten et al., 2017).

Many authors on this topic advise the following points to be considered and implemented into handovers:

- Consider any barriers – for example, the MDT may use different language or terms, and this can cause confusion – use one shared language.
- Involve the patient – they have valuable points to offer during this process and can contribute in a positive way. Include them in the informal and formal aspects of handover, allow the patients to ask and answer questions as well as clarify points.
- Privacy is a priority – maintain confidentiality. Sensitive information should not be shared at the bedside, but shared in a more appropriate way. Create a safe and comfortable space for patients.
- Handover should be structured – the World Health Organization recommend using SBAR (Situation, Background, Assessment, Recommendations) to structure handovers. An accurate, structured format that is understood by all is key. (SBAR format does not include patient involvement, this must be factored in.)

Whilst there can be variations in handovers in primary and secondary care, in different fields and settings, some of the fundamental principles outlined above remain the same. Always check the receiver understands the information being given. You should always involve the patient, because '[e]vidence suggests that communication improves when nursing handover involves the patient and is carried out using a structured format' (Mascioli et al., 'Improving Handoff Communication', cited in NICE, 2018: 5).

Table 3.5 SBAR format

S - Situation	I am (name), (X) nurse on ward (X). I am calling about (patient X). I am calling because I am concerned that... (e.g. BP is low/high, pulse is XX, temperature is XX, Early Warning Score (NEWS2) is XX).
B - Background	Patient (X) was admitted on (XX date) with... (e.g. MI/chest infection). They have had (X operation/procedure/investigation). Patient (X)'s condition has changed in the last (XX mins). Their last set of clinical observations were (XX). Patient (X)'s normal condition is... (e.g. alert/drowsy/confused, pain free).
A - Assessment	I think the problem is (XXX). And I have... (e.g. given O2 /analgesia, stopped the infusion) OR I am not sure what the problem is but patient (X) is deteriorating OR I don't know what's wrong but I am really worried.
R - Recommendations	I need you to... Come to see the patient in the next (XX mins) AND Is there anything I need to do in the mean time? (e.g. stop the fluid/repeat the observations)

GO FURTHER

Read the following documents that outline the benefits and pitfalls of handovers:

Raeisi, A., Rarani, M.A. and Soltani, F. (2019). 'Challenges of patient handover process in healthcare services: A systematic review', *Journal of Education and Health Promotion*, 8 (1): Article #173. https://www.ncbi.nlm.nih.gov/pmc/articles/PMC6796291/ (accessed October 10, 2022).

National Institute for Health and Care Excellence (NICE) (2018) *Chapter 32 Structured Patient Handovers: Emergency and Acute Medical Care in Over 16s: Service Delivery and Organisation.* https://www.nice.org.uk/guidance/ng94/evidence/32.structured-patient-handovers-pdf-172397464671 (accessed October 10, 2022).

Instigating change in healthcare can be a complex and lengthy process. It is fair to say that whilst evidence suggests best practice, this may not yet be evident in all areas. Improvements can still be made in many areas. Handovers following these fundamental principles are not yet standard practice (Ruhomauly et al., 2019). Recent evidence also suggests that in a modern healthcare system, where available and possible, handovers should utilise digital processes. Your own experiences may be that you have witnessed several of the methods mentioned.

SBAR increases safety, increases professionalism around communications and handover and helps facilitate interprofessional communication (Randmaa et al., 2014).

Breaking bad news

This is also an area of communication that can cause anxiety when you are a student nurse or even early registrant. It is key to begin with a definition of bad news.

> Bad news is defined as any information which adversely and seriously affects an individual's view of their future. (Buckman, 1992)

When we begin to analyse this definition, what is evident is that what constitutes bad news is individual to the recipient. How someone responds to bad news can be influenced by multiple factors.

Historically, breaking bad news was seen as the point where the doctor sat with the patients to discuss a distressing diagnosis, poor prognosis, or treatment options. The role of the nurse during this time was to merely be present and offer support following the conversation (Warnock, 2014). This is dated and more recently this view has been challenged as too simplistic and not representative of a modern healthcare system or the roles of each professional involved. Authors in this area have proffered 'bad news' as not one single interaction but several (Narayanan et al., 2010).

EXAMPLE OF INCIDENTS SEEN AS BAD NEWS

- Explaining and giving information of needed complex treatments, for instance renal dialysis; oncology therapies.
- Discussing updates with family members where a patient's condition may not be improving.
- Informing loved ones that a patient has deteriorated or died.
- Discussing palliative care processes with patients.
- Advising patients they may need care and support at home on discharge.

Whether something is considered bad news relies on how it is perceived by the receiver, this therefore will differ between individuals. Several points will impact and influence this communication interaction. For instance, the patients' expectations; their values and beliefs; their current situation; their previous experiences. How the information is delivered can also be an influential factor. Whether news is perceived as good, bad or neutral, the receiver must be taken into consideration by the person giving the information. Being prepared helps.

(LOWER LEVEL) BAD NEWS IN A MODERN HEALTHCARE SYSTEM

- Restricted visiting times - routine for staff to some degree but can have significant detrimental effects on patients.
- Delays in discharges - receiving medications to take home late.
- Services not in place for the patients - again routine to staff (perhaps desensitisation has occurred) but devastating for patients.

It is key, before delivering bad news to patients, to have some understanding of how this information may affect them. Understandably, recent writings in this area see communication as a process and not an isolated event. Keeping patients and relatives informed can help alleviate the impact of some bad news. The difference between regular updates of a patient and their condition versus a sudden phone call or interaction with no warning can have a significant impact.

Communication skills already discussed are important in how well prepared the healthcare professional may be, as well as how the patient receives and processes the information given. Baile et al. (2000) discuss a protocol for breaking bad news – SPIKES. SPIKES is a detailed framework used in speciality areas, primarily in oncology, but the format can be adapted for other settings. Certainly, key learning points can be taken from each of the six steps, which are:

- **S**etting up the interview
- **P**erception of condition/seriousness
- **I**nvitation from the patient to give information
- **K**nowledge: giving medical facts
- **E**motions are explored both empathetically and sympathetically
- **S**trategy and summary

(after Baile et al., 2000)

GO FURTHER

Watch this YouTube video that outlines SPIKES being used:

FrontLine Communication (2020) 'Breaking Bad News over the phone SPIKES model', Front Line Communication (YouTube video), May 16. https://www.youtube.com/watch?v=wIUrzfLDrIg (accessed October 10, 2022).

It is important to point out that while SPIKES is used as an example, other models and frameworks are available and used in a variety of settings. Explore these as further background reading.

ACTIVITY: COMMUNICATION SKILLS

Considering the SPIKES 6 Steps Framework, think about how you would prepare for a conversation where a registrant has to explain a patient's deterioration to a loved one. Consider this in the context of your chosen field of study.

The way in which staff members are involved in breaking bad news can be affected by several factors. Their clinical setting, their specific role and their level of experience will all impact their involvement. Authors in this area recognise breaking bad news as an extremely difficult experience for both parties. There is strong evidence to suggest staff can be reluctant to engage in these communication interactions for fear it may be too difficult for the patient or the staff member. However, this reluctance has significant negative impact on patients, and no positive outcomes are recognised when staff avoid this communication.

Many areas of the nurse's role are difficult and challenging; this is one of them. Whilst it can be difficult to gain experience as a student due to the sensitive nature and appropriateness of students being present, it is an area you can explore and discuss with both academic and practice staff. Listening to their experiences can help you.

It can be difficult to engage in difficult communications. We may want to avoid it; we may subconsciously avoid it. The following table looks at some of the barriers encountered when difficult communications are avoided.

Table 3.6 Potential outcomes of not engaging in difficult communications

Patient satisfaction is greatly reduced.

Patients may have false hope, or extreme confusion and fear.

It denies patients the opportunity to be involved and make decisions.

Patients lack trust in healthcare professionals.

Breaks down relationships rather than builds them.

Patients and family feel isolated, there is a lack of transparency, undue stress is caused on family relationships and dynamics.

Staff stress and burnout.

The process of breaking bad news is uncomfortable and complex. It requires knowledge on the part of the communicator, and must be done well. There is no second chance to get it right as miscommunication can have long lasting effects. When this is done well it can be a positive experience for patients and those close to them and can serve to help them deal with life changing events.

STUDENT VOICE

I remember my first placement shift; I was so overwhelmed by the amount of information that I did not understand. Handover, medical notes, conversations in the office – I had no idea what people were talking about. I also had no idea how I would begin to learn this. This really affected my confidence for a long time. I started to ask questions, and question whether the terms should even be used. If patients cannot understand them, why should we use them. I learned there are times, when talking to colleagues that this language may have a place, but not everywhere.

Aisha, 2nd year, Adult Health

CHAPTER SUMMARY

As this chapter has outlined, communication is a vast topic and one that you will continue to grow, develop skills, and gather new knowledge in. You will observe countless communication events and interactions during your studies, use critical thought and analysis on your observations, good and bad, to help you develop and use guided reflection to help in this area.

Some challenges in communications we discussed are:

* **Using abbreviations or jargon** – you will have noticed during your placement experiences that a whole new language is used. Whether its abbreviations, terminology, or specialised terms: this can be overwhelming at the start. Some abbreviations can have more than one meaning and very often the patient has a different one again – this is not ideal or effective or safe. Most health boards have a recognised abbreviation list that can be used, and staff must not veer from it. If there is ambiguity about abbreviations or terms then it should be clarified for all in the team, including the patient.

- **Time constraints** – this is a well-documented barrier. Competing demands faced by staff can make time feel like a luxury in modern healthcare environments. It can be useful to remember that saying hello to a patient, a smile or social conversation does not need to be time consuming. Interruptions and diversions are one of the biggest constraints to effective communication. If you are distracted by something more urgent when you are with someone it is important to recognise it with the patient, or the team. Explain to them and arrange to resume the conversation timely and realistically. Assure patients that their concerns or feelings are important and make a point to return to them as soon as you can.
- **Environment** – some environments can be more overwhelming than others. It can be difficult to facilitate a calm and quiet environment all the time. As staff or students, you become familiar with sounds and the sensory overload of your environment, but patients and visitors rarely get used to it. It remains overwhelming to them. This can be even more of a challenge to those with hearing or other sensory impairments, cognitive impairments, or any barriers to concentration levels.
- **Pain** – information often needs to be obtained from patients when they are in pain, or distressed. We need to be mindful of how this will affect the communication interaction. The patient is unlikely to find it easy to participate in the communication. Ask yourself – 'do we need to do this now?' If the answer is no, ensure the patient's pain is addressed and return another time. If the answer is yes, and this should be a clinical need and not because now fits into our routine or our to do list, then again, acknowledge how the patient is feeling and ensure the pain is addressed by an appropriate member of staff before beginning.
- **Embarrassment** – this can be on either side, patient or staff member. We can anticipate embarrassment to some degree and seek to reduce it. Transparent, open interactions can alleviate it. When managing embarrassment, consider your own body language and non-verbal communication, ensure it is positive. Seek to avoid judgemental questions, for example 'You don't smoke more than ten a day, do you?' could be perceived as judging the person; instead ensure you remain open 'How many cigarettes do you smoke a day?'. Reflecting on and being aware of our own assumptions or prejudices is important in communication. Take time to consider how these might influence the interaction. Amoah et al. (2019) conducted an exploratory study that recognised how a person's cultural background and lifestyle behaviours affected their communications. They also recognised how nurses' misconceptions of a patient significantly impact communication. Being consciously aware of our own values, beliefs and judgements can help us address them so that they do not negatively affect our relationships with patients.

These challenges are not new to nurse or other healthcare education. More recent changes and improvements see this area being addressed in pre-registration nurse education, with many higher education institutions taking a more inter-professional approach to their programmes and teaching. You may already have experience of this. Educating professionals together who will ultimately work together is an evidence-based approach and has many benefits, not just in communication. In addition to this, communication education is often delivered using a simulation-based education approach. Immersing students in authentic situations and experiences that match clinical experience has a long list of research-based benefits.

ACE YOUR ASSESSMENT

Q1   How should you start conversations with patients or colleagues?

a   Welcome them, introduce yourself ("Hello, my name is…") and ask what the person would like to be called.

b   Welcome them, addressing them using the person's name from your notes.

c   Introduce yourself and explain your role. Ask the person's name and how they would like to be addressed. Orientate them to their surroundings and inform them of what to expect.

Q2   What are the benefits of a good handover?

a   Improves communication
b   Improves safety
c   Can provide structure for colleagues
d   All of the above

Q3   What acronym can be used when breaking bad news?

a   SPOKES
b   SPIKES
c   SPAKES

Q4   What does jargon mean?

a   Professional healthcare language
b   Technical language. Abbreviations only healthcare staff understand
c   The abbreviations used when writing notes

Q5   What does S B A R stand for?

a   Situation, Background, Assessment, Recommendations
b   Situation, Background, Assessment, Reason for admission
c   Situation, Basics, Assessment, Recommendations

Answers

1   C
2   D
3   B
4   B
5   A

GO FURTHER

National Institute for Health and Care Excellence (NICE) (2018) 'Emergency and acute medical care in over 16s, Quality statement 4: Structured patient handovers'. https://www.nice.org.uk/guidance/qs174/chapter/Quality-statement-4-Structured-patient-handovers (accessed October 10, 2022).

Makaton video: CBeebies | Mr Tumble Nursery Rhymes Playlist. (2017) CBeebies (YouTube video), July 11. https://www.youtube.com/watch?v=iyIDg6m4gAO (accessed October 10, 2022).

british-sign.co.uk (n.d.) 'Fingerspelling alphabet'. https://www.british-sign.co.uk/fingerspelling-alphabet-charts/ (accessed October 10, 2022).

REFERENCES

Ali, M. (2018) 'Communication skills 3: Non-verbal communication', *Nursing Times*, 114 (2): 41–2. https://cdn.ps.emap.com/wp-content/uploads/sites/3/2018/01/180117-Communication-skills-3-Non-verbal-communication.pdf (accessed October 10, 2022).

Amoah, V.M.K., Anokye, R., Boakye, D.S., Acheampong, E., Budu-Ainooson, A., Okyere, E., Kumi-Boateng, G., Yeboah, C. and Afriyie, J.O. (2019) 'A qualitative assessment of perceived barriers to effective therapeutic communication among nurses and patients', BMC Nursing, 18(4). doi: 10.1186/s12912-019-0328-0

Bach, S. and Grant, A. (2011) *Communication and Interpersonal Skills for Nursing* (2nd edition). Exeter: Learning Matters.

Baile, W.F., Buckman, R., Lenzi, R., Glober, G., Beale, E.A. and Kudelka, A.P. (2000) 'SPIKES – A six-step protocol for delivering bad news: Application to the patient with cancer', *The Oncologist*, 5 (4): 302–11. doi.org/10.1634/theoncologist.5-4-302

Bottomley, J. and Pryjmachuk, S. (2019) *Communication Skills for Your Nursing Degree*. St Albans: Critical Publishing.

Buckman, R. (1992) *How to Break Bad News: A Guide for Health Professionals*. Baltimore, MD: Johns Hopkins Press.

Entwistle, N.J. (2018) *Student Learning and Academic Understanding: A Research Perspective and Implications for Teaching*. Amsterdam: Elsevier.

Huxley, C.J., Atherton, H., Watkins, J.A. and Griffiths, F.E. (2015) 'Digital communication between clinician and patient and the impact on marginalised groups: A realist review in general practice', *The British Journal of General Practice: The Journal of the Royal College of General Practitioners*, 65 (641): e813–e821 .

Merten, H., van Galen, L.S. and Wagner, C. (2017) 'Safe handover', *BMJ*: Article #359. doi.org/10.1136/bmj.j4328

Montague, E. (2013) 'Nonverbal interpersonal skills in clinical encounters', *Journal of Participatory Medicine*, 14 (5): e33.

Narayanan, V., Bista, B. and Koshy, C. (2010) '"BREAKS" protocol for breaking bad news', *Indian Journal of Palliative Care*, 16 (2): 61–5. https://www.ncbi.nlm.nih.gov/pmc/articles/PMC3144432/ (accessed October 10, 2022).

National Institute for Health and Care Excellence (NICE) (2018). *Chapter 32 Structured Patient Handovers: Emergency and Acute Medical Care in Over 16s: Service Delivery and Organisation*. https://www.nice.org.uk/guidance/ng94/evidence/32.structured-patient-handovers-pdf-172397464671 (accessed October 10, 2022).

National Institute for Health Research (NIHR) (2021) *Annual Report 2019/2020*. Leeds: NIHR. https://www.nihr.ac.uk/documents/about-us/our-contribution-to-research/research-performance/NIHR_Annual_Report_19_20.pdf (accessed October 10, 2022).

Randmaa, M., Mårtensson, G., Leo Swenne, C. and Engström, M. (2014) 'SBAR improves communication and safety climate and decreases incident reports due to communication errors in an anaesthetic clinic: A prospective intervention study', *BMJ Open*, 4 (1): e004268. doi.org/10.1136/bmjopen-2013-004268

Ruhomauly, Z., Betts, K., Jayne-Coupe, K., Karanfilian, L., Szekely, M., Relwani, A., McCay, J. and Jaffry, Z. (2019) 'Improving the quality of handover: Implementing SBAR', *Future Healthcare Journal*, 6 (Suppl 2): 54.

Warnock, C. (2014) 'Breaking bad news: Issues relating to nursing practice', Nursing Standard, 28 (45): 51–8.

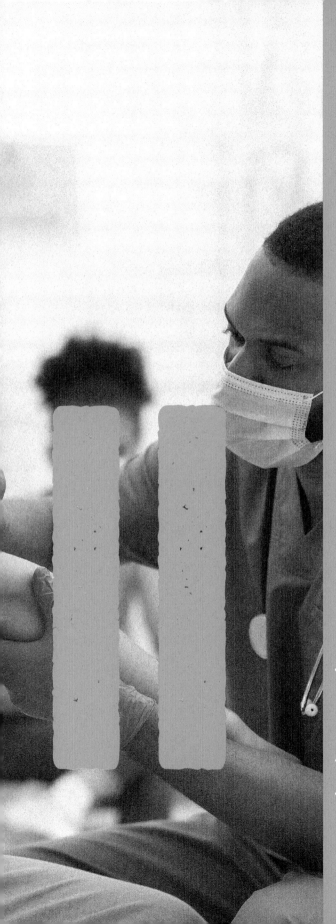

CLINICAL SKILLS FOR NURSING CARE

4 HISTORY TAKING AND
   EXAMINATIONS   71

5 DIGNITY, COMFORT,
   REST AND SLEEP   119

6 HYGIENE AND SKIN
   INTEGRITY   135

7 NUTRITION AND
   HYDRATION   171

8 BLADDER AND BOWEL
   HEALTH   209

9 MOBILITY AND SAFETY   251

10 RESPIRATORY CARE   283

11 PREVENTING AND
   MANAGING INFECTION   313

12 END OF LIFE CARE   349

13 MEDICATION
   ADMINISTRATION   375

HISTORY TAKING AND EXAMINATIONS

4

LEE GAUNTLETT AND PETER SEWELL

─────── LEARNING OBJECTIVES ───────

After reading this chapter, you should be able to:

- Identify signs of ill health and distress by conducting a comprehensive patient history
- Identify signs of self-harm and assess suicide risk by conducting a comprehensive mental health history
- Undertake a whole-body systems assessment including respiratory, circulatory, neurological, musculoskeletal, and cardiovascular examinations
- Perform an Electrocardiogram (ECG)
- Perform venepuncture and cannulation
- Record vital signs and document them appropriately

STUDENT VOICE

INTRODUCTION TO HISTORY TAKING

Patients present to healthcare professionals for a myriad of reasons; they may have a worsening illness or symptoms, may need reassurance, or may need to talk to someone about mental anguish they are suffering. Regardless of the specific motivation, patients often seek understanding and an explanation for what they are experiencing, turning to healthcare services for our expertise.

History taking is about listening to the patient's story; to their symptoms, their concerns and their expectations. It is often the part of clinical examination which is focused more on the 'art' of medicine, rather than solely the science of illness. Not all patients are the same and indeed, each patient will recount their individual story in a unique way. The nuances of history taking are complex and it develops with practice, however a standardised approach to history taking allows even the most inexperienced practitioner to glean a wealth of important information which may have consequences through the patient's individual journey.

PATIENT HISTORY TAKING FORMAT

> Understanding the complexity and processes involved in history taking allows nurses to gain a better understanding of patients' problems. Care priorities can be identified, and the most appropriate interventions commenced to optimise patient outcomes. (Fawcett and Rhynas, 2012: 41)

Patients do not present their symptoms in a predictable manner, nor do they all express specific symptoms in a similar way. As a result, taking a history can often seem daunting to many nursing students. To aid this, many healthcare professionals use a standard approach to history taking, often disguised in their patient questioning.

History taking is typically split into six distinct sections:

1 Presenting Complaint
2 History of Presenting Complaint
3 Past Medical History
4 Drug History
5 Social History
6 Impression/Diagnosis

Each section has its own objectives and allows a 'logical' approach to structure the consultation with the patient. You will note this medical model places the presenting complaint at the forefront of the history process.

Presenting complaint (PC)

The presenting complaint (PC) describes the specific reason the patient has sought help. While it is often tempting to over-complicate this with more symptoms and detail, ideally this should be restricted to a few words or a phrase. For example, 'chest pain' or 'laceration to right arm'. Many patients will present with a mix of acute and chronic symptoms – and it is often difficult for the patient (and an experienced healthcare practitioner) to separate these in a meaningful way. The role of the presenting complaint is to 'set the scene' for the remainder of the discussion with the patient, narrowing the scope of the history to the issue at hand.

History of presenting complaint (HPC, HxPC)

The history of presenting complaint is an opportunity to delve deeper and gather detailed information about the patient's reason for attendance. It is important to ask open ended questions, so the patient can tell you their story in their own words. Often, patients will not provide information in a structured or logical format, so it's important to let them say what they feel is important, with follow-up questions for clarity.

It is often logical to ask about the chronology of the symptom(s) and to build a timeline of how symptoms began and how they have progressed. Some symptoms appear insidiously over weeks to months, slowly increasing in intensity, while others appear quickly and suddenly. Often, multiple symptoms will appear at once. It's important you enquire about all new symptoms in a consistent way to ensure details are not missed. For example:

- When did you first notice the pain?
- Has the dizziness always been the same, or does it change depending on the things you're doing?
- Does anything make the bleeding worse?
- Do you have any other symptoms?

For any presenting complaint with pain, it's good to have a logical framework for questioning. Please see 'Pain Assessment' later in this chapter for more information.

Once questioning has been exhausted, it's good practice to ask a standard set of questions (often referred to a **systems review**) which are a general list of questions which aim to gain any additional information omitted by the patient (or symptoms which they may deem not important to mention or may have forgotten).

Example systems review questions:

- Any headache/visual changes?
- Any loss in taste or smell?
- Any nausea and vomiting?
- Any sore throat or lumps/bumps in neck?
- Any chest pain or palpitations?
- Any shortness of breath?
- Any cough/sputum?
- Any abdominal pain?
- Any fever/rigor?
- Any change in urination – such as burning/stinging?
- Any change in bowel habit?
- Any blood noted in stool?
- Any limb weakness?
- Any limb swelling?

As you can see, these questions are produced in a 'head-to-toe' order but use a non-nuanced 'scatter-gun' approach to history taking. This should only be done for completeness and not form the basis of the primary history of presenting complaint. The questions may need to be worded in a more specific way, if the patent has limited understanding; for example, 'has anything been different when you go to the toilet', 'does it hurt when you wee?'.

Past medical history (PMHx)

The past medical history is a misnomer; this is the section in which a healthcare professional enquires about aspects of a medical, surgical, neurological and psychological/mental health history which may be related to the patient's current symptom(s). This is not simply an exercise in constructing a long list of medical conditions but allows an opportunity to build a much broader picture of the patient, allowing exploration of previous or concurrent conditions which are being managed.

Often, existing chronic conditions have a degree of influence on acute symptoms. For example, a presenting complaint of 'painful leg' may seem innocuous enough at first glance. Has the patient had a trip or a fall? Do they have an existing wound? However, if further questioning illustrated the patient had diabetes, peripheral neuropathy and hypertension, a skilled healthcare practitioner may be concerned the issue could be related to a vascular insufficiency, venous ulceration, or acute infection. This would prompt a different approach to the remainder of the history and examination.

Some patients will struggle to articulate their past medical history. Individuals with a learning disability, children or elderly patients may be unable to provide any significant insight with direct questioning, however if asked 'have you been to hospital before?', or 'what did you last see your doctor for?' may provide some clues (as may involving their carer, chaperones or advocate). Non-native English speakers might experience difficulty with this too.

In relation to the past medical history of children, it's good practice to enquire about birth. For example:

- Vaginal or caesarean section birth
- Term or premature birth
- Low/high birth weight
- Were there any complications at birth? Did the child require the special care baby unit?

Furthermore, it may also be appropriate to enquire about early development, asking the following:

- Did the child meet all their developmental milestones?
- Any concern from health visitors?
- Any concerns from school/teachers regarding the patient?
- Has the child had their vaccinations?

Drug history (DHx, Meds)

A drug history should be thoroughly explored, including prescribed drugs, their doses and frequency of administration. Patients will often struggle to recall specific drugs and doses, but may say things like 'I take a tablet for my blood pressure, and one for my cholesterol'. While lacking detail, it can provide clues to medical conditions they may have omitted in the questioning of their past medical history! It is important to also discuss over-the-counter (OTC) medications, herbal remedies, and vitamin supplements.

A much more difficult topic to approach is recreational drugs (which is often overlooked). Drugs of abuse/addiction may significantly contribute to mortality and co-morbidities but may also play a significant role in the presentation. Ensure that all patients are asked specifically if they take any non-prescription medications and ensure it is documented. Some patients may need help with their addiction during the admission, so early identification of these needs is essential.

Social history (SH, SHx)

The social history is concerned with reaching beyond the presenting symptoms or episode of illness, to gain a much wider perspective on the patient, which may significantly contribute to the management of the patient.

It's good practice to ask about profession (or retired profession), smoking and alcohol status (as well as duration/amount smoked). Professional background can often have a significant influence on diagnosis and treatment, as some occupations have significant risk for a range of pathologies. For example, miners may be more prone to respiratory conditions, builders may have been exposed to asbestos and have fibrosis of the lungs, and patients working in the farming industry may be more likely to suffer from rarer pathogens driving their infections.

It's important to also understand what the patient's day-to-day life is like; and how much functional ability they have, and how much support they require in the community. Ask them about their hobbies and interests, as well as the more mundane aspects of life, such as how they get to the toilet!

ASSESSMENT OF PAIN

It is estimated that chronic pain affects between 35.0% and 51.3% of the UK adult population (Fayaz et al., 2016), with acute pain affecting up to 84% of hospitalised patients (Gregory and McGowan, 2016). Despite its commonality, the exact mechanisms of pain transmission are poorly understood.

There are many approaches to pain assessment in a clinical setting. The most widely used in UK medical practice is the SOCRATES mnemonic:

- **S**ite – where is the pain?
- **O**nset – when did the pain begin, was it sudden or gradual? Was it during activity or at rest?
- **C**haracter – how would you describe the way the pain feels?
- **R**adiation – does the pain travel to another part of the body?
- **A**ssociation – is the pain linked to another symptom?
- **T**ime course – does the pain follow a pattern? Is the pain always the same?
- **E**xacerbating/relieving factors – does anything make the pain worse, or better?
- **S**everity – how bad is the pain?

The SOCRATES assessment provides a logical framework for pain evaluation. The severity can typically be assessed with a numerical pain scale (0–10) by asking the patient to assign a score their pain, with 0 suggesting no pain at all, and 10 being the worst pain they can imagine. While inaccurate and subjective, the pain severity scale can be used to assess the response of analgesia or can indicate further clinical deterioration of a patient.

PAIN ASSESSMENT IN CHILDREN

Assessing pain in children can often be difficult. Their age or level of development will vary the responses gained from clinical questioning. It may be more appropriate to use the child's own language to engage them in discussion, for example 'does your tummy hurt?' or 'where is the ouchy?'. Some children will struggle to interact with a stranger, so it may be more suitable to involve a parent/carer or even a child's favourite toy to help glean important clinical information, for example 'can you point on mummy where it hurts?' or 'can you point on the teddy where it's sore?'

There is a tendency to under-estimate pain in children, especially those who are socially withdrawn or have other developmental issues. It's important that pain is assessed on a regular basis and that the child is believed. Being dismissive of pain can fester distrust, making further interaction much more challenging.

One tool to aid assessment is the Wong-Baker Pain rating scale (Wong-Baker Faces Foundation, 2020), shown in Figure 4.1.

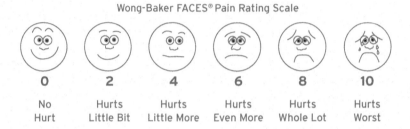

Wong-Baker FACES® Pain Rating Scale

0	2	4	6	8	10
No Hurt	Hurts Little Bit	Hurts Little More	Hurts Even More	Hurts Whole Lot	Hurts Worst

Figure 4.1   The Wong-Baker Pain Rating Scale

Source: Wong-Baker FACES Foundation (2020). Wong-Baker FACES® Pain Rating Scale. Retrieved 19 July 2022 with permission from www.WongBakerFACES.org. Originally published in Whaley & Wong's *Nursing Care of Infants and Children.* © Elsevier Inc.

The tool features six images of faces, each with worsening pain (and ever-more distressed facial expressions) reading from left to right. The images can be presented to a child, and they may be able to point at the face which corresponds to how they feel. While subjective, this tool can aid assessment and the response of analgesia or intervention. The Wong-Baker Pain Rating Scale is designed to be used in children above three years of age.

PAIN ASSESSMENT WITH PATIENTS WITH COMMUNICATION DIFFICULTIES

When a patient has cognitive difficulties, be it from acute medical or mental health illness or from a learning disability, gaining an accurate understanding of their level of pain can be challenging. In this situation it may be suitable to talk to a friend or relative, or even a group of individuals who knows the patient well. While they may not be able to give you detailed information on specific symptoms such as pain, bowel habits or fever, they may be able to tell you how the patient's behaviour has changed. For example, they may tell you about a long period of decline, which may be suggestive of a deterioration in an existing medical condition, or they may tell you about a sudden acute change, which is more suggestive of an acute pathology. Furthermore, they may be able to give you subtle clues which may prompt further investigation, such as:

- 'She's been running to the toilet more often lately'
- 'There has been a big change in their behaviour around mealtimes'
- 'He's been really thirsty and drinking pints of water'
- 'She's not really eaten in weeks'

This will give you the basis for further questions or investigations.

THE PSYCHIATRIC/MENTAL HEALTH HISTORY

The standard medical model of history taking has some validity for use in psychiatric patients, indeed many patients with primary mental health concerns may also have concurrent medical conditions which need to be considered and managed. However, the psychiatric history asks very different questions, which can be difficult for newly qualified or inexperienced staff to remember.

GO FURTHER

The I-AM-A-STAR framework was developed by Mansel et al. (2018) as an aide-memoire for nursing students to recall the components of the mental state examination. It is freely available to access and easy to follow: https://cronfa.swan.ac.uk/Record/cronfa38823 (accessed January 30, 2023).

Signs of Suicide/Self Harm

Self-harm is a provocative topic – for some, self-harm is something they are embarrassed or ashamed of and will often attempt to keep the signs of injury hidden from view. For others it stirs the emotions and can prompt recall of major traumatic experiences which drove them to express their mental anguish into physical pain. It can therefore be a difficult topic to approach, especially within a brief consultation with a patient.

Questioning about self-harm should be performed at an appropriate point within the history process – typically after a good rapport has been established and once the patient has begun to engage with the questioning. Some patients may lead the conversation to talk about self-harm spontaneously, while others may need encouragement.

Types of self-harm

- **Cutting or burning the skin.** This can often be concealed on the thighs, upper arms, or chest wall. Some patients may have extensive horizontal scarring to the forearms, and this can easily be concealed in long-sleeved jumpers or jackets.
- **Punching and striking themselves/other objects**. This can be seen with abrasions to the hands or knuckles (if striking walls etc.).
- **Hair plucking**. Often seen with extremes of emotional stress, patients may pull out their own eyelashes, eyebrows, and hair.
- **Poisoning**. The most common forms of drug poisoning in the UK are paracetamol overdoses. While a widely available over-the-counter medicine, paracetamol toxicity can cause coagulation disorders, bleeding, and liver failure.

Suicidal Ideation (SI)

Suicidal ideation (SI) is a broad term which encompasses the various form of contemplation an individual may possess about suicide (Harmer et al., 2022). Most people who have suicidal ideation (suicidal thought) do not go on to take their own life, however those with suicidal ideation are at a slightly increased risk of suicide compared to those who do not. Complicating the matter further is the transitory nature of the thoughts; feeling of suicide may wax and wane depending on specific circumstances. For example, if the patient has received bad news or is undergoing significant emotional distress, suicidal thoughts may intensify.

Examples of questions to assess suicidal ideation:

- In the past few weeks, have you thought life wasn't worth living?
- Have you ever thought about taking an overdose of tablets?
- How often do you think about killing yourself?

Suicide Risk Assessment

According to the Office of National Statistics (ONS) there were 6,507 suicides in the UK in 2018. The reasons behind suicide and attempted suicide are multifactorial and complex. What is clear is that there is a gender bias; males are more likely to take their own life than females, attributed amongst other reasons, due to more 'lethal' methods chosen. Females are much more likely to self-harm than men and are more likely to seek medical or psychiatric help.

Despite falling death rates in recent years, suicide rates are increasing in the under 25s (Office for National Statistics (ONS), 2019), perhaps precipitated by difficult socio-economic conditions, which may be further precipitated by the lockdowns and economic difficulties caused by the global Coronavirus pandemic.

When a patient presents to a healthcare setting with attempted suicide or self-harm, it is important to recognise this encounter as an opportunity to talk to the patient, gather information and refer the patient to appropriate services which can offer support. The difficulty is predicting which individuals will escalate their suicide attempts and likely come to the most harm. One assessment tool commonly used in general practice and the acute care setting is the SADPERSONS scale (Patterson et al., 1983). Designed to be used by non-mental health practitioners, the scale can help the assessor quickly decide if an intervention is required.

Criteria	Score
Sex: Male	+1
Age: <19 or >59 years old	+1
Depression or Hopelessness	+2
Previous Suicide Attempt	+1
Ethanol (Alcohol or Drug Use)	+1
Rational Thinking Loss (patient is lacking insight, psychotic illness)	+2
Single, Widowed or Divorced	+1
Organised or Serious Attempt (i.e., suicide note, bought equipment)	+2
No Social Support (alone, isolated)	+1
Stated Future Intent (plans to repeat suicide attempts)	+2

Figure 4.2   **Modified SADPERSONS Scale (suicide risk calculation)**

Source: Evaluation of suicidal patients: The SAD PERSONS scale, Patterson et al, (1983)

Based on the responses to the questions, a score is calculated:

- 0–5: Patient is low risk. They may be safe to be discharged (depending on individual circumstances and local policy).
- 6–8: Patient is medium risk. They may require input from mental health services.
- >8: Patient is high risk. They will require input from mental health services and admission to a place of safety is likely.

ACTIVITY: PAUSE AND REFLECT

It's not easy to discuss suicide or self-harm with a patient. You should always remember that it is not our place to judge a patient's actions; nor to dismiss the emotional turmoil they might find themselves in.

Imagine a point in your life where you have been low, for example suffering from financial difficulties or grieving for the loss of a loved one. Would you have asked for help? Would you feel able to talk to a healthcare professional? Would you want to open-up and answer potentially intrusive questions about your thoughts and feelings? Would you openly admit to self-harm or suicidal ideation?

'We' in the healthcare profession are not immune to a mental health crisis. We could easily find ourselves struggling in life and needing help.

FULL BODY ASSESSMENT

This comprehensive clinical examination involves:

1. Gait Assessment
2. Chest Auscultation
3. Cardiovascular Auscultation
4. Gastrointestinal Examination
5. Cranial Nerve Examination
6. Upper Limb Neurological Examination
7. Lower Limb Neurological Examination

WATCH THE VIDEO

UNDERTAKING A WHOLE-BODY SYSTEMS ASSESSMENT

Watch along as you read through this step by step procedure by scanning the QR code with your smartphone camera or via https://study.sagepub.com/rowberry.

WATCH THE VIDEO

ASSESSMENT DIFFERENCES ON DARK SKIN

Watch along as you read through this step by step procedure by scanning the QR code with your smartphone camera or via https://study.sagepub.com/rowberry.

GAIT, ARMS, LEGS AND SPINE ASSESSMENT: DISCUSSION

While it would be beyond the scope of this book to examine every bone or joint in the musculoskeletal system; it is important that you are equipped with a basic framework for assessing some important functions which are critical to the patient's performance of the activities of daily living.

KEY TERMS

Activities of Daily Living (ADLs): collectively describes the fundamental skills to care for one self. They include personal hygiene, dressing, eating, continence and mobility.

Gait: the person's manner of walking.

GAIT ASSESSMENT: STEP BY STEP

- Ask the patient if they can walk unaided or have any difficulties with mobility. If they do, make suitable adjustments to this examination.
- Ask the patient to walk away from you, then back to you over a distance of a few meters. Pay attention to their gait by looking at the level of their hips.
- Look at an asymmetry in hip/leg movement which may suggest difficulty or pain.
- Look at stride length and foot placement (are they walking on their heels or tip toes?).
- Look at their shoes, are the soles of the shoes worn in a particular way?

ARMS ASSESSMENT: STEP BY STEP

- Ask the patient to put their hands behind their head. This tests shoulder abduction and external rotation, as well as power of the upper limbs (resisting gravity).
- Ask the patient to put their arms out and turn their palms downwards (arm pronation).
- Ask the patient to turn their palms up (arm supination).

- Ask the patient to grip your index fingers and to squeeze tightly (power grip).
- Ask the patient to touch each finger to the thumb on the same side (precision grip).

These maneuvers will allow you to broadly comment on the power, coordination, and range of movement of the upper limbs. If a patient possesses the ability to perform these tasks, they are more likely to be able to feed themselves and complete basic personal hygiene. Look carefully for difficulty, signs of pain or limited range of movement.

LEGS ASSESSMENT: STEP BY STEP

While patient is lying down (if tolerated):

- Passively flex and extend the knee, looking for range of movement and discomfort.
- Passively flex the patient's hip and knee joint to 90° and then rotate their foot laterally.
- Palpate the patella (kneecap) and tap to examine if large effusion.   ·
- Look at soles of feet for deformation/callous formation.

SPINE ASSESSMENT: STEP BY STEP

Lumbar flexion

- Place two fingers of the same hand on the patient's lumbar spine (spinous processes).
- Ask the patient to bend forward.
- As they do, fingers should move apart as spine flexes forward and the gap between spinous processes increases.

Note any abnormal findings and document as per local policy.

CHEST AUSCULTATION: INTRODUCTION

Chest auscultation (listening of sounds) is a routine examination performed by a range of health professionals, in a variety of settings. It is a simple examination which the majority of patients are familiar with and able to tolerate well.

The examination is performed with the lung anatomy in mind; we have two lungs, each split into lobes - there are three lobes on the right side, with two lobes on the left. To allow all lobes to be examined thoroughly, auscultation is conducted on the patient's anterior chest wall, posterior chest wall, and beneath each axilla.

GO FURTHER

This webpage produced by Lumen Learning offers extensive open educational resources, which are of a high quality and easy to follow: https://courses.lumenlearning.com/suny-ap2/ (accessed October 11, 2022).

WATCH THE VIDEO

UNDERTAKING CHEST AUSCULTATION

Watch along as you read through this step by step procedure by scanning the QR code with your smartphone camera or via https://study.sagepub.com/rowberry.

CHEST AUSCULTATION: STEP BY STEP

- Ensure you have explained the process of chest auscultation to the patient and gained verbal consent (or a best interest decision is in place) to conduct the examination.
- Ideally the patient's chest should be fully exposed, so the examination should be conducted in a closed room or behind curtains to maintain dignity. Furthermore, a blanket could be used to protect the patient's modesty to loosely cover the chest wall and lifted for placement of the stethoscope.
- Hold the diaphragm of the stethoscope between the index and middle finger of your dominant hand.
- Place the stethoscope onto the patient's chest, using gentle pressure. The stethoscope should be in contact with the chest for a full cycle of inspiration and expiration.
- Ask the patient to breathe through their mouth and ask them to fully inhale and fully exhale in each auscultation position.
- Auscultate the anterior chest wall in four different positions:
  - Apical zone (above clavicle)
  - Upper zone (below clavicle, mid-clavicular line, 2nd–3rd intercostal space)
  - Mid zone (lateral to sternum, level of hilar structures)
  - Lower zone (lung bases, lateral to mid-clavicular line)
  - Compare side-to-side, e.g. apical zone on right to apical zone on left
- Once anterior auscultation is complete, ask patient to flex arms, with hands on hips, opening the axillary chest wall.
- Auscultate the axilla in two different positions (comparing side-to-side):
  - Upper zone (mid-axilla line, just below arm pit)
  - Lower zone (mid-axilla line, superior to lowest palpable rib)
- Auscultate the posterior chest wall – ask the patient to sit forward (assistance may be needed). Auscultate in four different positions (comparing side-to-side).

- o   Apical zone (above scapula)
- o   Upper zone (medial to scapula - ask patient to fold arms to open scapula)
- o   Mid zone (below scapula)
- o   Lower zone (lung bases)
- Once the examination is complete, ensure you cover the patient and instruct them to dress. Clean your stethoscope and wash your hands as per local policy.

Special considerations

When auscultating the chest of a small child or infant, the lack of physical space makes it difficult to auscultate in so many anatomical locations. It may be more appropriate to listen in two or three different anterior positions in this instance.

Breast tissue can overlie the anterior lung bases and disrupt stethoscope positioning. It is acceptable to auscultate on the breast directly, however this may dampen sounds from the lung bases. It is suitable to ask the patient to lift their breasts if it aids the clinical examination.

Some patients will be unable to sit forward and allow full examination of the posterior chest wall. It is suitable to ask a colleague to assist the patient to sit forward. If this is not possible, the posterior examination can be omitted, if the omission is documented clearly in the patient notes.

Auscultation findings

When listening to sounds generated by respiration it is important to listen to the inspiratory and expiratory phase, comparing one lung to the other. It is important to note:

- **Respiratory rate** – Is it slow? (known as bradypnoea < 12 per minute) often seen opiate toxicity, hypercapnia (high blood CO_2 levels) or due to intracranial pathologies. A fast rate >25 breaths per minute (tachypnoea) can be caused by acute infection, asthma, and pulmonary oedema.
- **Breathing pattern** – A normal breathing pattern should be smooth, with inspiration half the duration of expiration. Inhalation and expiration should be rhythmical. Excessive work of breathing and deep inhalation can be associated with metabolic disorders, such as diabetic ketoacidosis.
- **Chest symmetry** – Is the right and left side of the chest rising and falling together? One side not rising could suggest serious pathology, such as a haemothorax or pneumothorax. Paradoxical chest wall movement (a portion of the chest wall rising when the chest is falling) can suggest a 'flail segment', caused by multiple broken ribs.

Wheeze

A wheeze by definition is a 'whistling sound', often heard as a high-pitched continuous noise, louder than the breath sounds which generate it. A wheeze is suggestive of a limitation in airflow and is often associated with asthma and respiratory infections. While even the most inexperienced practitioner can hear a wheeze, it takes more practice and a nuanced approach to allow a comprehensive description of the wheeze itself.

When auscultating a wheeze, the practitioner should address the following questions:

- Is the wheeze present in inspiration, expiration or both phases? An expiratory wheeze is more common in asthmatics (typically after exercise). An inspiratory wheeze however could be caused by severe asthma, or a physical airway obstruction (foreign body, or mass). A wheeze in both the inspiratory and expiratory phase is more common with COPD.
- Is the wheeze monophonic (one sound), or polyphonic (multiple sounds)? A monophonic wheeze is generally due to obstruction or compression of the large airways, while a polyphonic wheeze is more typical of obstruction in the smaller airways.
- Is the wheeze located in one area, or widespread? A wheeze located in a single area could be more suggestive of a foreign body or mass (such as a tumour), while a widespread wheeze is more suggestive of asthma/COPD.

Crackles

Crackles are discontinuous sounds, often briefly occurring on auscultation. They are not 'musical' like a wheeze and can also be described as coarse or fine. They are present in a wide range of medical conditions such as pneumonia, atelectasis (lung collapse), interstitial lung disease and pulmonary oedema.

When auscultating a crackle, the practitioner should address the following questions:

- Is the crackle present in inspiration, expiration or both phases?
- Do the crackles occur throughout the lungs, or only at the bases?
- Are the sounds transmitted to the upper airway, or only audible in the lung bases?
- Are the sounds altered after a cough?

Pleural rub

Pleural rub is audible friction between the two pleural linings, caused by pleural thickening and inflammation. The sound is non-musical and often described as a 'grating sound' or 'creaking'. Commonly accompanied with pain on respiration.

Stridor

Stridor is a loud, high pitched noise, often heard from the larger airways (so more audible in the neck and upper airways), **without** a stethoscope. Stridor is often caused by airway obstruction limiting flow and can often be classed as an airway emergency needing immediate escalation of patient treatment.

CARDIOVASCULAR AUSCULTATION: DISCUSSION

Cardiovascular auscultation (listening of sounds) is a routine examination performed by a range of health professionals in a variety of settings. It is suitable to be conducted alongside the respiratory examination.

The examination is performed with the heart anatomy in mind; we have four heart chambers and four valves which are located beneath the rib cage. The valves are auscultated beneath specific rib spaces whilst the examiner also palpates the carotid pulse. This allows the relationship between the pulse and the cardiac sounds to be correlated.

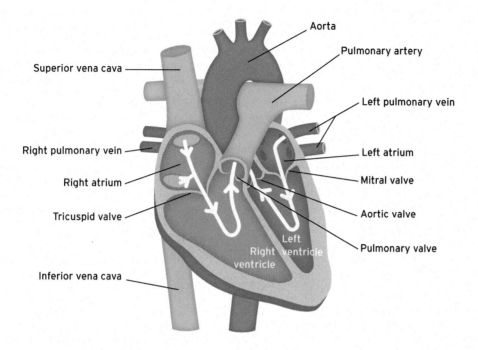

Figure 4.3   Chambers of the heart and blood flow around the heart

CARDIOVASCULAR AUSCULTATION: STEP BY STEP

- Ideally the patient's chest should be fully exposed, so the examination should be conducted in a closed room or behind curtains to maintain dignity. Furthermore, a blanket could be used to protect the patient's modesty to loosely cover the chest wall, and lifted for placement of the stethoscope.

- Palpate (feel) the radial pulse, assess rate and rhythm (for one minute).

- Compare radial pulses by palpating each pulse simultaneously, looking for any sign of radial-radial delay between them.

- Ask patient to open mouth and look at tongue/oral mucosa (it may be suitable to use a pen torch and tongue depressor for this step; you may need to action the movement required for some patients to understand what is required here).

- Hold the diaphragm of the stethoscope between the index and middle finger of your dominant hand and place the stethoscope onto the patient's chest, using gentle pressure. While palpating the carotid pulse with your non-dominant hand, auscultate the anterior chest wall in four different positions:

  o   2nd intercostal space, right sternal edge (aortic valve)

  o   2nd intercostal space, left sternal edge (pulmonary valve)

  o   5th intercostal space, right sternal edge (tricuspid valve)

  o   5th intercostal space, mid clavicular line (mitral valve)

- Check lower limbs for signs of peripheral oedema; press on the ankles and lower legs. See if your finger marks remain in the skin.

- Once the examination is complete, ask the patient to cover themselves or redress.

- Document your examination findings.

Cardiovascular examination – clinical findings

Heart sounds are complex and take years of practice to reliably auscultate and describe with accuracy. This section will aim to give you an appropriate *introduction* to heart sounds but is by no means exhaustive in content.

Heart valves only make a sound when they close. This sound is often described as a 'lub-dub', after an approximation of the noise which is heard.

- The first heart sound (called S_1) is the 'lub' sound. This is caused by closure of the mitral and tricuspid valves at the start of **systole**.
- The second heart sound (called S_2) is the 'dub' sound. This is caused by closure of the aortic and pulmonary valves at the start of **diastole**.
- Sometimes the S_2 sound can be split (caused by respiration), making a 'd-dub' sound. This is a normal finding.

ACTIVITY: CRITICAL THINKING

Palpation of the carotid pulse during auscultation of the heart valves allows the examiner to orientate the pulse to the 'lub-dub' sound. The 'lub' and 'dub' sounds are so similar, it's easy to get them confused! The carotid pulse indicates **systole** so the corresponding sound will be S_1 (the lub). Without carotid palpation, the examiner may incorrectly hear the 'dub' sound and associate this to S_1. Why would confusing S_1 ('lub') and S_2 ('dub') be a problem? (See 'Have a go' below for the answer.)

Valve pathologies – basic explanation

At the start of the S_1 ('lub') phase the mitral and tricuspid valves are firmly **closed**. During the S_1 ('lub') phase, the aortic and pulmonary valves are **open,** and blood is flowing across the valves. Additional sounds in the S_1 ('lub') phase are caused by turbulence. But **what** is causing the turbulence and **where** in the heart is it occurring?

Turbulence (added sounds) in the S_1 ('lub') phase can mean broadly two things:

1   Either the mitral or tricuspid valves are leaky (known as **regurgitation**)
2   Either the aortic or pulmonary valves are tight (known as **stenosis**)

Conversely, at the start of the S_2 ('dub') phase the aortic and pulmonary valves are firmly **closed**. During the S_s ('dub') phase, the mitral and tricuspid valves are **open,** and blood is flowing across the valves. Additional sounds in the S_2 ('dub') phase are caused by turbulence.

Turbulence (added sounds) in the S_2 ('dub') phase can mean broadly two things:

1   Either the aortic or pulmonary valves are leaky (known as regurgitation)
2   Either the mitral or tricuspid valves are tight (known as stenosis)

To differentiate the added sounds further, we compare the sound to the valve position it was heard in:

- 2nd intercostal space, right sternal edge (aortic valve)
- 2nd intercostal space, left sternal edge (pulmonary valve)
- 5th intercostal space, right sternal edge (tricuspid valve)
- 5th intercostal space, mid clavicular line (mitral valve)

ACTIVITY: HAVE A GO

Identifying heart sounds

If an added sound is heard on heart auscultation, ask yourself the following questions:

- Was it heard in S_1 or S_2?
- In which of the four auscultation areas was the added sound the loudest?

If it was loudest in S_1:
   Either the mitral or tricuspid valves are leaky (known as regurgitation)
   or
   Either the aortic or pulmonary valves are tight (known as stenosis)
   As it was heard in the 2nd intercostal space, right sternal edge (over the area of aortic valve) it's likely to be the **aortic valve** which is to blame. As the sound occurred in S_1, it must be **aortic stenosis**, as in S_1 (systole) the aortic valve is open, and blood is flowing across the valve.
   You can now see why identifying the 'lub' and the 'dub' by palpation of the carotid pulse is critical to identify possible pathologies and their origin.

Oedema

Often noted as swelling in the feet and ankles, oedema is an abnormal collection of fluid between the cells of the body (Knott, 2018). While oedema is a normal inflammatory process for localised injury (such as a small laceration or insect bite), frequent or permanent oedema is an abnormal finding. You may hear oedema noted as 'pitting'; this is the formation of indentations after an examiner presses on the oedematous skin. This can be a sign of heart failure or liver failure amongst a wide range of other pathologies.

ACTIVITY: CRITICAL THINKING

If a patient has extensive pitting oedema in their lower limbs, it's clear that there is an excess of fluid pooling in the legs. But where else could it accumulate?

   It's important to remember that fluid tends to pool in that position due to gravity, and if a previously ambulant patient becomes bed-bound, this fluid may begin to accumulate in other tissues, such as the buttocks, back, pelvis and groin. If a patient with peripheral oedema becomes breathless, this could suggest fluid is pooling in the lung bases (known as pulmonary oedema). This will need specific treatment focused on fluid removal and dilation of the pulmonary vessels. Simple bronchodilator inhalers (such as salbutamol) and antibiotics may not provide any benefit.

CASE STUDY

Mr Pillai, 68-year-old patient with cough and shortness-of-breath

Mr Pillai has been treated on a medical ward for one week for confusion, thought to be secondary to a urinary tract infection. IV fluids have been given as he has been refusing oral intake and has been receiving IV antibiotics in-line with local policy. While confused, Mr Pillai is calm and permitting observations. He is obese, with a background of hypertension, diabetes, and heart failure.

Over the past 24 hours, the patient has seemed more short-of-breath. He now needs oxygen via nasal cannula to maintain saturations of 94% and he has a productive cough. The remainder of the observations show a tachycardia and tachypnoea. Blood pressure and temperature are within normal limits.

You decide to conduct a respiratory and cardiovascular examination. Chest expansion is equal, however there are loud crackles heard at both lung bases. There is no wheeze. You try and listen to the patient's heart sounds, but the crackles from the lungs are muffling the sounds. You look at the patient's legs and feel that their ankles are swollen.

Questions

1   What do the lung crackles suggest?
2   What do the swollen ankles suggest?
3   Is there any aspect of the current treatment regime that may be making the current situation worse?
4   Does this patient need escalation to the medical team?

In this scenario, the patient is suffering from a compromised respiratory and cardiovascular system due to heart failure. The crackles at both lung bases (pulmonary oedema), with productive cough and pedal oedema are all suggestive of fluid overload, likely worsened by well-meaning IV fluid and antibiotics for a urinary tract infection. Hospital acquired respiratory infection is a possibility, however that is likely to produce purulent sputum and a pyrexia, with the absence of pedal oedema.

There is significant deterioration visible, and the need for oxygen and tachypnoea are worrying 'red flag' signs which need to be escalated urgently to the medical team. Furthermore, the doctors should review the current IV fluid regime to prevent further fluid accumulation and worsening deterioration. This patient may need diuretics to remove the excess fluid pooling in the lungs and lower limbs.

GASTROINTESTINAL EXAMINATION: DISCUSSION

The gastrointestinal examination consists of abdominal palpation (assessing pain or masses and denoting the liver edge) followed by auscultation. The abdomen can be divided into either four or nine regions (see below) and the examiner palpates superficial structures in each zone in turn, before repeating the process again with a firmer palpation technique to assess deeper structures. Palpation should be performed with a flat palm, with the examiner intermittently looking at the patient's face to assess for signs of pain or discomfort.

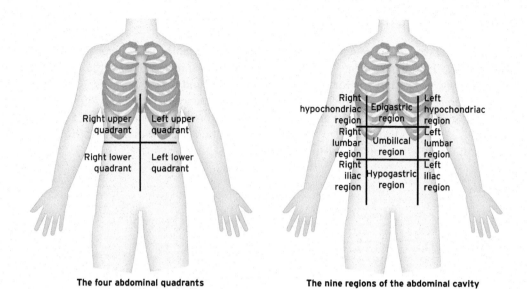

The four abdominal quadrants   The nine regions of the abdominal cavity

Figure 4.4   The quadrants and regions of the abdomen

For examination purposes, the abdominal cavity is arbitrarily split into regions; some prefer the simplicity of four zones (upper right, lower right, upper left, lower left), while more experienced practitioners split the abdomen into nine zones. Regardless of the examiner's preference, it doesn't matter which method you choose, as neither has any more beneficial effect to the quality of examination, assessment, or patient outcomes.

GASTROINTESTINAL EXAMINATION: STEP BY STEP

This gastrointestinal examination in this chapter represents a 'partial' examination, with a number of elements omitted for simplicity and to make it suitable for undergraduate students.

- Ensure you have explained the process of abdominal palpation to the patient and gained verbal consent to conduct the examination. Ideally the patient's abdomen should be fully exposed (from nipples to groin), so the examination should be conducted in a closed room or behind curtains to maintain dignity. The patient should be lying flat on their back (if tolerated).
- Examine for signs of jaundice (yellowing) in the eyes.
- Ask the patient if they have any abdominal pain before starting palpation. Start **away** from the painful area.
  - Palpate with a flat hand, the four areas of the abdomen, superficial **and** deep.
  - Palpate up from the right lower quadrant to the right costal margin to find the liver edge. This is typically performed as the patient breaths in (as inspiration will lower the diaphragm and thus causes the liver edge to descend). While the abdomen is normally soft, the liver edge should produce a noticeable density change as the examiner palpates. If felt, make a note of the liver distance from the right costal margin (for example, 2cm from margin).
- Auscultate the abdomen in each of the four quadrants - note bowel sounds in each quadrant.
- Once the examination is complete, ask the patient to cover themselves or redress. Document your examination findings.

Abdominal examination findings

A 'normal' abdomen should be soft, non-tender with no discernible masses palpable. Bowel sounds (the noise made by the movement of the intestines) should be present. But what is a normal bowel sound? How often should they occur and what should they sound like?

A book is unable to teach you this! It is difficult to define and will vary from person-to-person. The sound itself is an 'echo' through the abdominal wall and will vary in tone based on a multitude of factors, such as patient's body mass, last meal, last bowel motion (that's without considering the many pathological factors which can affect them).

ACTIVITY: HAVE A GO

Take a stethoscope and try and auscultate your own abdominal bowel sounds, then compare them with the bowel sounds of a family member or friend. Start to build up a picture of what is 'normal' outside of clinical practice, so when you begin to assess patients, you can quickly identify sounds which are normal, and those which are not!

KEY TERMS

Bowel ischaemia: damage to the bowel, caused by a restriction of blood flow to bowel tissue.

Bowel obstruction: mechanical or functional obstruction of the intestines which prevents the normal movement of faeces/products of digestion.

Inflammatory bowel disease: a group of intestinal disorders that cause inflammation of the digestive tract. For example, Crohn's disease or ulcerative colitis.

As the gastrointestinal examination is conducted, the examiner should think about a multitude of clinical findings, outlined below:

- **Jaundice** – The abnormal yellowing of skin (often seen earliest in the sclera of the eyes, which should be white, and changes to a yellow colour). It is caused by hyperbilirubinaemia (high bilirubin levels) which is often a consequence of biliary tree obstruction, liver disease or chronic alcohol abuse.
- **Tenderness** – A common clinical finding in the abdominal examination. It's important to note the characteristics of the pain and examine in detail the position of the pain and its response to palpation. Pain in the right upper quadrant may be related to the liver, gallbladder, or bile ducts, while pain in the left upper quadrant may be related to the stomach, pancreas, or spleen. Pain which is described as more superficial may relate to structures near the abdominal wall, or the wall itself (such as hernias). Pain on palpation often indicates the presence of an underlying abdominal pathology.
- **Guarding** – This is **voluntary** tensing of the abdominal muscles when pain is provoked by palpation, which is a normal response mechanism; when we are in pain, we tense the abdominal wall muscles to prevent the painful area beneath being palpated! **Involuntary** guarding, however, is an abnormal examination finding. This is unprovoked tensing of abdominal wall muscles and can be a sign of significant intra-abdominal inflammation.

- **Palpable masses** – Make a note of the anatomical location and try to describe the mass:
    - Is it superficial or deep?
    - Is it large or small? (Can you estimate its diameter?)
    - Does it have a regular or irregular shape?
    - Is it painful to palpation, or painless?
    - Is it pulsatile or non-pulsatile?
    - On auscultation, can you hear bowel sounds within it?
    - Is it fluctuant? (feels fluid filled?)

Remember, in some patients, faecal matter may be palpable as an intra-abdominal mass.

- **Abdominal distension** – An abnormally swollen abdomen, often caused by pressure from within the abdominal cavity. Can be associated with simple pathologies, such as constipation, overeating or excessive wind. More worryingly, distension can be caused by bowel obstruction, gastrointestinal bleeding, or ascites from liver failure. The findings of distension must be correlated with other clinical findings in the overall clinical context.
- **Bowel sounds:**
    - **Hyperactive** – Loud gurgling or rumbling, widespread sounds. Increased frequency. Can be heard in early bowel obstruction, but commonly with increased gastric transit (diahorrea or laxative use).
    - **Tinkling bowel sounds** – Sounds like a drip of water from a dripping tap hitting a metal bathtub! Can be a sign of bowel obstruction.
    - **Hypoactive** – Soft, low gurgling. Brief at times. Long gaps between sounds. Can be a sign of slowed gastrointestinal transit (constipation) often a result of medication use (such as opiates).
    - **Absent** – No audible bowel sounds after >3 mins of auscultation. This can be caused by bowel ischaemia or failure, anaesthesia or as a consequence of inflammatory bowel disease.

Any worrying findings on abdominal examination should be escalated appropriately using local guidelines.

CASE STUDY

A 14-year-old child with abdominal pain

A 14-year-old patient is bought to the A&E department by their mother. The child appears distressed, holding their lower abdomen and complaining of pain. The discomfort has been present for 24 hours and worsening. You find it difficult to gain a detailed history, with the patient often looking towards their mother to assist with answering questions. The mother states the child has vomited twice before arriving at the department. Initial observations show a respiratory rate of 24 breaths per minute, pulse of 110pbm, with a blood pressure of 128/58 and a temperature of 38.0 degrees.

You perform an abdominal examination. When you palpate the lower right quadrant, the child tenses, screams out in agony and pushes your hand away. You attempt auscultation of the abdomen and hear normal bowel sounds.

Questions

1   Are there any signs from the history which may be concerning?
2   Are there any 'red flags' or worrying signs which need urgent escalation?
3   What simple bedside tests may aid the management of this patient?

(Continued)

In this example, the child is looking towards their mother to answer the history questions. This is not necessarily a sign of concern. It may be due to a nervous disposition, or due to pain or distress from the unfamiliar questions and situation. Worsening abdominal pain should always be treated seriously and has a multitude of causes which need to be investigated.

Prompt completion of observations is vital to help determine clinical severity and need for escalation. Remember that children have different observational parameters to an adult, and the respiratory rate, pulse rate and blood pressure in this example are all normal for a child of that age. Therefore, in this case, there are no red flags!

There are some simple bedside tests which should be routinely conducted. For instance, urine should be taken, and a urine dipstick test should be performed to exclude a urinary tract infection. Furthermore, a pregnancy test should be conducted on a female child of this age (typically girls >12 years old), however this will need discussion with the parent/carer as well as consent from them. This can often be a difficult subject to approach and will test your communication skills!

It would be sensible to take a blood sample from this patient – however cannulation of children is typically performed by doctors.

There are a range of conditions which can cause pain of this nature, such as constipation, menstrual cramps, urine infections, inflammatory bowel conditions and ectopic pregnancy to name a few! The abdominal examination findings in this example are consistent with an appendicitis; however, the A&E clinicians need to re-examine the patient and request appropriate tests before referral to the surgical team.

CRANIAL NERVES EXAMINATION: DISCUSSION

Anatomy and physiology recap

The cranial nerves are 12 paired nerves which descend directly from the brain. Broadly speaking, they allow transmission of signals from the brain to areas of the head and neck (Drake et al., 2010). The nerves are labelled with roman numerals and have names (some of which relate to their function).

Cranial nerves (and their function):

 I   Olfactory nerve (smell)
 II   Optic nerve (sight, pupil reaction)
 III   Occulomotor nerve (eye movement, pupil reaction)
 IV   Trochlear nerve (eye movement)
 V   Trigeminal nerve (splits into three nerves, see Figure 4.5; provides sensation to face, power to muscles of mastication)
 VI   Abducens nerve (lateral eye movement)
 VII   Facial nerve (facial muscle movement, taste to anterior of tongue)
 VIII   Vestibulocochlear nerve (hearing)
 IX   Glossopharyngeal nerve (sensation to oropharynx, taste to posterior of tongue)
 X   Vagus nerve (speech, parasympathetic supply to heart, stomach, and intestines)
 XI   Hypoglossal nerve (movement of tongue)
 XII   Accessory nerve (some neck muscle movement)

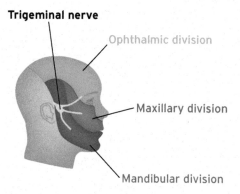

Trigeminal nerve

Ophthalmic division

Maxillary division

Mandibular division

Figure 4.5 Divisions of the trigeminal nerve

As you can see from the list above, the cranial nerves have multiple functions, and in some cases more than one function per nerve. It is beyond the scope of this examination to interrogate a patient's hearing or sight in-depth; indeed, these are specialist examinations, performed by skilled practitioners with a variety of dedicated equipment. The purpose of the cranial nerve examination is to briefly review each cranial nerve to determine if there is a **gross abnormality** which would need further investigation. For example, if hearing loss was noted, this may prompt referral to audiology services.

In clinical practice, the cranial nerve examination (or parts of it) is on patients presenting with suspected stroke, head injury, facial masses and suspected head and neck cancer.

CRANIAL NERVES EXAMINATION: STEP BY STEP

- Ensure you have gained verbal consent to conduct the examination. Ideally the patient should be sitting opposite the examiner on a chair. You will need some additional equipment, such as a pen torch, cup of drinking water, book/reading chart, tongue depressor and a piece of gauze/cotton wool.
- The examination reviews each nerve in numerical order.
- Olfactory (I) – Difficult to assess in clinical practice.
  - Ask patient if any changes in taste or smell. Any significant changes may prompt further specialist investigations.
- Optic (II) – Difficult to assess without specialist equipment.
  - Ask the patient if they can read a sentence of text from a book or magazine. If there are any gross visual changes noted, the patient may require formal review by an ophthalmologist or optician.
  - Use pen-torch to assess pupil response to light. Ask the patient to stare straight ahead or at a fixed point behind you. Briefly shine the torch light into an eye and examine if you can see a suitable pupil response. Normally, the pupil will constrict to the introduction of light, and dilate as the light is moved away. Test both eyes, comparing side to side.
- Occulomotor (III), Trochlear (IV), Abducens (VI)
  - Ask the patient to open their eyes as wide as possible, then ask them to close them. Note closure/opening of the eye lids. Compare side to side for discrepancy.

(Continued)

- o   Ask the patient to look straight ahead. Bring your raised index finger in front of the patient's vision, approx. 30cm from their face. Ask them to stare directly at your finger and to follow it with their eyes. Move your finger slowly horizontally, then laterally (typically to make a H shape), to test all movements of the eyes. Again, compare side to side.
- Trigeminal (V)
    - o   The trigeminal nerve splits into three separate nerves, each of which supplies a different region of the face with sensation. Ask the patient to close their eyes and tell you when they feel touch to their face. Using a gauze swab or cotton ball, press lightly and briefly at six different positions (three on each side of the face) and compare side to side. The three positions are:
    - o   Forehead, directly above eye socket
    - o   Cheeks, directly below eye socket
    - o   Jaw
- Test the power of the masseters (muscles of mastication) by asking the patient to clench their teeth, while you palpate anterior to the angle of the jaw. As they clench, you should feel the muscle belly bulge beneath your fingers.
- Facial (VII)
    - o   Ask the patient to raise their eyebrows (look surprised). Mirroring of these facial expressions may be required for those who have difficulty with descriptions.
    - o   Ask the patient to show you their teeth (jaw closed).
    - o   Ask the patient to shut their eyes tightly.
- Vestibulocochlear (VIII) – Difficult to assess in clinical practice.
    - o   Whisper a set of numbers into one ear (for example 7, 6, 3), while rubbing the lobe of the other ear. Ask the patient to repeat the numbers. Repeat on the other ear. If any gross deficit is found, this may need further review by an audiologist or ENT doctor.
- Glossopharyngeal (IX), Vagus (X)
    - o   Ask patient to open their mouth widely. Use tongue depressor to gently depress the tongue down so you can visualise the soft palate (posterior roof of the mouth) and uvula. Look for asymmetry. Once you have completed a brief inspection, ask the patient to say 'ahhh' and note phonation of the sound, plus any deviation of the uvula.
    - o   Ask patient to cough and swallow a small volume of water. Any difficulty may require a formal swallowing assessment by an appropriate practitioner.
- Hypoglossal (XII)
    - o   Ask patient to open mouth, examine tongue for symmetry and wasting. Normally, the tongue should be symmetrical and smooth.
    - o   To test tongue power (with the patient's mouth closed), ask them to push their tongue into the side of their cheeks and to hold the position. The examiner should push on the bulging cheek while asking the patient to resist the motion. Both sides should be tested and compared.
- Accessory (XI)
    - o   Ask patient to shrug their shoulders, and keep them there, while you apply downward pressure. Note any asymmetry or restriction of movement.
    - o   Once the examination is complete, document the findings, using the twelve cranial nerve names (or roman numerals) as headings.

NEUROLOGICAL EXAMINATION: DISCUSSION

The neurological examination assesses the patient's upper and lower limbs separately. This is because the examination can often be quite lengthy, but primarily because the examiner is assessing the limbs comparing side-to-side. The structure of both examinations are as follows:

1   Tone
2   Power
3   Sensation
4   Coordination
5   Reflexes

Tone is the resistance felt when a limb is moved passively (without the patient voluntarily moving the limb). To test this, a limb is moved by the examiner with the patient instructed to 'relax and not resist the movement; or told 'let your arm go floppy'. The examiner is trying to feel muscular tone across the joints. Hypertonia (increased tone) feels like the muscles are tight and there is resistance to the movement. This can suggest an upper motor neuron lesion (a lesion between the brain and spinal cord). Hypotonia (decreased tone) feels like the muscles are extremely weak. This can suggest a lower motor neuron lesion (a lesion in the nerves travelling peripherally from the spinal cord).

    Power is a test strength of an individual muscle. In testing the muscle, by association we test the supplying nerve. It is measured using the Medical Research Council (MRC) scale developed in 1943. Despite the age of the research the scale was derived from, it is still widely used in clinical practice across the UK. To test power, the patient is asked to hold a limb in a given position and resist the examiner's attempts to move the limb.

    For example, the patient is asked to flex their arms at their elbow, with the examiner trying to straighten (extend) the arms. If able to resist, the muscle (in this example the bicep) is given a score MRC 5. If the patient cannot resist the examiner moving the limb, but can raise it, this would score MRC 3. If the patient is unable to lift the arm at all, and there appears to be no movement of the muscle, this would score MRC 0.

MRC Scale for Muscle Power	
0	No muscle contraction seen.
1	Muscle contraction is visible but there is no movement of the joint.
2	Active joint movement is possible with gravity eliminated.
3	Movement can overcome gravity but not resistance from the examiner.
4	The muscle group can overcome gravity and move against some resistance from the examiner.
5	Full and normal power against resistance.

Figure 4.6   MRC Scale for Muscle Power

Source: Used with the permission of the Medical Research Council

ACTIVITY: HAVE A GO

Assessing a patient's muscle power using MRC scoring

For the following examples, what MRC score would you attribute to the patient?

1   A patient has suffered a dense stroke resulting in a left sided weakness. On asking the patient to lift their left arm, you see some fasciculations of muscle movement, but the arm does not move.
2   In a supine position, an elderly patient struggles to lift their right leg up off the bed. When you place your hand on the quadriceps muscle above the right knee, they are unable to lift the limb as they did before.

Answers

1   MRC score 1 out of 5 (patient only has a flicker of movement in the limb).
2   MRC score 3 out of 5 (patient can lift leg to overcome gravity, but not resistance).

Testing **sensation** is multimodal as there are many complex pathways which transmit sensation signals. As a recap of anatomy and physiology, the spinal cord consists of ascending and descending tracts. The ascending tracts are sensory pathways which carry somatosensory information from the peripheries to the brain. Within these tracts there are multiple further divisions, however for the purpose of this chapter, we will look at only two divisions:

1   **Dorsal column** – these relay signals for position sensation, vibration, and **soft touch**.
2   **Spinothalamic tracts** – these relay signals for **pain** and temperature sensation.

To broadly assess both pathways, we will test the dorsal column by asking the patient if they can feel the **soft touch** of a gauze swab or cotton ball on their skin and test the spinothalamic tract by using a pin (or neuro-tip) to test **pain** sensation. Sensitivity of touch must be considered here for those who have sensory issues.

GO FURTHER

This webpage produced by KENHUB provides an excellent overview of spinal cord anatomy and tracts, with some fantastic images and explanations: www.kenhub.com/en/library/anatomy/ascending-and-descending-tracts-of-the-spinal-cord (accessed October 11, 2022).

The next question is, *where on the body do we test these pathways?* There are many nerves which run from the dorsal column and spinothalamic tracts to the peripheries which makes things much more complicated to examine. To add some order, we can split these nerves into anatomical segments called 'dermatomes'. A dermatome is an area of skin supplied by a single spinal nerve. The dermatome is named after the spinal nerve which supplies it. For example, C6 (cervical nerve 6), T7 (thoracic nerve 7), S4 (sacral nerve 4).

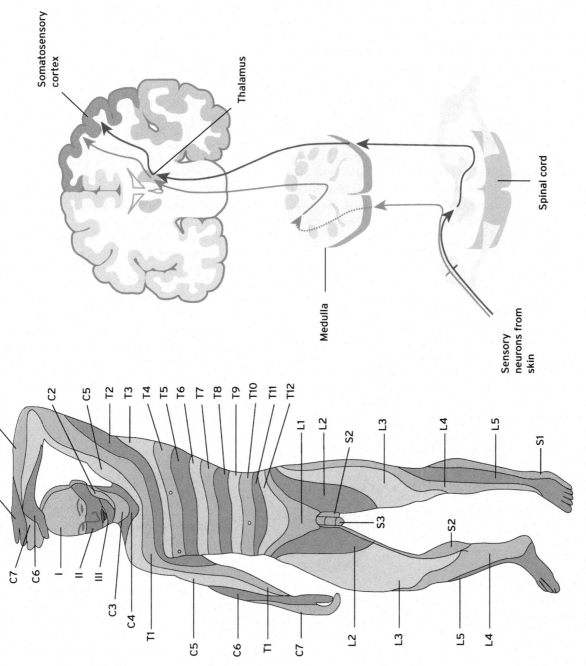

Figure 4.7 Dermatomes of the human body

We aim to test all dermatomes in each limb. In the arms there are six dermatomes (C4, C5, C6, C7, C8, T1) and in the legs there are five dermatomes (L2, L3, L4, L5, S4). It is important to note that the posterior lower limb dermatomes (S1, S2, S3) have been omitted from the examination. Testing sensation and pain around the anus is deeply unpleasant and should not routinely be performed. If there is any suspicion of damage to these nerves, it should be escalated to a doctor who may wish to perform a rectal examination.

If a patient confirms a loss of sensation, it's important to note the modality (soft-touch or painful stimuli) and the dermatome in which this occurred. There may be multiple dermatomes affected in a limb. If there is any ambiguity, the test can be repeated.

Coordination is primarily a test of cerebellar dysfunction (as the cerebellum controls movement, coordination, and balance). Due to the complexity of the movements, coordination testing also tests power and proprioception to some degree.

To test coordination in the upper limbs, ask the patient to touch each finger on one hand to their thumb on the same hand. For the lower limbs, ask the patient to tap their feet against the end of the bed or against the examiner's hand. If coordination is poor on a given side, it can suggest a cerebellar injury. Remember, the test is very crude and subjective in nature. There is commonly a discrepancy in coordination, particularly in the hands, due to one hand being dominant.

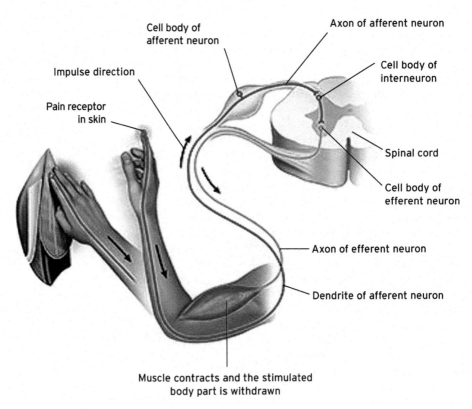

Figure 4.8   The reflex arc

Reflexes test the somatic (muscle) reflex arc; the pathway that links sensory neurones to the spinal cord. The striking of a tendon hammer to the brachioradialis tendon (wrist) or patellar tendon (knee) should provoke a response from the spinal cord – the limb should move rapidly, with suppression from the brain coming shortly after. The examiners should see a small but brief movement; the arm will supinate (turn), while the lower leg will extend at the knee.

An abnormal reflex is one which is diminished or suppressed, or conversely one which is greatly exaggerated (hyperreflexia). Hyperreflexia can suggest an upper motor neurone lesion as signals are missing from the brain which should supress the reflex response. It's important to note that an absent or diminished reflex could be due to examiner error (incorrect anatomical striking, or poor tendon hammer technique), or due to the patient tensing or expecting the strike. It is good practice to ask the patient to let the limb 'go floppy' prior to striking with the tendon hammer.

KEY TERMS

Dermatome: an area of the skin supplied by nerves from a single spinal root.

Extension: enlargement or lengthening of a limb, by movement of the joint.

Flexion: bending of a limb or joint.

UPPER LIMB NEUROLOGICAL EXAMINATION: STEP BY STEP

- Ensure you have gained verbal consent to conduct the examination. Ideally the patient's arms and shoulders should be exposed. The examination should be conducted in a closed room or behind curtains to maintain dignity. The patient should be lying at a slight incline.

- **Tone** – Ask the patient to relax their arms by their side. One-by-one, hold each arm and extend and flex the arm at the shoulder, the elbow, and at the wrist. It is also good practise to supinate and pronate (turn) the wrist joint. Compare side-to-side.

- **Power** – Ask the patient to hold their arms/hands in the following positions and to resist your attempts to move the limb ('don't let me move you'):

  o Shoulders abducted; elbows flexed (think of chicken wings!). Press downwards to assess power of shoulder muscles (nerves C5/C6).

  o With arms by their side, ask the patient to flex their elbows, with the knuckles facing out- wards (think of a boxer stance!). Push against the forearms to test the strength of the triceps and pull against the forearms to test the strength of the biceps (nerves C7/C8).

  o With arms outstretched and fists clenched (palms down) hold each of the patient's fore- arms to stabilise them, then pull down on the wrist, then push up on the wrist to test wrist flexion and extension (nerves C7/C8).

  o Ask the patient to grip the examiner's extended index fingers and squeeze. This tests grip strength (nerve C8).

  o With arms outstretched (palms down), ask the patient to abduct their fingers (splay their fingers widely). Try and squeeze the fingers together (nerve T1).

- **Sensation** – Using two modalities (soft touch and pain sensation) test dermatomes C4, C5, C6, C7, C8, T1 on each limb, comparing side to side. **One** point of touch per dermatome is sufficient. **It may be useful to have a dermatome map at hand**.

  o Soft touch – Use a gauze swab or cotton ball. With their arms in a relaxed position by their side, ask the patient to close their eyes and to tell you if they can feel each touch in turn.

(Continued)

Press the gauze swab/cotton ball lightly, but briefly on the skin. Remember to go side to side, comparing the sensation at one part of the right arm, with the left.

o   Pain - Use a pin, blunt needle, or Neuro-Tip. With their arms in a relaxed position by their side, ask the patient to close their eyes and to tell you if they can feel each touch in turn. Press the pin lightly, but briefly on the skin. Remember to go side to side, comparing pain sensation at one part of the right arm, with the left. Once complete, make sure you tell the patient they can open their eyes again!

- **Coordination** - Ask the patient to touch each finger on one hand to their thumb on the same hand.

- **Reflex** - Ask the patient to keep their arms relaxed, by their side. Gently grasping the patient's wrist, strike **your** hand with the tendon hammer over the radial head (the prominent bone on the lateral surface of the wrist); the impact should cause the brachioradialis reflex, and the wrist should turn. Do not strike the patient's radial head directly, as this can be extremely painful!

- Once the examination is complete, ask the patient to cover themselves or redress and document your examination findings using the five examination headings (tone, power, sensation, coordination, and reflexes).

LOWER LIMB NEUROLOGICAL EXAMINATION: STEP BY STEP

- Ensure you have gained verbal consent to conduct the examination. Ideally the patient's legs should be fully exposed. The examination should be conducted in a closed room or behind curtains to maintain dignity. The patient should be lying at a slight incline.

- **Tone** - Gently rock each leg from side to side, by pushing on the bulky part of the thigh. Look down the leg as you do this; the knee and ankle in turn should also rock with the upper leg.

- **Power** - Ask the patient to keep their legs/ankles in the following positions and to resist your attempts to move the limb ('don't let me move you'):

o   Ask the patient to perform a straight leg raise (hip flexing, while keeping their leg straight), then push downwards above the knee (nerves L1/L2).

o   Ask the patient to bend their knee. Place your hand anteriorly below the knee (on the lower leg) and ask them to push you away. After, with knee bent, put your hand behind the lower leg and ask them to pull you towards them (nerves L3/L4).

o   Put your hand on the top of the patient's foot (the dorsum) and ask them to flex the ankle while you press downwards. After, place your hand under the foot and ask the patient to extend the ankle and try to push you away (nerves L2/S1).

o   Hold the patient's toe in a neutral position and ask them to flex and extend the toe (nerve S1).

- **Sensation** - Using two modalities (soft touch and pain sensation) test dermatomes L2, L3, L4, L5, S4 on each limb, comparing side to side. **One** point of touch per dermatome is sufficient. **It may be useful to have a dermatome map at hand.**

o   Soft touch - Use a gauze swab or cotton ball. With their legs in a relaxed position, ask the patient to close their eyes and to tell you if they can feel each touch in turn. Press the gauze swab/cotton ball lightly, but briefly on the skin. Remember to go side to side, comparing the sensation at one part of the right leg, with the left.

o Pain – Use a pin, blunt needle, or Neuro-Tip. With their legs in a relaxed position, ask the patient to close their eyes and to tell you if they can feel each touch in turn. Press the pin lightly, but briefly on the skin. Remember to go side to side, comparing pain sensation at one part of the right leg, with the left. Once complete, make sure you tell the patient they can open their eyes again!

- **Coordination** – Place your hands near the soles of the patient's feet and ask them to tap your hands with their feet (rapidly extending and flexing the ankle joint). Alternatively, you could ask the patient to tap the foot of the bed. Aim for 5–10 'taps' per foot before asking the patient to stop. Compare side to side.

- **Reflexes** – Ask the patient to keep their legs relaxed. Test the reflex on one leg at a time by gently placing your non-dominant hand underneath the patient's leg, within the popliteal fossa (behind the knee), so the knee is slightly elevated from the bed and slightly flexed. With your other hand palpate the patella tendon (just below the kneecap). Once identified, strike the tendon once with the tendon hammer. If the reflex is triggered, the knee should extend briefly.

- Once the examination is complete, ask the patient to cover themselves or redress and document your examination findings using the five examination headings (tone, power, sensation, coordination, and reflexes).

CONDUCT ROUTINE INVESTIGATIONS

Introduction to an Electrocardiogram (ECG)

An Electrocardiogram (often known as a 12-lead ECG, or ECG) is a simple bed-side test which is used to check the heart's rhythm by detecting the electrical signals produced by the heart. An ECG is quick to perform, relatively inexpensive and can be performed by a range of trained healthcare personnel.

An ECG can help detect:

- Heart arrythmias (abnormal heartbeat), where the heart beats too slow (bradycardia), too fast (tachycardia) or in an irregular manner.
- Heart attacks (myocardial infarction), where a blockage in a coronary artery causes a partition of the cardiac muscle to become damaged.
- Heart enlargement (muscle hypertrophy), often a symptom of a failing heart.
- Coronary artery disease, where coronary arteries become narrowed by a build-up of fat along the vessel walls, preventing flow of blood.
- Electrolyte disturbance/toxins, which can alter the heart's rhythm or rate in a specific way.

An ECG is now routinely performed on most acutely unwell patients, regardless of whether their presenting complaint is related to cardiac pathology. The test is also used extensively in mental health services to assess changes in heart rhythm associated with commonly used anti-depressant or antipsychotic medications.

How to perform an ECG

There are three broad types of ECG which are routinely performed:

1 A resting ECG carried out while the patient is lying flat (supine).
2 A stress or exercise ECG, often carried out with the patient performing an exercise on a treadmill or bike.

3   An ambulatory ECG, often carried out at home over a longer period (typically 24–48 hours). The patient will wear a small ECG monitor, which is often carried in a small satchel.

A standard 12-lead ECG takes recordings from 10 electrodes which are split into two groups:

1   Six precordial electrodes (named $V_1 - V_6$) which are attached to the anterior thorax.
2   Four limb leads (RA, LA, LL, RL) which are attached to the arms and legs.

ACTIVITY: CRITICAL THINKING

What does the term '12-lead' actually mean?

A common misconception among inexperienced healthcare practitioners concerns the term '12-lead'. The 'leads' are not the wires that connect the machine to the patient but refer to the 'views' of the heart the machine produces. Remember, on a standard 12-lead ECG machine, there are 10 wires which are connected to the patient, which provide 12 views (leads) of the heart!

Accurate placement of the ECG electrodes is extremely important as misplacement can cause changes in the ECG morphology which could potentially lead to erroneous interpretations of the results. It is therefore crucial that healthcare professionals undertaking an ECG are well versed in finding specific anatomical landmarks on their patients.

KEY TERMS

Angle of Louis or **sternal angle**: the joint formed between the manubrium and the sternum. It is often easy to palpate (feel) and indicates the approximate position of the second rib.

Anterior axillary line: an imaginary line which passes vertically downwards from the anterior axillary fold (the anterior start of the armpit crease).

ECG morphology: the form, shape, or structure of the ECG waveform.

Intercostal space: the space between two ribs.

Medial malleolus: bony prominence on the medial side of the ankle.

Mid-axillary line: an imaginary line originates in the axilla (or armpit) and passes vertically downwards.

Precordial: the region of the thorax immediately in front of or over the heart.

WATCH THE VIDEO

Watch along as you read through this step by step procedure by scanning the QR code with your smartphone camera or via **https://study.sagepub.com/rowberry**.

ECG PROCEDURE: STEP BY STEP

- Expose the patient's thorax (chest), wrists and ankles.
- Ensure the patient is lying supine (on their back), with their arms by their side and legs uncrossed. The patient's head can be raised on a pillow, or by raising the head of the bed. It is important the patient is lying in a comfortable and relaxed position before the electrodes are placed.
- In line with local policy ensure skin is prepared. Ensure any hair which may prevent electrode adhesion is removed.
- Electrode placement:
  - Identify the angle of Louis/sternal angle.
  - Place electrode V_1 and V_2 either side of the sternum at the angle of Louis (2nd intercostal space).
  - Skip the V_3 electrode for now, we will place that later.
  - From the 2nd intercostal space on the left side of the sternum, count down to the 4th intercostal space and place your finger there. With your other hand, draw an imaginary straight line down from the middle of the left clavicle until it is level with your finger marking the 4th intercostal space. At this point place electrode V_4.
  - Imagine a diagonal line running from electrode V_2 and V_4 – at the midpoint of this line place electrode V_3.
  - Place the 5th (V_5) electrode in the anterior axillary line, 5th intercostal space.
  - Place the 6th (V_6) electrode in the mid-axillary line, 5th intercostal space.
  - Place RA electrode to the radial side of the right wrist, and the LA electrode to the radial side of the left wrist.
  - Place RL electrode to the right medial malleolus, and the LL electrode to the left medial malleolus.
- Connect all ECG to placed electrodes.
- Electrocardiograph machinery varies based on manufacturer, therefore operate according to manufacturer's instructions and local policy.
- Ensure a qualified practitioner interprets ECG findings.

GO FURTHER

Jackson, M. (2022) 'How to Read an ECG', Geeky Medics, July 23. https://geekymedics.com/how-to-read-an-ecg/ (accessed October 11, 2022).

(Continued)

This excellent website demonstrates how to read an ECG using a systematic approach. It features extensive step by step explanations and handy diagrams to aid understanding. If you want to put your ECG interpretation knowledge to the test, you can also check out an ECG quiz also available on the website!

ACTIVITY: COMMUNICATION SKILLS

While often considered a 'routine' test, an ECG could be considered by some to be quite invasive as the patient is required to have their bare chest exposed for a period. Consent to perform the investigation must be sought before conducting the ECG and the attendance of a chaperone must be offered. Bras will need to be removed (as they will prevent accurate electrode placement). Always ensure that a sheet or blanket is available and can be placed over the patient's chest once electrodes are placed.

Breast tissue can overlie the areas of electrode placement and can give a poor test result due to electrical impedance through the tissues. It is preferable in this situation to place the pre-cordial (chest) leads under the breast, rather than on its surface. This however will require the breast to be lifted. Furthermore, scarring from previous surgeries, wounds, or skin lesions may also prevent portions of skin being used. In these situations, place the electrode as close as possible to its designated spot and ensure the clinician reviewing the ECG results is aware of the unconventional electrode placement.

How would you ask a patient to prepare for an ECG?

- How will you ask the patient to expose their chest?
- How would you ask a patient to remove their bra?
- How would you ask a patient if you can place electrode stickers beneath their breast?

Venepuncture

WATCH THE VIDEO

VENEPUNCTURE

Watch along as you read through this step by step procedure by scanning the QR code with your smartphone camera or via https://study.sagepub.com/rowberry.

VENEPUNCTURE: STEP BY STEP

- Introduce yourself to the patient and clarify patient's details (to ensure you have the correct patient) and gain consent to perform venepuncture.

- Check if the patient has an allergy (for example, to latex gloves), and check to ensure the patient does not have any medical conditions which would prevent a particular limb from being used (for example, arterio-venous fistula, lymphoedema, stroke or recent mastectomy). Furthermore, venepuncture should not be conducted on an arm which has an intravenous infusion attached as this may alter blood composition and skew results.

- Position the patient so they are sitting/lying comfortably. Expose the patient's arm ready to conduct the procedure. It sometimes helps to place a pillow under the patient's arm for comfort and to help extend the arm at the elbow.

- The antecubital fossa is a common location for venepuncture (targeting the median cubital vein). Apply tourniquet approximately 4–5 finger widths above this site.

- Palpate the target vein to see if it is suitable – an ideal vein has a 'bounce' to it. Hard or rigid veins should be avoided as these may be scarred or inflamed.

- Once a target has been identified, wash hands (in-line with local policy) and don gloves.

- Clean the target venepuncture site as per local policy and leave to dry.

- Anchor vein from below with non-dominant hand, gently pulling downwards on the skin.

- Insert the prepared venepuncture needle at approximately 30 degrees with the bevel facing upwards. You should feel a sudden reduction in resistance as the needle enters the vein.

- Attach each blood bottle in the correct order of draw to the needle and allow them to fill completely before moving to the next bottle.

- Once all required bottles have been filled, release the tourniquet and remove it.

- Withdraw the needle from the patient's arm and apply a dressing (such as cotton wool or gauze).

- Invert the blood bottles as per local policy. Discard sharps and clinical waste in their appropriate receptacles.

Cannulation

WATCH THE VIDEO

CANNULATION

Watch along as you read through this step by step procedure by scanning the QR code with your smartphone camera or via https://study.sagepub.com/rowberry.

CANNULATION: STEP BY STEP

The exact procedure/equipment will vary greatly across clinical locations. Students are advised to consult local policy prior to undertaking this skill.

(Continued)

- Introduce yourself to the patient and clarify patient's details (to ensure you have the correct patient) and gain consent to perform cannulation.
- Check if the patient has an allergy (for example, to latex gloves), and check to ensure the patient does not have any medical conditions which would prevent a particular limb from being used (for example, arterio-venous fistula, lymphoedema, stroke or recent mastectomy).
- Position the patient so they are sitting/lying comfortably. Expose the patient's arm ready to conduct the procedure. It sometimes helps to place a pillow under the patient's arm for comfort and to help extend the arm at the elbow.
- The antecubital fossa is a common location for venepuncture (targeting the median cubital vein). Apply tourniquet approximately 4–5 finger widths above this site.
- Palpate the target vein to see if it is suitable – an ideal vein has a 'bounce' to it. Hard or rigid veins should be avoided as these may be scarred or inflamed.
- Once a target has been identified, wash hands (in-line with local policy) and don gloves.
- Clean the target canulation site as per local policy and leave to dry.
- Anchor vein from below with non-dominant hand, gently pulling downwards on the skin.
- Insert the prepared cannula needle at approximately 30 degrees with the bevel facing upwards. You should feel a sudden reduction in resistance as the needle enters the vein.
- Observe the cannula chamber and wait for a flashback of blood to confirm position within the vein.
- Withdraw the introducer needle slightly and lower the cannula angle, so the cannula is almost level with the patient's skin.
- Carefully advance the cannula whilst simultaneously withdrawing the introducer needle until the cannula is fully inserted beneath the skin, and the needle is almost removed.
- Release the tourniquet and carefully place some sterile gauze directly underneath the cannula hub to catch any blood loss as you remove the introducer needle.
- Gently apply pressure to the proximal vein close to the cannula tip to occlude the vessel and prevent bleeding.
- Pull the introducer needle backwards until it is completely removed. Dispose of the introducer needle immediately into an appropriate sharps container.
- Place the cannula cap onto the cannula hub (from the port you withdrew the introducer needle from).
- In-line with local policy, apply adhesive dressing to secure the cannula to the patient's skin.
- Discard clinical waste in an appropriate receptacle.

IDENTIFYING SIGNS OF DETERIORATION

Over recent decades there has been increasing emphasis placed on the nurse's ability to detect the early signs of deterioration in a patient's condition. Early identification of deterioration allows for timely commencement of treatment and can prevent a cascade of decline which can result in critical illness or death.

Identification of a deteriorating patient relies on the use of careful structured observation and timely reporting of abnormalities. Historically the emphasis in nursing has been placed on identification of the deteriorating patient in the hospital setting, but it is equally important in all care settings. Secondary care providers have for some time been utilising 'track and trigger' assessment tools to aid them in the early detection of the deteriorating patient. The NICE guidance on care of the acutely unwell patient in hospital (2007) recommends the use of these systems in all hospital patients and all staff must be competent in undertaking and interpreting these observations and must be able to recognise and respond promptly to the acutely unwell patient.

Clinical signs of a patient who may be deteriorating towards critical illness are usually very similar, because the deterioration will quickly cause changes to crucial physiological systems of the body: respiratory, cardiovascular, and neurological systems. Because of this, close observation of respiratory rate, heart rate, blood pressure, oxygen saturations (and the amount of oxygen the person is receiving), new requirement for oxygen supplementation and consciousness levels will often provide early indication of a deteriorating patient. Additionally, monitoring temperature will help to identify whether infection or sepsis might be causing the deterioration.

'Early warning systems' provide a structured approach to assessing the patient using these observations, with a focus on the signs and symptoms of potentially life-threatening acute illness. These systems usually provide a scoring system which allows the clinician to quantify simplistically how unwell the patient is. The score can then be used as a guide to what action needs to be taken next (when to undertake the next set of observations and whether to refer to senior nursing or medical clinicians). There are several different variations of these early warning systems; it is important that you are familiar with the system used in your clinical area. NEWS2 is the most recent version of a well-recognised national warning system in the UK, that is widely used currently (Royal College of Physicians, 2017).

Many hospitals rely on healthcare support workers to undertake the routine observations that are the foundation of early identification of a deteriorating patient. It is important that a member of staff, who has the skills and training to interpret the results of the observations, will be responsible for reviewing these observations very soon after they are done and taking appropriate action in response to these. Additionally, staff who are undertaking observations should be trained to report any significant abnormality or change in observations to the responsible clinician immediately.

When interpreting the observations, it is important that the patient's normal 'baseline' is considered. For example, a patient with chronic lung disease (for example, COPD) may normally have oxygen saturations of 88% when they are in the best of health. If this is the case, then the appropriate response to this observation is likely to be different to the same finding in a young, normally healthy patient. It may be appropriate to not score on an early warning system for a chronically abnormal observation, but this should be discussed with a senior or experienced clinician first.

It is also vital that the clinician taking observations and calculating the NEWS2 score completes the *full set* of observations and that they are undertaken on admission and then at the frequency designated by the NEWS2 score. Without ensuring observations are completed in full and at the time designated by the previous NEWS2 score, it is possible that a patient's condition may deteriorate to a state of critical illness or cardiac arrest without being noticed by healthcare staff. The responsible nurse may be held accountable for this if early warning systems have not been adhered to.

Whilst taking accurate observations is the basis for detecting a deteriorating patient, observing trends in a patient's behaviour and observations is also important. Early signs of deterioration can sometimes be recognised intuitively by a carer or relative of a patient; they may just sense something is wrong without knowing what. It may be possible for someone who knows the patient well to detect deterioration even before physiological signs are apparent, therefore it is important that this insight is not ignored.

The following provides a guide to help you identify objective signs of a deteriorating, but it is not a replacement for common sense, intuition and asking for a review by a more senior clinician if you are unsure or concerned.

NEWS2 key		FULL NAME		
0 1 2 3		DATE OF BIRTH		DATE OF ADMISSION

		Score	
	DATE		DATE
	TIME		TIME

A+B Respirations Breaths/min

Range	Score
≥25	3
21–24	2
18–20	
15–17	
12–14	
9–11	1
≤8	3

A+B SPO₂ Scale 1 — oxygen saturation (%)

Range	Score
≥96	
94–95	1
92–93	2
≤91	3

SpO₂ Scale 2† — oxygen saturation (%)
Use scale 2 if target range is 88–92% eg in hypercapnic respiratory failure
† ONLY use Scale 2 under the direction of a qualified clinician

Range	Score
≥97 on O₂	3
95–96 on O₂	2
93–94 on O₂	1
≥93 on air	
88–92	
86–87	1
84–85	2
≤83%	3

Air or oxygen?

	Score
A=Air	
O₂ L/min	2
Device	

C Blood Pressure mmHg — Score uses systolic BP only

Range	Score
≥220	3
201–219	
181–200	
161–180	
141–160	
121–140	
111–120	
101–110	1
91–100	2
81–90	3
71–80	
61–70	
51–60	
≤50	

C Pulse Beats/min

Range	Score
≥131	3
121–130	2
111–120	
101–110	1
91–100	
81–90	
71–80	
61–70	
51–60	
41–50	1
31–40	
≤30	3

D Consciousness — Score for NEWS2 onset of confusion (no score if chronic)

	Score
Alert	
Confusion	
V	3
P	
U	

E Temperature °C

Range	Score
≥39.1°	2
38.1–39.0°	1
37.1–38.0°	
36.1–37.0°	
35.1–36.0°	1
≤35.0°	3

NEWS2 TOTAL	TOTAL
Monitoring frequency	Monitoring
Escalation of care Y/N	Escalation
Initials	Initials

Figure 4.9 NEWS2

Source: Royal College of Physicians (2017) *National Early Warning Score (NEWS) 2: Standardising the assessment of acute-illness severity in the NHS. Updated report of a working party.* London: RCP.

Assess consciousness level (the AVPU score)

AVPU, which is an acronym which stands for Alert, Voice, Pain and Unresponsive, is a tool for allowing rapid assessment of a patient's level of consciousness (Romanelli and Farrell, 2022). There are numerous other tools widely used in clinical practice to assess consciousness level (for example the Glasgow Coma Scale), however they tend to require a higher level of expertise to perform, and unlike the AVPU score, are not a parameter featured on the NEWS2 chart.

To assess a patient's AVPU score, simply judge which one of the following four statements apply to the patient:

- **Patient is ALERT** – the patient is aware and can respond to the environment around them.
- **Respond only to VOICE** – the patient's eyes open to direct verbal stimulus (not opened spontaneously).
- **Respond only to PAIN** – the patient's eyes are not open spontaneously and there is no response to verbal stimuli. When painful stimuli is applied, the patient may move, groan or cry out directly.
- **Are completely UNRESPONSIVE** – the patient does not respond to any stimulus.

If the patient is V, P or U then seek help immediately.

Take and document the respiratory rate

A normal respiratory rate (in a healthy individual) is 12–20 breaths per minute (Chourpiliadis and Bhardwaj, 2021). A respiratory rate higher or lower than this might be the caused by an acute pathology.

A high respiratory rate is a normal response to physical exercise, however if it continues at rest that it may be a sign of deterioration due to underlying pathophysiology. The respiratory rate is a very sensitive indicator of deterioration and is often the first sign that someone is beginning to deteriorate (Kelly, 2018).

To record a respiratory rate, use a watch/timer and count the number of breaths (the number of times the patient's chest rises and falls) the patient takes for a full minute. A raised respiratory rate doesn't necessarily indicate respiratory pathology. Increasing the respiratory rate is the body's first and most rapid mechanism for responding to acidosis which can be caused by a range of conditions.

GO FURTHER

There is an extensive open access article from the Nursing Times which discusses how to take a respiratory rate in detail. Please see the link below:

Wheatley, I. (2018) 'Respiratory rate 3: How to take an accurate measurement', *Nursing Times*, 114 (7): 21–2. https://cdn.ps.emap.com/wp-content/uploads/sites/3/2018/06/180627-Respiratory-rate-3-how-to-take-an-accurate-measurement-1.pdf (accessed October 11, 2022).

Take and document the heart rate

Heart rate is a sensitive indicator of a deteriorating patient. A high heart rate (> 100 beats per minute) is referred to as tachycardia. Low heart rate (< 60 beats per minute) is referred to as bradycardia.

A high heart rate is a normal response to physical exercise, however if it continues at rest then it may be a sign of deterioration due to underlying pathophysiology. There are numerous factors which can influence the heart rate. They include:

- **Dehydration** – with reduced blood volume, your heart has to work harder to maintain circulation. Dehydration often causes a tachycardia.
- **Infection** or **inflammation** – it is a normal physiological response for your heart to pump faster in response to infection or inflammation, in an attempt to deliver more oxygenated blood to organs and tissues, supporting the immune response.
- **Medications** – these can be prescription and non-prescription medications and may have a wide variety of effects on the heart. For example, 'Beta-blockers' such as Bisoprolol will slow the heart and can sometimes cause bradycardia. Conversely, amphetamines will increase heart rate as well as causing coronary artery spasm (causing chest pain).
- **Arrythmias** – such as atrial fibrillation (AF) will cause changes in the heart rate.
- **Thyroid pathology** – a hyperactive thyroid can cause tachycardia, while an underactive thyroid can cause bradycardia.
- **Anxiety** or **panic attack** – can cause significant tachycardia.

It is acceptable to use a pulse oximeter to take heart rate routinely, however it may be imprecise. If the patient is deteriorating and not on a cardiac monitor, it is advisable to take the radial pulse manually, as this will give you a precise measurement and allow you to assess the character and rhythm of the pulse.

TAKING A PULSE RATE: STEP BY STEP

- Wash hands (as per local policy) and greet the patient.
- Explain the procedure to the patient and gain consent to continue.
- Position the patient in a comfortable position either sitting or lying on a bed. Choose an appropriate arm to measure the pulse.
- Using your index or middle finger, palpate the patient's radial pulse (found on the lateral side of the wrist, in line with the thumb). Press firmly with the 'pulp' of your fingers.
- Using a clock, watch or timer, count each 'beat' of the radial pulse for 60 seconds.
- Once complete, thank the patient and document your findings.

Take and document the blood pressure

Blood pressure is often one of the last observations to become abnormal in a deteriorating patient, as the body can compensate very well for a deteriorating blood pressure in a number of ways, in particular by increasing heart rate and contractility and by vasoconstriction.

Ideally check blood pressure on both arms on all occasions. If the first result is abnormal, then always check blood pressure in both arms.

If blood pressure is unrecordable or very low when using an automatic blood pressure device, feel for a radial pulse – if it is not palpable this confirms the blood pressure is very low (and there is not a mechanical fault). You can also check an unrecordable or very low blood pressure reading by using a manual sphygmomanometer, but this should not delay seeking help to manage the low blood pressure.

TAKING A BLOOD PRESSURE: STEP BY STEP

Korotkoff sounds (Korotkov, 1905) are audible noises which are generated through the process of conducting a manual blood pressure reading. The blood pressure cuff constricts the upper arm vessels, causing production of the sounds. A nursing student listening with a stethoscope will be able to hear these Korotkoff sounds, with the **first** and **final** Korotkoff sounds being of particular importance as these are used to denote where systolic and diastolic readings are taken.

Despite being in use for over 100 years, the underlying physiology of the Korotkoff sounds are not fully understood, however there are two main schools of thought, that they are produced by fluid turbulence through the compressed vessel, or through arterial wall oscillations (Campbell et al., 2021)

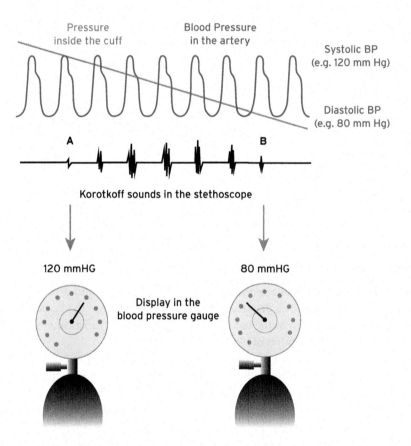

Figure 4.10   **Korotkoff sounds when taking a manual blood pressure**

Source: Wikimedia Commons/PhilippN (CC BY-SA 3.0)

- Wash hands (as per local policy) and greet the patient.
- Explain the procedure to the patient and gain consent to continue.

(Continued)

- Position the patient in a comfortable position either sitting or lying on a bed. Choose an appropriate arm to take a blood pressure reading. Sites which have an intravenous cannula or wound should be avoided. Furthermore, blood pressure readings should not be taken from limbs which have an arterio-venous fistula, lymphoedema or from the same side as a mastectomy.
- Gather equipment. All devices should be clean, calibrated and ready for use.
- Ensure the cuff is the correct size for the patient. If the cuff is too large, it can underestimate the blood pressure.
- Locate the patient's brachial artery (medial side of the upper arm) – wrap the cuff around the patient's bare arm with the cuffs lower edges around 2cm above the brachial pulse. The cuffed arm should be at the level of the patient's heart to ensure an accurate reading.
- Ensure the patient is at rest and ask them not to talk or eat. Ensure their legs are uncrossed.
- Locate the radial pulse and palpate it while inflating the cuff. When the radial pulse can no longer be felt, deflate the cuff, ensuring that you take note of the reading on the manometer (this is the approximate systolic reading).
- Place the stethoscope into your ears, and position the diaphragm of the stethoscope over the patient's brachial pulse. Inflate the cuff to 20mmHg above the approximate systolic previously noted.
- Slowly deflate the cuff while simultaneously listening for the first Korotkoff sound (a tapping sound that denotes the systolic reading) and the Korotkoff sound disappearing (this denotes the diastolic reading). Once the Korotkoff sounds are absent, fully deflate the blood pressure cuff.
- Thank the patient, decontaminate the equipment (as per local policy) and document the blood pressure findings.

Taking and documenting the oxygen saturations

A pulse oximeter is used to measure oxygen saturations and placed onto a peripheral part of the body; usually a finger, toe or ear. The device emits light which passes into the tissue and measures the amount absorbed by haemoglobin in the blood. Using a complex mathematical formula, the device is able to calculate the oxygen saturation of blood.

Pulse oximetry is non-invasive and well tolerated by patients, however it is also prone to errors and has several drawbacks nursing students should be aware of. For example, cold peripheries and movement artifacts (such as rigors or seizure activity) can produce inconsistent readings. Furthermore, the use of nail varnish or false nails can block the light emitted by the device, causing erroneous readings.

Having low oxygen saturations can be a sign of acute deterioration, however it is important to consider whether low oxygen saturation levels are normal for an individual patient as a result of chronic disease. In NEWS2 there are two sections for scoring for oxygen saturations, one is for patients with hypercapnic respiratory failure, who need oxygen saturations titrated to 88–92%. The decision to use this oxygen saturation scoring, rather than standard scoring, should be made by a competent clinical decision maker (RCP, 2017).

Once the decision on which oxygen saturation part of the NEWS chart is to be used has been made, the other should be crossed through.

TAKING OXYGEN SATURATIONS: STEP BY STEP

- Wash hands (as per local policy) and greet the patient.
- Explain the procedure and gain consent to continue.
- Ensure the patient is comfortable, in a sitting position or lying on a bed.
- Select an appropriate finger to place the pulse oximeter on – ensure there is no nail varnish or dirt covering the nail.
- Switch on the pulse oximeter and place on desired finger.
- Ask the patient to remain still while the oximeter calculates the oxygen saturation. Once a consistent reading is displayed, document this appropriately.

Taking and documenting the temperature

Tympanic thermometers are generally used in the UK, because of the ease of use and reasonable level of accuracy. In a hospital setting, temperatures greater than 38 degrees centigrade should be referred to a suitably qualified practitioner for consideration of blood culture sampling (the exact temperature threshold for referral may differ in healthcare settings).

TAKING THE TEMPERATURE: STEP BY STEP

The exact method of use will depend on the brand of the tympanic thermometer. Always follow the manufacturer's instructions and local guidelines.

- Ensure the tympanic thermometer is switched on, clean and calibrated for clinical use.
- Wash hands (as per local policy) and greet the patient.
- Explain the procedure and gain consent to continue.
- Ensure the patient is comfortable, in a sitting position or lying on a bed.
- Place a disposable cover over the probe end.
- Place the probe into the ear canal and gently advance until the probe seals the opening of the ear canal. At the same time, use your other hand to pull **gently** on the patient's ear in a backwards and upwards direction. This will straighten the ear canal and make passage of the probe easier for a more accurate measurement.
- Press the record button to record the tympanic temperature.
- Remove and dispose of the tympanic thermometer cover in a suitable clinical waste receptacle.
- Thank the patient and document the findings.

WATCH THE VIDEO

TAKING AND RECORDING VITAL SIGNS

Watch along as you read through this step by step procedure by scanning the QR code with your smartphone camera or via https://study.sagepub.com/rowberry.

Calculating the Early Warning Score (NEWS2)

Once a full set of observations has been completed, a nursing student will need to record each finding on the NEWS2 chart. Figure 4.11 shows each physiological parameter on the left column, followed by the NEWS2 score it receives in the corresponding row.

ACTIVITY: HAVE A GO

A full set of observations are conducted on Mrs Rushesha, a 62 year old female who has presented to A&E. Mrs Rushesha is alert and orientated. She has a respiration rate of 23, with oxygen saturations of 95% on room air. Mrs Rushesha has a blood pressure of 96/52, with a regular pulse of 102bpm, with a fever of 38.3 degrees.

1   What will Mrs Rushesha's NEWS2 score be?

Answer

Mrs Rushesha's NEWS2 score would be 7

NEWS2: Additional points to consider

- If the patient is receiving oxygen supplementation, then an additional score of 2 should be applied.
- The new SpO_2 Scale 2 should be used for patients with 'a prescribed oxygen saturation requirement of 88–92%' (Royal College of Physicians, 2017). This should only be used in patients with confirmed respiratory failure with hypercapnia (high carbon dioxide levels) and the decision to use the SpO_2 Scale 2 should be made (and documented) by a responsible practitioner or doctor.
- If the patient is alert, it is important to assess if they have a 'new confusion' by asking staff or relatives 'does the patient seem confused to you?' or 'is the patient more confused than normal?'. A new confusion would score 3 on NEWS2, prompting escalation.

Chart 1: The NEWS2 scoring system

Physiological parameter	Score 3	Score 2	Score 1	Score 0	Score 1	Score 2	Score 3
Respiration rate (per minute)	≤8		9-11	12-20		21-24	≥25
SpO$_2$ Scale 1 (%)	≤91	92-93	94-95	≥96			
SpO$_2$ Scale 2 (%)	≤83	84-85	86-97	88-92 ≥93 on air	93-94 on oxygen	95-96 on oxygen	≥97 on oxygen
Air or Oxygen?		Oxygen		Air			
Systolic blood pressure (mmHg)	≤90	91-100	101-110	111-219			≥220
Pulse (per minute)	≤40		41-50	51-90	91-110	111-130	≥131
Consciousness				Alert			CVPU
Temperature (°C)	≤35.0		35.1-36.0	36.1-38.0	38.1-39.0	≥39.1	

Figure 4.11   NEWS2 matrix

Source: https://www.rcplondon.ac.uk/projects/outputs/national-early-warning-score-news-2

- If one of the parameters cannot be completed (for example, if a patient refuses to have their blood pressure taken), then the NEWS2 score must still be calculated and documented as incomplete. A patient may trigger for escalation on a single parameter, or on the total score, even if incomplete.

NEWS2 – escalation of care

The NEWS2 score will designate:

- When the next set of observations should be carried out
- If additional support should be sought and which healthcare providers should provide this
- The urgency of referral for additional support
- The most suitable environment in which the patient should be cared for (in hospital, in critical care etc.)

It is vital that directions based on the NEWS2 score are followed exactly.

Any parameter which scores red (for example, a respiratory rate of 30, or new confusion) would require an urgent ward-based review of the patient. This could be by a nurse practitioner, ward doctor or on-call doctor. If however the total (aggregate) score is >7, this will require an emergency response.

Chart 2: NEWS2 thresholds and triggers

NEWS2 score	Clinical risk	Response
Aggregate score 0–4	Low	Ward-based response
Red score Score of 3 in any individual parameter	Low-medium	Urgent ward-based response*
Aggregate score 5–6	Medium	Key threshold for urgent response*
Aggregate score 7 or more	High	Urgent or emergency response**

* Response by a clinician or team with competence in the assessment and treatment of acutely ill patients and in recognising when the escalation of care to a critical care team is appropriate.

** The response team must also include staff with critical care skills, including airway management.

Figure 4.12   NEWS2 matrix (2)

Source: https://www.rcplondon.ac.uk/projects/outputs/national-early-warning-score-news-2

CHAPTER SUMMARY

This chapter was designed to give nursing students a comprehensive overview of numerous aspects of patient assessment and introduced numerous clinical skills, for example:

- Patient history taking (including suicide risk assessment), along with specific questioning to allow assessment of pain using a standardised approach.
- A full systems assessment, including a basic musculoskeletal examination, followed by extensive respiratory, cardiovascular, gastrointestinal, and neurological examinations.
- The conduction of simple investigations and procedures, such as the recording of an electrocardiogram (ECG) and venepuncture.
- The completion of a full set of observations and recording of findings on a NEWS2 chart so patient care can be escalated based on clinical need.

The information provided is not exhaustive for any individual topic but will serve as a basis for further reading.

ACE YOUR ASSESSMENT

Q1   The acronym SOCRATES is used to aid the assessment of pain. What does each letter stand for?

   a   Site, Onset, Character, Radiation, Association, Time course, Exacerbating/relieving factors, Severity

   b   Source, Onset, Character, Referred pain, Aggravating factors, Time course, Exacerbating/relieving factors, Severity

   c   Symptoms, Onset, Character, Relieving factors, Additional pain, Time course, Exacerbating factors, Source

Q2   In chest auscultation, which high-pitched continuous noise is suggestive of a limitation in airflow and is often associated with asthma and respiratory infections?

    a   Inspiratory stridor

    b   Expiratory wheeze

    c   Unilateral coarse crackles

Q3 Which heart valve allows blood flow from the left atrium to the left ventricle?

    a   Pulmonary valve

    b   Mitral valve

    c   Tricuspid valve

Q4 The abdomen can be arbitrarily divided into four or nine regions to aid clinical examination. A patient presents with pain approximately over the liver. Which region will this be within? (use either the four or nine quadrant model)

    a   Right upper quadrant/right hypochondriac region

    b   Right lower quadrant/right iliac region

    c   Left upper quadrant/left hypochondriac region

Q5 Which Korotkoff sound denotes the systolic blood pressure?

    a   First sound

    b   Second sound

    c   Final sound

Answers

1   A

2   B

3   B

4   A

5   A

GO FURTHER

Life In the Fast Lane ECG library (https://litfl.com/ecg-library) provides a wealth of information about ECG's, including a basic overview of how to conduct the ECG, as well as detailed diagrams and waveforms featuring various pathology.

REFERENCES

Campbell, M., Sultan, A. and Pillarisetty, L. (2021) 'Physiology, Korotkoff sound', StatPearls, June 25. https://www.ncbi.nlm.nih.gov/books/NBK539778/ (accessed October, 11, 2022).

Chourpiliadis, C. and Bhardwaj, A. (2021) 'Physiology, respiratory rate'. StatPearls, September 20. https://pubmed.ncbi.nlm.nih.gov/30725991/ (accessed October, 11, 2022).

Drake, R. L., Vogel. W. and Mitchell, A.W. (2010) *Grey's Anatomy for Students* (2nd edition). Philadelphia, PA: Elsevier.

Farre, A. and Rapley, T. (2017) 'The new old (and old new) medical model: Four decades navigating the biomedical and psychosocial understandings of health and illness', *Healthcare (Basel)*, 5 (4): Article #88.

Fawcett, T. and Rhynas, S. (2012) 'Taking a patient history: The role of the nurse', *Nursing Standard*, 26 (24): 41–6.

Fayaz, A., Croft, P., Langford, R.M., Donaldson, L.J. and Jones, G.T. (2016) 'Prevalence of chronic pain in the UK: A systematic review and meta-analysis of population studies', *BMJ Open*, 6 (6). doi.org/10.1136/bmjopen-2015-010364

Gregory, J. and McGowan, L. (2016) 'An examination of the prevalence of acute pain for hospitalised adult patients: A systematic review', *Journal of Clinical Nursing*, 25 (5/6): 583–98.

Harmer, B., Lee, S., Duong, H. and Saadabadi, A. (2022) 'Suicidal ideation', PubMed - StatPearls Publishing, May 2. https://pubmed.ncbi.nlm.nih.gov/33351435/ (accessed October 11, 2022).

Kelly, C. (2018) 'Respiratory rate 1: Why measurement and recording are crucial', *Nursing Times*, 114 (4): 23–4. https://www.nursingtimes.net/clinical-archive/respiratory-clinical-archive/respiratory-rate-1-why-measurement-and-recording-are-crucial-26-03-2018/ (accessed October 11, 2022).

Knott, L. (2018) 'Oedema - Swelling', Patient, December 28. https://patient.info/signs-symptoms/oedema-swelling (accessed October 11, 2022).

Korotkov, N. (1905) 'Concerning the methods of blood pressure measurement (from the clinic of S. P. Fedorov)', *Proceedings of the Emperor's Military Medical Academy St Petersburg*, 11: 365–7.

Kotsovolis, G. and Kallaras, K. (2010) 'The role of endothelium and endogenous vasoactive substances in sepsis', *Hippokratia*, 14 (2): 88–93.

Mansel, B. and Bradley-Adams, K. (2018) '"I AM A STAR": A mnemonic for undertaking a mental state examination', *Mental Health Practice*, 21 (1): 21–6.

National Institute for Health and Clinical Excellence (NICE) (2007) *Acutely Ill Patients in Hospital: Recognising and responding to deterioration* (CG50), nice.org.uk, July 25. https://www.nice.org.uk/guidance/cg50 (accessed October 14, 2022).

Office for National Statistics (ONS) (2019) 'Suicides in the UK: 2018 registrations', ons. gov.uk, September 19. https://www.ons.gov.uk/peoplepopulationandcommunity/birthsdeathsandmarriages/deaths/bulletins/suicidesintheunitedkingdom/2018registrations (accessed October 11, 2022).

Patterson, W.M., Dohn, H.H., Bird, J. and Patterson, G.A. (1983) 'Evaluation of suicidal patients: The SAD PERSONS scale', *Psychosomatics*, 24 (4): 343–5 & 348–9.

Romanelli, D. and Farrell, M. (2022) 'AVPU Score', StatPearls. https://www.ncbi.nlm.nih.gov/books/NBK538431/ (accessed October 11, 2022).

Royal College of Nursing (RCN) (2022) 'Infection prevention and control – Sepsis', RCN, August, 17. https://www.rcn.org.uk/clinical-topics/infection-prevention-and-control/sepsis (accessed October 11, 2022).

Royal College of Physicians (RCP) (2017) 'National Early Warning Score (NEWS) 2', rcplondon.ac.uk, December 19. https://www.rcplondon.ac.uk/projects/outputs/national-early-warning-score-news-2 (accessed October 11, 2022).

DIGNITY, COMFORT, REST AND SLEEP

5

SARAH TAIT AND LOUISE GILES, WITH SARAH KINGDOM-MILLS (LEARNING DISABILITIES CONTRIBUTION)

NMC STANDARDS COVERED IN THIS CHAPTER

ANNEXE B NURSING PROCEDURES

3.1 Observe and assess comfort and pain levels and rest and sleep patterns
3.4 Take appropriate action to ensure privacy and dignity at all times
3.5 Take appropriate action to reduce or minimise pain or discomfort
3.6 Take appropriate action to reduce fatigue, minimise insomnia and support improved rest and sleep hygiene

---

LEARNING OBJECTIVES

After reading this chapter, you should be able to:

- Take appropriate action to ensure dignity for everyone at all times
- Observe and assess rest and sleep patterns and take appropriate action to reduce fatigue, minimise insomnia and support improved rest and sleep hygiene
- Observe and assess comfort; take appropriate action to reduce or minimise discomfort
- Use appropriate bed-making techniques including those required for people who have limited mobility or who are unconscious

INTRODUCTION

Within this chapter we will introduce you to some essential elements around patient care that include dignity, comfort, assessment of rest and sleep and sleep hygiene.

Observing dignity is essential for establishing a nurse–patient relationship (RCN, 2022).

A person's comfort and ability to rest can have a profound effect on their recovery from illness or treatment and nurses are in a privileged position to positively impact their experience of care. This is achieved through paying close attention by observing and assessing the person and agreeing the plan of care with them.

DIGNITY

What is dignity?

Dignity is one of the most important things to the human spirit. It means *being valued and respected for what you are*, what you believe in, and how you live your life. Dignity is concerned with how people feel, think and behave in relation to the worth or value of themselves and others. To treat someone with dignity is to treat them as being of worth, in a way that is respectful of them as valued individuals.

When dignity is present, people feel in control, valued, confident, comfortable, and able to make decisions for themselves (NMC, 2018). When dignity is absent people feel devalued, lacking control and comfort. They may lack confidence and be unable to make decisions for themselves. They may feel humiliated, embarrassed, or ashamed.

Dignity applies equally to those who have capacity and to those who lack it. Everyone has equal worth as human beings and must be treated as if they are able to feel, think and behave in relation to their own worth or value (RCN, 2022).

The Amsterdam Declaration recognised dignity as one of the main rights for patients (WHO, 1994). Being treated with dignity and involved in decision-making is associated with positive outcomes, such as high patient satisfaction (Beach et al., 2005). In a review of the World Health Organization (WHO)'s general population surveys in 41 countries, most participants selected dignity as the second most important domain in care – only 'promptness of care' was more highly rated (Valentine et al., 2008).

The concept of dignity can be hard to pin down, but Nordenfelt and Edgar (2005), in their European study, described four different types of dignity. These are as follows:

- **Menschenwürde** – this is the basic dignity of all human beings. Simply by being human we are all entitled to this and even if someone lacks the ability to think, move or communicate, it is important to remember that a human being should always be treated in a way that maintains human dignity.
- **Dignity as merit** – this type of dignity is conferred upon someone because of their title, rank or what they have done in their life regarding their deeds or merits. For example, if a resident or patient has a professional status such as a doctor or a title, taking this away from them takes away their dignity and sense of self-worth.
- **The dignity of morality** – this refers to somebody's own moral code and beliefs. We might not agree with or have the same view as an individual's moral code, but we must respect it.
- **The dignity of personal identity** – ignoring somebody's personal identity and humiliating them or abusing them because of this robs them of their dignity. We all have a right to maintain our own individuality, and ignoring this or actively ridiculing somebody's beliefs goes against the concept of dignity.

Although these concepts may seem academic, if you work in care you can probably see when unthinking actions about residents and patients cross the line into taking somebody's dignity away.

—————————————————— **GO FURTHER** ——————————————————

Read the following fact sheet on Deprivation of Liberty Safeguards (DoLS) from Age UK:

Age UK (2022). *Factsheet 62: Deprivation of Liberty Safeguards.* https://www.ageuk.org.uk/
globalassets/age-uk/documents/factsheets/fs62_deprivation_of_liberty_safeguards_fcs.pdf
(accessed October 12, 2022).

ACTIVITY: PAUSE AND REFLECT

Consider the following:

1   What are Deprivation of Liberty Safeguards?
2   Who do Deprivation of Liberty Safeguards apply to?
3   What is a deprivation of liberty?

What does dignified care look like? How do we ensure it is maintained?

People should receive care from competent nurses who have the knowledge, skills, and desire to provide a high standard of care which meets their patients' individual needs, and they should be encouraged to speak up straight away if they see nurses providing poor care or behaving in a way that causes them distress. Nurses should be trustworthy, dependable and show empathy, compassion and kindness (NMC, 2018).

When receiving care it must make the person feel valued and treated as an individual, by nurses who listen to what they have to say, take time to communicate in the way that is best for the individual, and find out from them, and others who are important to them, how they want to be cared for, provide care in a way that respects their right to privacy and dignity, work together with them, and the people who are important to them, by making sure that their wishes are taken into account when decisions are being made.

Wherever a person receives care from a nurse, they should feel they are in safe hands, believe that their individual needs are being met in a fair, non-judgmental and respectful way and be confident that the nurses and any required equipment are available. Patients/clients/service users should be in no doubt that the nurses are committed to ensuring a high standard of care is provided.

ACTIVITY: WHAT'S THE EVIDENCE?

The principles of nursing practice describe what everyone from nursing staff to patients can expect from nursing.

Each of the eight principles were developed by the Royal College of Nursing (RCN) in partnership with the Department of Health (DoH), the Nursing and Midwifery Council (NMC), patients, the public and healthcare staff.

The principles describe what constitutes safe and effective nursing care, and cover the aspects of behaviour, attitude and approach that underpin good care. The first principle states that nurses and nursing staff treat everyone in their care with dignity and humanity – they should understand their individual needs, show compassion and sensitivity, and provide care in a way that respects all people equally.

Principle A
Nurses and Nursing staff treat everyone in their care with dignity and humanity - they understand their individual needs, show compassion and sensitivity, and provide care in a way that respects all people equally.

Principle B
Nurses and nursing staff take responsibility for the care they provide and answer for their own judgements and actions - they carry out these actions in a way that is agreed with their patients, and the families and carers of their patients, and in a way that meets the requirements of their professional bodies and the law.

Principle C
Nurses and nursing staff manage risk, are vigilant about risk, and help to keep everyone safe in the places they receive healthcare.

Principle D
Nurses and nursing staff provide and promote care that puts people at the centre, involves patients, service users, their families and their carers in decisions and helps them make informed choices about their treatment and care.

Priniciple E
Nurses and nursing staff are at the heart of the communication process: they assess, record and report on treatment and care, handle information sensitively and confidentially, deal with complaints effectively, and are conscientious in reporting the things they are concerned about.

Principle F
Nurses and nursing staff have up-to-date knowledge and skills, and use these with intelligence, insight and understanding in line with the needs of each individual in their care.

Principal G
Nurses and nursing staff work closely with their own team and with other professionals, making sure patients' care and treatment is co-ordinated, is of a high standard and has the best possible outcome.

Principle H
Nurses and nursing staff lead by example, develop themselves and other staff, and influence the way care is given in a manner that is open and responds to individual needs.

Figure 5.1   Royal College of Nursing (RCN) Principles

Source: RCN (2020)

---------------------------------- GO FURTHER ----------------------------------

The RCN have created a series of short films that highlight how the principles can be put into practice. These are available to watch on the RCN website, or via the following link: https://www.rcn.org.uk/professional-development/principles-of-nursing-practice/principles-of-nursing-practice-films (accessed October 12, 2022).

Every nurse must abide by the NMC *Code* (2018). Those accessing care are advised as to what to expect in the NMC's publication 'Care and respect every time', available here:

https://www.nmc.org.uk/globalassets/sitedocuments/nmc-publications/nmc-care-and-respect.pdf (accessed October 12, 2022).

PAIN AND COMFORT

Comfort is being in the position of physical or mental ease and freedom from pain, whether physical or emotional pain. Physical pain tends to be a sensation that is delivered via the nervous system. For example, when there is tissue damage, messages are sent to the brain via the nervous system to alert that there is injury, causing a body part to hurt, to ultimately try to prevent further damage. Emotional pain is of a psychological nature that is usually intense and emerges from a non-physical source, caused by the actions of another being, or because of grief, trauma or associated mental illness. Although emotional pain is often dismissed as less severe than physical pain, it is essential that it is not ignored. A mental health nursing student has said 'Patients often say that physical pain is easier to deal with than emotional pain.' Whereas physical pain can be pinpointed to a specific injury, when someone suffers with emotional pain, it can be difficult to identify the source and thus treat. Consequently, to deal with emotional pain, a person will often resort to self-injurious behaviour to take their mind off the emotional pain, giving them a physical pain to focus on instead.

Emotional pain can materialise as physical pain. Babbel (2018) refers to somatisation, where she indicates that emotional problems can emerge as pain in various parts of the body, for instance, stress and tension could present as a headache or where an individual is carrying the 'weight of the world on their shoulders,' this could present as shoulder pain. Anyone can experience somatic symptoms, the most common being the physical symptoms of anxiety (stomach-ache, heart racing); it is important that we understand that the person is not feigning illness and that their symptoms are very real. Emotional pain and physical pain are generally viewed as different, often with emotional pain being viewed as less serious. However, it is claimed that as a result of certain neurological structures, similarities can be identified between emotional and physical pain, thus pain should be perceived as a spectrum of pain, rather than a definitive physical or emotional pain (Biro, 2010; Eisenberger, 2012).

Managing pain

It is imperative that pain relief is appropriate to allow a person to rest, be comfortable and to be able to sleep. It is important to recognise that pain is unique to the individual and that how individuals respond to pain will be different. To determine the degree of pain, an assessment must be established. The NICE Chronic Pain Guidelines (2021) suggest a person-centred assessment, and also advise to consider the cause of pain and to develop an individualised care and support plan. There is a range of analgesic treatments that can help individuals overcome their pain. However, in the first instance, non-pharmacological pain management should be considered, including exercise programmes, psychological therapies, acupuncture, or electrical physical modalities. This would be followed with pharmacological methods of pain management. However, care and consideration is required when administering medications that are associated with dependence and many analgesic medications have dependency tendencies.

Comfort is a state of physical ease and freedom from pain, and whilst when nursing people we cannot always ensure they are pain-free, we are aiming to ease or alleviate a person's grief or distress. This can be seen when considering the case study below.

CASE STUDY

Providing dignified care

Ewan is 80 years old and has lived alone since their life partner died three years ago. Ewan has maintained independent living with the support of their children who live locally and see or speak with their father daily. Ewan takes medication for arthritic pain and hypertension and has a fine tremor that sometimes makes it difficult to attend to buttons and zip fasteners.

Ewan was admitted to the Emergency Department with chest and back pain along with nausea and dizziness. Investigations were conducted, including blood tests, x-rays, ultrasound scans and a CT scan to eliminate concerns about a potential aneurysm dissection and ultimately to diagnose shingles around his back and chest.

Ewan was initially very concerned about the pain and the number of investigations being undertaken and had raised anxiety, further compounded by a recent bereavement in the same hospital.

The nurse's approach was one that ensured that Ewan felt supported and cared for by explaining all the processes and maintaining privacy and dignity throughout all the examinations and investigations – it was the nurse's attention to helping Ewan get undressed and put on a hospital gown that led to identification of the rash.

Ewan talked about the gentleness of the nurse's approach and that at no point was there any impatience in assisting them as their tremor seemed worse than usual which meant they needed more help in dressing and undressing, in attending to personal care needs and with holding a cup so that they could take a drink and any prescribed analgesia. The application of dressings was performed with care to prevent further pain and ensure comfort once Ewan was dressed prior to discharge. Ewan said that the nurse took time to listen to all concerns and anxieties and once the diagnosis was made, the nurse was attentive to Ewan's wish to go home and to contact their son and daughter-in-law so that they could come to collect them. Ewan was particularly pleased that the nurses' concern extended to the family and took the time to explain what had happened and reassured them.

Rest and sleep

Rest and sleep mean different things to different people. That is why it matters to provide individualised care and consider what makes each person unique and doing everything you can to put their needs first (RCN, 2022).

CASE STUDY

Rachel

Rachel was admitted to the ward after attempting to take her own life. Rachel lost her partner Sandra a year ago to cancer and has visited the GP on a few occasions suffering with depressive symptoms. Rachel's main symptom insomnia has been having a negative effect on her mood and her negative mood has been having a negative effect on her ability to sleep. This bidirectional relationship between poor sleep and depression is having an intense effect on her recovery and Rachel is asking the nurse for support to improve her sleep.

What is sleep?

Sleep is 'a periodic state of physiological rest during which consciousness is suspended' (Collins Dictionary, 2020). Sleep is thought of as a natural occurrence and is said to take up to a third of each individual's time during a lifetime (Mandal, 2020).

Typically, the body and mind shut down and the body's command system becomes inactive, allowing our muscles and consciousness to rest. However, it differs from that of a coma, where a person appears to be sleeping but is unresponsive to pain and any stimulation.

When sleeping, the person's responsiveness to external stimuli is reduced, but they can be awakened and will respond to pain, noise, and any stimulation, unlike being unconscious. While sleeping, our brain acts as a filter to external stimuli and decisions are made whether to respond to those stimuli or not. This filtering process is essential in protecting us from danger or threats to our lives and to respond to noises that are important to us (Micic and Zajamsek, 2021).

Sleep covers several phases and is not defined as one constant state – simply put, it can be divided into REM (Rapid Eye Movement) and NREM (Non-Rapid Eye Movement) – for your own deeper learning please explore this further. These phases change as the night progresses and can be interrupted because, for example, we hear a noise or alter our position.

To function adequately, both mentally and physically, healthy sleep patterns are essential. It is evident that good quality healthy sleep improves the immune system and influences the maintenance of a healthy diet, as well as positive mental wellbeing.

Healthy sleep improves the function of our brains, leading to better concentration levels, positive thinking, learning, creativity and memory. Contrastingly, poor sleep can have a detrimental effect and contribute to various public health issues such as obesity and poor mental health, resulting in foggy thinking, depression, and low energy (Fry, 2022).

What constitutes 'a good night's sleep'?

Most of us recognise that when we have a bad night's sleep, it affects the rest of the day, including our energy levels, our concentration span, our mood and overall wellbeing. However, there are more scientific ways to measure the quality of our sleep, from simple questionnaires gathering subjective, personal data to polysomnography which gathers objective data through the measurement of limb movements, eye movements, brain waves and oxygen levels during the sleep process.

The number of times an adult wakes during the night, the time it takes them to fall asleep plus other factors all impact on the quality of sleep gained. Studies conducted by Della-Monica et al. (2018) indicated that more awakenings during the night pertains to poor sleep, and higher REM periods for individuals equated to better quality sleep. Their study included adults aged 20–84 and while age appeared not to influence sleep quality, there were some variances reported between males and females.

Internal and external factors can also influence sleep quality. The comfort of the environment as well as the temperature and external noise all have an impact. These may be in the individual's control and can be altered in a positive way to promote sleep quality. There have been many studies conducted into the use of phones or other blue light devices before sleeping, mainly finding these have a negative impact on sleep and should be avoided. Not being able to switch off from our thoughts of family, work or other worries appears in many large sleep studies.

Simple changes to our environment and pre-sleep routine can in fact positively influence the quality of sleep adults experience. We will look at how these factors impact patients' sleep when they are in hospital later in this chapter.

Benefits of developing a bedtime routine

Children with a consistent effective bedtime routine are thought to have improved attention, cognition, inhibition and perform better in educational institutions (Kitsaras et al., 2018). Yet, an optimal sleep routine is also said to benefit adults. A bedtime routine can help the individual separate night from day and help clear the mind and initiate a relaxed state to enable sleep. There is a section on sleep hygiene towards the end of this chapter with ideas of how to incorporate a bedtime routine.

For babies, parents need to teach them how to develop a sleep routine by using certain methods consistently. A recognised awake in the day, asleep at night pattern does not show in babies until around the four-month mark. Any parental training should wait until this point. Babies of this age learn through routine. Soothing practices at bedtime are usually factored into parents' processes. They will cry when falling to sleep and parents will make a choice on 'cry it out' or not as a preference to them in their situations.

To aid a sleep routine, parents need to be flexible in terms of what suits them and their baby. There are various methods that are said to help encourage a sleep routine, some of which are mentioned below. However, a consistent routine that helps the baby learn the difference between night and day can be beneficial.

Examples of a helpful routine:

- Consistent bedtime
- A bath and dress for bed
- Cuddles with a night-time feed
- A story
- A lullaby
- Consistent comforting parting words, 'Good night, sweet dreams' and a kiss.

KEY TERMS

Bedtime fading: this is where the actual time of bedtime changes and is lengthened by 10–15 minutes each time, when the baby learns to fall asleep very soon after going to bed, this then becomes the actual time for bedtime.

Chair method: the baby is prepared for bed and the parent sits in a chair next to the baby's cot after the baby is put to bed. When the baby falls asleep, the parent leaves the room, if the baby wakes up, the parent has to re-enter the room and sit back in the chair, until the baby falls asleep again. Each night, the chair should be moved further and further from the cot until eventually the chair is outside of the bedroom.

Graduated crying – Ferber method: this is where parents let the baby cry but check in regularly, leaving longer periods of time between the checking-in periods. It is recommended that there is no dialogue or picking up if choosing this method. This routine continues for a period of time, and can vary from baby to baby, until the baby has learned to fall asleep by themselves.

There is research behind each of these methods and they are recommended as part of a routine more so than choosing to have no routine for babies' bedtime. This is a new skill for babies to learn and when they are receiving attention and love during waking hours, these methods are thought not to cause any harm to development (Gagne, 2020).

The amount of sleep that a baby or infant needs will depend on their age ranging from 16 hours during day and night for a newborn – approx. 50% during the day and the same during the night – to 13 hours for a two-year-old with only one or two hours of sleep happening during the day. Their sleep cycle also differs compared to adult's sleep: babies have significantly less REM sleep (dream sleep) than adults.

What is the evidence about the amount of sleep we need?

On average an adult requires between 7.5 and 9.5 hours of sleep a night, and it is thought that a sleep routine is most important as this tends to prevent disruption and causing sleep problems. Teens need approximately 8–10 hours while an older adult will need approximately 7–8 hours.

Taking time throughout the day to catch up on sleep on a regular basis can disrupt one's natural sleeping patterns. However, the exact number of hours needed for an individual is also dependent on genetics as well as age.

These are 'general guidelines' and will be affected by:

- Other health issues, as some people are at higher risk at night from other illnesses.
- Have energy levels changed, perhaps a more physically demanding job – or vice versa.
- Is there already a history of sleep disturbances?
- Work including high levels of concentration, or is it emotionally demanding?
- Having a high caffeine (or other stimulant) intake during the day.

Most adults will have a personal preference as to whether they prefer to be 'up with the lark' or are a 'night owl' and knowing this about oneself can help when devising a healthy pre-sleep and sleep routine.

Sleep deprivation/insomnia

Many people are affected by sleep deprivation, complaining that they do not sleep well or at all. Being deprived of sleep rarely results in death, yet a lack of sleep has an abundance of consequences that may result in death, for example, increasing the risk of accidents and such like.

Self-assessment of symptoms for sleep disturbances or insomnia can sometimes be a good place to start when an individual reports this.

Symptoms of insomnia include:

- Lying awake unable to fall asleep
- Constantly waking during the night, sleeping for very short periods
- Difficulties falling back to sleep after waking
- Feel tired all day, mood is low
- Poor concentration during waking hours

Some potential causes of insomnia:

- Room temperature that does not meet your preference
- Too much noise
- Too much light
- Shift work
- Uncomfortable bed

- Stress and anxiety
- Stimulants or drugs

Individuals can look to alter factors in their control but should seek medical advice if symptoms persist or are beyond their control. For people who have a learning disability, it may be that the people who know them best are able to notice changes in behaviours that can affect sleep patterns and thus put things in place to improve matters.

Sleep disturbances/disorders

Insomnia is seen as a sleep disturbance or disorder. Other sleep disturbances include:

- Narcolepsy – falling asleep suddenly and uncontrollably during the day.
- Sleep apnoea – abnormal breathing patterns during periods of sleep (many different types and can be dangerous for patients).
- Restless leg syndrome – an uncomfortable and sometimes painful feeling in the legs causing an urge to move the legs around constantly, resulting in poor sleep quality.

CASE STUDY

Obstructive sleep apnoea

Mo Jamil is a 47-year-old male with a two-year history of obstructive sleep apnoea. The sleep apnoea presented itself when Mo Jamil complained of extreme tiredness, sleepiness during the day and limited ability to concentrate. Up until the point of diagnosis, Mo Jamil thought he was having approximately eight hours sleep a night, however he said that this was never enough. He also noticed a significant increase in his weight over a period of a year and on awakening in the morning would have a headache and a sore throat.

From a time in his early twenties, Mo Jamil was told by friends/family that he snored badly at night. Mo Jamil attributed the snoring to the fact that he used to smoke, however having not smoked for several years, the snoring remained a problem. Mo Jamil's wife would never complain about the snoring, but Mo Jamil's children would often tell him that he would be snoring loudly, when sleeping or falling off to sleep.

Mo Jamil remembers falling asleep at meetings in work and being nudged awake by a colleague when a snore was released. He also remembers having to nap throughout the day over the past year or two and would joke with friends of a 'nana nap'. This became easier in Covid times as working from home meant that a sleep through the day was achievable.

Mo Jamil explained his symptoms to the GP; loud snoring, headaches, sore throat, smelly breath, tiredness throughout the day, weight gain, difficulty losing weight and showed the GP photos of his nose, which had been broken as a child and never fixed properly. Mo Jamil wondered if it was his nose that was disrupting the air flow for him as he was sleeping, which was then causing the above-mentioned symptoms.

The GP referred Mo Jamil to the Lung Function Clinic. At the clinic, the clinicians discussed a sleep study and sent Mo Jamil home with a monitor to record his heart rate and oxygen levels whilst sleeping. The study concluded that Mo Jamil had a reading of 14 on the Apnea-Hypopnea

Index (AHI). A reading of 14 indicates a mild to moderate level of breathing and sleep disturbance, meaning Mo Jamil was stopping breathing around 14 times a night. Due to an AHI of 14, Mo Jamil was informed that the most effective form of treatment would be a CPAP (Continuous Positive Airway Pressure) machine.

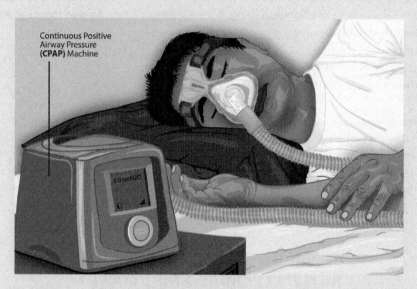

Figure 5.2   Continuous Positive Airway Pressure (CPAP) machine

Source: Wikimedia Commons/https://www.myupchar.com/en (CC BY-SA 4.0).

One year on, despite having a few difficulties early on with the mask sizing and amount of air pressure, Mo Jamil persevered with the CPAP and says that he would now find it difficult to live without a CPAP machine. His AHI is considerably lower at 3 and he has much safer levels of oxygen in his system. He says the difference to how he feels daily is astonishing. No longer does he suffer with daytime sleepiness, he has lost 10lb in weight and continues to lose weight having energy to exercise before or after work. Mo Jamil now awakes in the morning feeling refreshed and ready for the day ahead. He feels more able to keep on top of his workload and is able to concentrate for longer periods. Overall Mo Jamil is pleased with the treatment outcome of the CPAP and is generally feeling more positive.

Sleep disturbances or disorders must be diagnosed by an appropriate clinician; however, if patients report new signs and symptoms to you, you can hopefully recognise the significance of these and report them. The Epworth Sleepiness Scale (Johns, 2010) indicates four possible responses to a range of situations and is used to diagnose obstructive sleep apnoea when the person answers as honestly as possible a series of questions. The score guides them to seek medical review as a score greater than 10 indicates a possible sleep disorder.

Table 5.1   The Epworth Sleepiness Scale (Johns, 2010)

Situation	Responses
• Sitting & reading	**0 = would never doze**
• Watching television	**1 = slight chance of dozing**
• Sitting inactive in a public place e.g. cinema	**2 = moderate chance of dozing**
• As a passenger in a car for an hour without a break	**3 = high chance of dozing**
• Lying down to rest in the afternoon	
• Sitting and talking to someone	
• Sitting quietly after lunch (when you have not had any alcohol)	
• In a car while stopped at traffic	

A significant percentage of the adult population experience sleep disturbances and there are tentative studies that report they are more prevalent in adults with a mental health diagnosis resulting in an adverse effect on a person's quality of life (McCall et al., 2000).

Hombali et al. (2019) studied the links between mental health diagnosis and sleep disorders, concurring with the DSM that there are connections between the two and that accurate, in-depth sleep assessments should be conducted on a more widespread basis than is currently evident.

ACTIVITY: PAUSE AND REFLECT

Consider the following:

1   Have you seen sleep assessments completed in areas you have attended for clinical placements? If yes, what did this entail and how was the data gathered then used?
2   If you have not seen sleep assessments, how do you feel these would impact patients if they were conducted more regularly?

SLEEP QUALITY FOR PATIENTS IN HOSPITALS

CASE STUDY

Mrs Kaur

Mrs Kaur was admitted to the ward three nights ago and has been complaining to the day staff that the staff on night duty and other patients make far too much noise for her to have sufficient sleep at night. She explains that she is taking daytime naps which she does not like to do but is unable to keep herself awake during the day. Mrs Kaur tells you that lights are left on at night, that there is banging echoing through the corridor, patients are shouting out for the nurse throughout the night and one particular staff member has worn very noisy shoes and has been heard speaking loudly back to the patient who was shouting. Mrs Kaur pleads with you to try to help her have a decent sleep.

This chapter has already explored the internal and external factors affecting a person's sleep quality in their own home. It is important to now consider the picture for patients in hospitals.

Hospitals, overall, are not quality sleep environments and the factors usually affecting a person are worries keeping them awake, too much light and too much noise. Morse and Bender (2019) indicate that despite knowing these factors, many areas do little to document patients' sleep patterns or alter the environment, where possible, to promote sleep.

Arguably, sleep for patients who are vulnerable or experiencing ill health is now even more important. Further understanding of why it is important, factors that affect sleep and how to improve things for patients in hospital is needed. It is inevitable that patients will be woken at times, for essential treatment or assessment, emergencies or when clinically necessary and most patients perhaps anticipate this as a side effect of being in a hospital environment. However, their recovery can be hindered, and measures should be taken to address this where possible.

Many published studies exist looking at noise levels in critical care, A&E and operating theatres and these environments hold little control over factors that affect patients due to the nature of activities and patient dependence in these areas. However, there are fewer published studies looking at general ward areas. Those that are available gathered data on the patient's perspective of disturbances and many cited ward equipment, staff conversations and other patients as the main sources. 40%–60% of patients in hospital report poor quality sleep on a regular basis. Additional research is needed in this area to fully understand what is avoidable and what can be altered to improve wards in relation to patients' sleep experiences. Documentation has been published by WHO that outlines acceptable noise levels for all general wards; studies published in this area report night-time noise levels exceeding WHO recommendations.

Many authors who write in this area conclude that assessment and documentation of patient's sleep should be recorded more frequently. There are areas and health boards that regularly assess inpatients' sleep quality and have taken measures to improve this experience for patients. You are likely to see a variation between areas in relation to sleep and sleep assessment; anonymously recording your observations may help increase your knowledge as well as allowing you to share best practice with areas that may be looking to improve in this area.

SLEEP HYGIENE

Sleep hygiene is not a new concept. It is an important area to gather knowledge as a student so that you may offer advice or practical help to patients you care for. This chapter has recognised the importance of sleep and the benefits quality sleep gives us. It has also recognised that at times, sleep disturbances are inevitable. However, advising patients on sleep hygiene and promoting quality sleep will be an important skill needed during your studies.

Advice points for promoting sleep hygiene:

- Try to wake and get up the same time each day.
- Make attempts to go to sleep at the same time also.
- Exercising during the day helps promote night-time sleep but avoid directly before going to bed.
- Where possible, control the bedroom environment in relation to light, temperature, odours and noise. This can be difficult in multi-person rooms in hospital settings.
- Avoid dated institutional practices such as switching on lights early in the morning as this may not be appropriate for all patients.
- Avoid blue light devices for an hour before bedtime.
- Try winding down and relaxing before going to bed, try relaxation techniques. Avoid intense conversations or activities at this time.

- Avoid stimulants, alcohol, smoking before going to bed.
- Avoid taking daytime naps – this affects night-time sleep quality.

CHAPTER SUMMARY

This chapter has introduced you to dignity, comfort, pain, rest and sleep. All of which are fundamental to promoting the health and recovery of our patients. Any observation of undignified care needs to be reported to the relevant personnel. The absence of dignified care goes against everything the Nursing Midwifery Council advocate (NMC, 2018) and ultimately leaves our patients feeling devalued, lacking in control and comfort. In providing dignified care and in ensuring safe and effective care, we will empower our patients to feel more confident and aid them in their journey to recovery or end of life.

To ensure the comfort of our patients, we need to understand their pain and be aware of the guidelines to pain management and not in all circumstances race to the medication cabinet. Yes, medication can help, but other forms of management can be explored which may suit the individual better and align with person-centred care.

In addition to ensuring dignified care and managing pain, we must ensure that our patients experience sufficient rest and sleep and that we find ways to help them improve the quality of their sleep. We can adopt various sleep assessment tools to identify sleep disorders and we can promote effective sleep hygiene methods. Ultimately, we need to be aware of the significance of sleep in relation to health.

ACE YOUR ASSESSMENT

Q1   How much sleep, on average, does an adult need?

    a   8–12 hours

    b   7.5–11 hours

    c   7.5–9.5 hours

Q2   Identify the correct sleep disorder names.

    a   Narcolepsy, restless leg syndrome, sleep apnoea

    b   Apnoea, painful limbs, full bladder

    c   Restless legs, restless arms, pain

Q3   What can be done to improve the sleep quality of patients in hospital?

    a   Pain-free, same bedtime, quiet music

    b   Avoid blue light, same bedtime, avoid naps

    c   Phone scrolling, avoid naps, hot drink

Q4   What does DoLS stand for?

    a   Deprivation of Liberties Safeguarding

    b   Depriving of Life Standards

    c   Deprivation of Living Standards

Q5   Identify correct examples of a helpful sleep routine for children.

    a   Lullaby, quiet play, bath

    b   Pyjamas, quiet play, light meal

    c   Bath, cuddles, story

Answers

1 C
2 A
3 B
4 A
5 C

REFERENCES

Babbel, S. (2018) *Heal the Body, Heal the Mind: A Somatic Approach to Moving Beyond Trauma*. Oakland, CA: New Harbinger.

Beach, C., Sugarman, J. and Johnson, R. (2005) 'Do patients treated with dignity report higher satisfaction, adherence and receipt of preventive care?', *Annals of Family Medicine*, 3 (4): 3318.

Biro, D. (2010) 'Is there such a thing as psychological pain? And why it matters', *Culture Medicine and Psychiatry*, 34 (4): 658–67.

Collins (2022) English Dictionary. https://www.collinsdictionary.com/dictionary/nglish/sleep (accessed October 12 2022).

Della Monica, C., Johnsen, S., Atzori, G., Groeger, J.A. and Dijk, D.J. (2018) 'Rapid eye movement sleep, sleep continuity and slow wave sleep as predictors of cognition, mood, and subjective sleep quality in healthy men and women, aged 20–84 years', *Frontiers in Psychiatry*, 9: Article #255. doi.org/10.3389/fpsyt.2018.00255

Eisenberger, N.I. (2012) 'The neural bases of social pain', *Psychosomatic Medicine*, 74 (2): 126–35. doi.org/10.1097/PSY.0b013e3182464dd1

Fry, A. (2022) 'What is healthy sleep?', Sleep Foundation, April 29. https://www.sleepfoundation.org/sleep-hygiene/what-is-healthy-sleep (accessed October 12, 2022).

Gagne, C. (2020) '6 most popular baby sleep-training methods explained', Today's Parent, March 6. https://www.todaysparent.com/baby/baby-sleep/most-popular-sleep-training-methods-explained/ (accessed October 12, 2022).

Hombali, A., Seow, E., Yuan, Q., Chang, S.H.S., Satghare, P., Kumar, S., Verma, S.K., Mok, Y.M., Chong, S.A. and Subramaniam, M. (2019) 'Prevalence and correlates of sleep disorder symptoms in psychiatric disorders', *Psychiatry Research*, 279: 11622. doi.org/10.1016/j.psychres.2018.07.009

Johns, M.W. (2010) 'A new perspective on sleepiness', *Sleep Biological Rhythm*, 8: 170–9.

Kitsaras, G., Goodwin, M., Allan, J., Kelly, M.P. and Pretty, I. A. (2018) 'Bedtime routines, child wellbeing & development', *BMC Public Health*, 18(1): Article #386.

Mandal, A. (2020) 'What is sleep?', News Medical Life Sciences, January 29. https://www.news-medical.net/health/What-is-sleep.aspx (accessed October 12, 2022).

McCall, W.V., Blocker, J.N., D'Agostino Jr, R., Kimball, J., Boggs, N., Lasater, B., Rosenquist, P.B. (2010) 'Insomnia severity is an indicator of suicidal ideation during a depression clinical trial', *Sleep Medicine*, 11(9): 822–7.

Micic, G. and Zajamsek, B. (2020) 'Curious kids: Why can't people hear in their sleep?' *The Conversation*, April 29. https://theconversation.com/curious-kids-why-cant-people-hear-in-their-sleep-132441 (accessed October 12, 2022).

Morse, A.M. and Bender, E. (2019) 'Sleep in hospitalized patients', *Clocks & Sleep*, 1 (1): 151–65. doi.org/10.3390/clockssleep1010014

NICE (2021) *Chronic Pain (Primary and Secondary) in Over 16s: Assessment of all Chronic Pain and Management of Chronic Pain*. NICE, April 7. https://www.nice.org.uk/guidance/ng193/resources/chronic-pain-primary-and-secondary-in-over-16s-assessment-of-all-chronic-pain-and-management-of-chronic-primary-pain-pdf-66142080468421 (accessed October 12, 2022).

Nordenfelt, L. and Edgar, A. (2005) 'The four notions of dignity', *Quality in Ageing and Older Adults*, 6 (1): 17–21.

Nursing and Midwifery Council (NMC) (2018) *The Code: Professional Standards of Practice and Behaviour for Nurses, Midwives and Nursing Associates*. London: NMC. https://www.nmc.org.uk/globalassets/sitedocuments/nmc-publications/nmc-code.pdf (accessed October 12, 2022).

Royal College of Nursing (RCN) (2022) 'Principles of nursing practice: 8 principles that apply to all nursing staff and nursing students in any care setting', RCN, September 29. https://www.rcn.org.uk/Professional-Development/Principles-of-nursing-practice (accessed October 12, 2022).

Valentine, N., Darby, C. and Bonsel, G.J. (2008) 'Which aspects of quality care are most important? Results from WHO's general population surveys of health system responsiveness in 41 countries', *Social Science and Medicine*, 66: 1939–50.

World Health Organization (WHO) (1994) *Declaration on the Promotion of Patients Rights in Europe*. Copenhagen: WHO Office for Europe. www.nurs.uoa.gr/fileadmin/nurs.uoa.gr/uploads/Nomothesia_Nosilefton/Evropaika_keimena/eu_declaration1994_1_.pdf (accessed October 12, 2022).

HYGIENE AND SKIN INTEGRITY

6

NICOLA TINGLE AND NERYS WILLIAMS, WITH SARAH KINGDOM-MILLS (LEARNING DISABILITIES CONTRIBUTION)

NMC STANDARDS COVERED IN THIS CHAPTER

ANNEXE B NURSING PROCEDURES

4.1 Observe, assess, and optimise skin and hygiene status and determine the need for support and intervention
4.2 Use contemporary approaches to the assessment of skin integrity and use appropriate products to prevent or manage skin breakdown
4.3 Assess needs for and provide appropriate assistance with washing, bathing, shaving and dressing
4.4 Identify and manage skin irritations and rashes
4.5 Assess needs for and provide appropriate oral, dental, eye and nail care and decide when an onward referral is needed
4.6 Use aseptic techniques when undertaking wound care including dressings, pressure bandaging, suture removal, and vacuum closures
4.7 Use aseptic techniques when managing wound and drainage processes

LEARNING OBJECTIVES

After reading this chapter, you should be able to:

- Understand the anatomy, physiology, and functions of the skin
- Assess and implement effective care for the patient in relation to hygiene needs, whilst promoting independence
- Effectively assess, prevent and manage common compromises to skin integrity
- Ensure aseptic management of wound dressings and some advanced wound care procedures

STUDENT VOICE

Assisting with personal hygiene and assessing skin is very personal and can be a bit intrusive. It is important that you put the patient at ease and maintain their dignity. Also, make the most of the time that you have with the patient because you can assess other things at the same time. When you are in a busy ward, it is the most quality time that you get with the patient – ask them questions, get to know them, assess their needs.

Johnson, 2nd year, Adult Health

INTRODUCTION

In this chapter, you will learn about the importance of hygiene and maintenance of skin integrity. Hygiene is a fundamental basic need, and some patients will inevitably need varying levels of assistance with this. There should be a careful balance between nurse assistance with personal hygiene, and promotion of independence. High standards of personal hygiene are important in maintaining physical, psychological, and social health; it prevents infection, maintains skin health and quality of life.

There are many factors which threaten skin integrity, particularly in higher risk groups with risks increasing proportionately with age, with underlying medical conditions and with polypharmacy. Chronic wounds are largely preventable, particularly within the healthcare setting. The methods for prevention are simple and require no complex interventions. The variety of compromises to the integrity of the skin are extensive, and beyond the scope of this chapter. Therefore, the focus of the second half of this chapter will be the assessment, prevention, and management of the two most common manifestations – pressure damage and moisture damage.

The skin is the largest organ of the human body, and serves many protective functions; care of the skin is a fundamental skill required within nursing. Breaches in skin integrity can at best cause minor discomfort for the patient; extreme cases of skin damage can lead to sepsis, loss of limbs or even loss of life. Prevention and management of skin integrity problems requires no complex interventions, and is the responsibility of everyone, with prevention always better than cure. Simple measures such as effective hygiene, management of incontinence, frequent repositioning and skin assessment can prevent onset of or prevent deterioration of existing skin integrity issues. There are adjuncts which can help in prevention of moisture lesions and pressure damage, but these should not be viewed as a replacement for basic nursing care.

ANATOMY AND PHYSIOLOGY RECAP

The skin

The skin is a complex organ, covering approximately 1.67 meters squared. It is the body's largest and heaviest organ (Figure 6.1); 15% of the total adult body weight is comprised of skin and its thickness ranges from <0.1mm at its thinnest part found on the eyelids, to 1.5mm at its thickest part which is found on the soles of the feet and palms of the hands. An average square inch of skin contains 650 sweat glands, 20 blood vessels, and more than 1,000 nerve endings (Yousef et al., 2022).

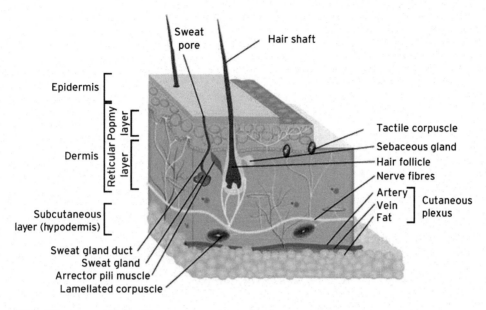

Figure 6.1 Structure of the skin

The skin is divided into several layers (Figure 6.2) including the epidermis which is composed mainly of keratinocytes. Beneath the epidermis is the dermo-epidermal junction, which is a multi-layered structure that anchors the epidermis to the dermis. The layer below the dermis, the hypodermis, consists largely of fat (Lawton, 2019).

Epidermis

The epidermis is the outer layer of the skin, defined as a stratified squamous epithelium. Humans shed around 500 million skin cells each day. The outermost parts of the epidermis consist of 20–30 layers of dead cells. Keratinocytes produce the protein keratin and are the major building blocks of the epidermis. The epidermis is avascular and therefore contains no blood vessels, it is entirely dependent on the underlying dermis for nutrient delivery and waste disposal through the basement membrane. The epidermis constantly makes new cells in its lower layers. Over the course of around four weeks, these cells make their way to the surface, become hard, and replace the shedding, dead cells (Kolarsick et al., 2011).

The primary function of the epidermis is to act as a physical and biological barrier to the external environment, preventing penetration by irritants and allergens. At the same time, it prevents the loss of water and maintains internal homeostasis. The colour of the skin comes from a pigment called melanin, which is produced by melanocytes. These are found in the epidermis and protect the skin from UV rays. The epidermis is composed of layers; most body parts have four layers, but those with the thickest skin have five (McLafferty et al., 2012).

The layers are:

- Stratum corneum (uppermost layer)
- Stratum lucidum (present in thicker skin only)
- Stratum granulosum
- Stratum spinosum
- Stratum basale (deepest layer)

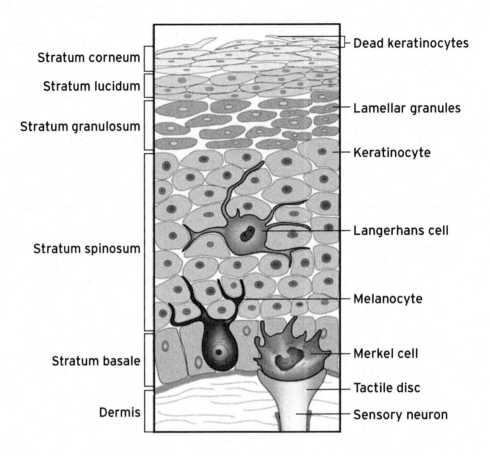

Figure 6.2 Layers of the skin

Dermis

The dermis forms the inner layer of the skin and is much thicker than the epidermis (1–5mm). It is situated between the basement membrane zone and the subcutaneous layer, and the main role of the dermis is to sustain and support the epidermis. The main functions of the dermis include:

- Protection
- Cushioning the deeper structures from mechanical injury
- Providing nourishment to the epidermis
- Wound healing

Hypodermis

The deepest layer of the skin is the subcutaneous tissue, the hypodermis, or the subcutis. It is not technically part of the skin, but it helps attach the skin to the bones and muscles. Subcutaneous tissue also provides the skin with nerves and blood supply. The hypodermis contains mostly fat, connective tissue, and elastin, which is an elastic protein that helps tissues return to their normal shape after stretching. The fat layer acts as protection, padding the bones and muscles whilst the high levels of fat help insulate the body and prevent a person from losing too much heat.

Functions of the skin

Skin is the 'sense-of-touch' organ that triggers a response if we touch or feel something, including things that may cause pain. This is important for patients with a skin condition, as pain and itching can be extreme for many and cause great distress.

One of the skin's important functions is to protect the body from cold or heat and maintain a constant core temperature. This is achieved by alterations to the blood flow through the cutaneous vascular bed. During warm periods, the vessels dilate and beads of sweat form on the surface. The secretion and evaporation of sweat from the surface of the skin also helps to cool the body. In cold periods, the blood vessels constrict, preventing heat from escaping.

The skin has a variety of other functions, including:

- Provides a protective barrier against mechanical, thermal and physical injuries and hazardous substances
- Prevents loss of moisture
- Reduces harmful effects of UV radiation
- Acts as a sensory organ (touch, detects temperature)
- Helps regulate temperature/thermoregulation
- An immune organ to detect infections
- Production of vitamin D

PATIENT EXPERIENCE

I always thought that pressure ulcers only happened to those people who were confined to bed. I have diabetes but apart from that, I am fit and well. I broke my leg and had to have surgery, and during that surgery I developed a pressure ulcer on my heel. Six weeks after discharge, I was readmitted to hospital with extreme pain in my leg, it had turned red and started to turn black in parts, I had sepsis. I ended up having a below knee amputation. A pressure ulcer brought an end to my career, my independence and meant that I could no longer care for my husband.

Anon

CLINICAL SKILLS RELATED TO HYGIENE AND SKIN INTEGRITY

Management of hygiene needs: Discussion

Communication

During personal hygiene, communication should underpin the interaction and facilitate the development of a rapport between the individual in receipt of care and yourself. It is an opportunity for you to provide undivided attention and can allow the individual to feel comfortable to share otherwise undisclosed thoughts and feelings, including details of themselves or circumstances that may otherwise remain untold. This requires the nurse to adopt good listening skills as much of the information disclosed can inform the nursing process of assessment, planning, implementation, and evaluation.

Developing an awareness of a patient's psychological needs and spending quality time with them allows you to note non-verbal cues, including the experience of pain through facial grimacing or establishing a general mood or emotion through noting changes in eye contact (eye contact and maintaining eye contact can be subjective and affected by a range of behaviours or conditions). It is also vital to be sympathetic to individual preferences and sensitive to individual choice. Some patients may prefer not to speak or communicate directly during procedures that are invasive, for example hygiene of intimate areas, therefore it is crucial you remain aware and are sensitive to these preferences.

When there is more than one team member involved in providing personal care, they must ensure that all conversations include and involve the individual in receipt of care and do not exclude them from the proceedings. The conversation should reflect the needs and experience of the patient, not the staff, whilst in the context of an acutely ill patient, it may be more appropriate to maintain verbal communication at a minimal level.

In the context of providing personal care to the unconscious patient, communication remains important. Whilst the patient may appear unaware of their surroundings, the importance of communication through non-verbal means, including touch, becomes of greater significance.

In some situations, it may be appropriate to include family in the process of assisting with personal hygiene needs. This can prove especially important when caring for children or individuals with learning disabilities (also termed intellectual disabilities). It can also prove significant in reducing levels of anxiety and allow family to feel involved in the process which can prove comforting and feel empowering.

Assessment

When assisting patients with meeting their personal hygiene needs there are several aspects to consider. Firstly, establish what the patient can do for themselves and encourage them to do as much as they can, aiding with tasks that they find difficult to achieve. Examples of this include encouragement to wash their own hands and face and to wash all areas that they can safely and comfortably reach. Prior to starting the process, ensure you have gained the patient's informed consent. Please refer to Chapter 3 to learn about gaining informed consent. Be mindful of how you obtain consent and ensure you have communicated your intentions clearly, allowing the patient to decide based on accurate information.

Dignity and privacy

Upholding and maintaining patient dignity and privacy should be at the forefront of your care and practice. Preventing the loss of dignity should underpin the intervention, and you should be mindful of the fact that many of the patients with whom you are working will find the experience invasive and potentially embarrassing. People who have been independent throughout their lives may find it difficult to come to terms with having to rely on such assistance that invades their personal space. Equally, providing care for a person of the same age as yourself can prove difficult for the recipient, who may experience a range of feelings including self-consciousness and embarrassment.

Be aware of the fact that you are providing care for people who are at a vulnerable point in their lives and as such your approach should be underpinned by respect and compassion. Remember, providing partial or full assistance to perform personal hygiene is not the sole domain of unregistered staff, it forms part of fundamental nursing care, and should be regarded as an opportunity to develop relationships, to communicate, to assess and note important changes or deterioration in the individual's condition.

Risk assessment

During the process, you should also complete a risk assessment and make decisions that relate to your approach in relation to Personal Protective Equipment (PPE). Please refer to Chapter 11 to learn about PPE. Be mindful of infection control policies and procedures and how the decisions you make might impact the self-esteem of the patient. Each area in which you work will have local policies and guidelines that relate to risk assessments. You should ensure that you are aware of the document's whereabouts, when and how to complete and how to implement the findings.

Spiritual and cultural preferences

Consider the needs of patients who have cultural and spiritual preferences and requirements. For example, fulfilling personal hygiene is important for meeting physical and spiritual needs within the Muslim community, and enabling individuals to access running water is an important aspect of providing appropriate and culturally sensitive care (Rassool, 2015). Religious and cultural practices and beliefs should also be taken into consideration when removing clothing for the purposes of providing or facilitating hygiene needs, and therefore you should develop self-awareness and cultural awareness to avoid insult or offense. Applying good communication skills is crucial in this context to ensure you have established the correct approach before proceeding.

CASE STUDY

Mr Aman

Religious and cultural awareness is a fundamental necessity in order to provide appropriate and effective nursing care. Consider the following case study and reflect on the approach you would adopt.

Mr Aman has been admitted onto a cardiac ward for routine surgery. The surgeon has asked for the patient to be prepared for theatre, and part of the preparation involves shaving the chest area. Mr Aman's Islamic religion requires he is not alone with the opposite sex and touch is prohibited unless between family members. Consider how you might facilitate the preparation required for the surgery. Consider also the religious and cultural needs of Mr Aman.

Remember, all actions should be underpinned by respect for the individual: establish how they would like to be addressed, communicate directly with them, establish how they would like to proceed and maintain the patient's centrality throughout.

ACTIVITY: COMMUNICATION SKILLS

Effective communication is essential to ensure patient dignity is maintained and to uphold patient centrality. Reflect on how you can maintain patient dignity throughout the process of undertaking or assisting with personal care when working with a patient who has communication needs. What type of communication skills would you adopt in this context? Consider the impact of non-verbal communication. Can non-verbal communication be as effective and powerful as verbal communication?

Consider a patient who has:

- Auditory hallucinations
- A hearing impairment
- Learning difficulties who has no verbal communication

Please note, the above examples are examples, and you may wish to use your own example.

Let's move onto step by step skills.

Bathing

BATHING: STEP BY STEP

When all preparations are made, including gaining informed consent, organising appropriate staffing levels and environment, it is necessary to gather all the required equipment for bathing a patient in bed. Ensuring you have prepared all necessary equipment will mitigate the need to halt proceedings and prevent unnecessary delay or loss of dignity. Be aware, this may be the first time the patient has experienced such care and may be feeling anxious about the process. Uphold dignity and privacy and maintain appropriate communication throughout the process.

EQUIPMENT

- A single used plastic bowl placed inside a plastic bag, or a single use disposable bowl depending on local policy.
- Towels, preferably the patient's own if available. Patients generally feel more comfortable when utilising their own belongings when performing personal hygiene, and the sight and feel of familiar belongings can aid the feeling of reassurance.
- You will require separate cloths/wipes for facial, torso, genital, and perineal areas.
- You will require soap or whichever solution is recommended by local policy, and toiletries, ensuring the products used are appropriate and that the patient is not allergic to any of the ingredients.
- Ask the patient what they would like to use, and which parts of the body they want washed with which particular items. Not all patients will want to wash their face with astringent soaps.
- Check the cultural, religious or spiritual preferences and establish how much the patient would like to do for themselves, encouraging them to be self-determined and as self-caring as possible.
- Gather either towels or light sheets to cover the parts of the body that are not being washed to maintain privacy and dignity.
- Use warm water and ensure to change the water when washing genital and perineal areas.
- You will also need to gather clean clothing or nightwear and clean bedding, and a receptacle for the collection of used or soiled clothes or bedding.

THE PROCESS

- Wash your hands and don appropriate PPE, including apron, and have gloves to hand for washing the genital and perineal regions.
- Ensure the curtains are fully drawn and the patient is lying in a comfortable and preferably semi recumbent position.
- Observe the patient for any signs of distress, anxiety or deterioration throughout the process.
- Arrange the furniture and equipment to enable easy reach and ensure that the patient's safety is maintained.

- Ensure easy access to the patient by removing unnecessary items and working within uncluttered space free of potential hazards including cables.

- Raise the bed to a working height that is safe for all members of staff, always ensuring the safety of the patient.

- Remove the patient's clothing having gained informed consent and maintain privacy and dignity by covering exposed areas with a towel or light sheet.

- Check the temperature of the water, ensuring it is neither too hot nor cold, aim for 35º–40º.

- Provide individualised care by establishing how much the patient will undertake and which areas they like to wash with soap.

- Wash, rinse off soap/solution and dry the patient's face, neck and ears.

- To reduce cross infection, a separate cloth should be utilised to wash the remainder of the patient's body.

- Wash, rinse and dry the patient's torso including upper limbs, chest and abdomen, followed by lower limbs and back, washing the limb furthest away from you first. To wash the patient's back, they will need to be safely rolled from side to side, taking this opportunity to remove soiled sheets and insert clean bedding. This action can cause some anxiety and therefore maintain good communication throughout offering reassurance whilst also upholding dignity and privacy.

- Wash the genital areas and perineal areas last, changing the water following washing of the perineal area. This will help prevent cross infection. Provide a disposable cloth and encourage the patient to wash their own pubic area to promote independence and dignity. Discard the cloth before moving onto washing the perineal region. If the patient has a catheter in-situ, clean the catheter at this point and discard the cloth immediately.

- Ensure the patient feels clean and dry in all areas before removing remaining soiled bed linen and remaking the bed with clean sheets.

- Throughout the process, observe the skin for any blemishes, rashes, discoloration or signs of trauma.

- If necessary, ask the patient whether they would prefer to have their hair washed as part of the process. If they would like to do so, gather the appropriate equipment, and complete this process.

- Then, offer the patient a brush or comb, however if they are unable to fulfil this task, brush or comb the patient's hair ensuring not to apply too much force as to cause pain, but ensure the removal of tangled hair. **Remember:** Not all hair will require a brush or comb. Hair type and style is individualistic, and it is important to recognise that different hair requires different grooming or treatment. Discuss with the patient how they prefer to care for their individual hair type and work with them to facilitate achieving the appropriate care. Hair care is discussed in greater detail in the Hair Care: Step by Step box below.

ACTIVITY: PAUSE AND REFLECT

- How did you feel when you participated in full personal hygiene for the first time?
- How would you do things differently in future if at all?
- How do you think the patient felt throughout the process?

Dressing

DRESSING: STEP BY STEP

- Always ask the patient what they would like to wear following bathing. It is important to include the patient in decisions about preferences and facilitate choice.

- Encourage the patient to dress in alternatives to nightwear during the day to avoid 'pyjama paralysis'. Enable and empower through providing choice and encourage the patient to do as much for themselves as possible.

- If the patient is not getting out of bed, it is likely that nightwear is most appropriate, however avoid using surgical gowns as this can undermine self-esteem and disempower individuals.

- Place soiled or used clothing in a patient property bag, labelled accurately, and place in the patient locker.

- Inform family, friends or carers of any laundry that needs to be undertaken and any requirement for clean clothing, including underwear, nightwear, and day clothing. It is also important that patients have access to appropriate footwear whilst in hospital. If the patient is unable to do so for themselves, speak with family, friends or carers and ask them to provide well-fitting and non-slip footwear. As the patient mobilises around the bed and ward area, it is crucial that they can do so safely. Loose or ill-fitting slippers and shoes can prove hazardous and lead to trips, slips and falls.

- Some underlying conditions will have an impact on a patient's ability to dress themselves, in which case they will rely on the nurse to assist them. It remains important to ensure the patient has a choice and should be encouraged to decide what they would like to wear. Conditions that have resulted in a dense weakness should be approached by dressing the weaker side first, this will allow the patient to push their dominant arm through sleeves and arm holes with greater ease.

- Assisting an adult to dress must be approached like all other fundamental needs. It should be underpinned by patience, compassion and understanding. It should be respectful of people's choice and should not undermine self-determination or disable. It can prove difficult for some to ask for help and you should approach the process with compassion always maintaining the individual's dignity.

Oral care

ORAL CARE: STEP BY STEP

ASSESSMENT

- Before undertaking the process of oral hygiene and mouth care, ensure you have gained informed consent.

- Any unexpected issues or problems you note during the procedure or an inability to undertake the intervention should be documented and assistance sought from other members of the multidisciplinary team such as the dental team, a specialist nurse or the speech and language therapist.

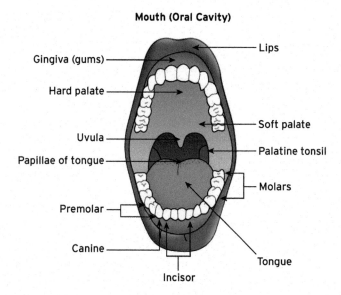

Figure 6.3   The mouth

Source: Wikimedia Commons

- Assessment should underpin the procedure and should alert the nurse to the needs of the patient, maintaining individualised care.
- Monitor the patient throughout for signs of distress, anxiety or changing condition.
- Establish if there is any relevant medical history or medication that might impact your ability to complete the process.
- The oral cavity, lips and teeth should be thoroughly assessed, looking for lesions, broken areas or signs of infection.
- A small pen torch is useful for use during an oral assessment. Poor oral hygiene, immuno-suppression and ill-fitting dentures can all lead to a common infection, Candida albicans (thrush). This fungal infection presents as small white spots, coating the patient's tongue, mucosa and at times the palate. If you suspect the patient has developed this infection, it should be reported and documented, and treatment started as soon as possible.
- An initial assessment should be followed by ongoing reassessment. As with all aspects of care, firstly establish how much the patient can and would like to do for themselves.
- Enable them to achieve as much as they can without assistance, offering support and encouragement, and if available offer the use of adapted toothbrushes with wider handles for example for use by patients who have reduced dexterity because of an underlying condition.

DEPENDENT PATIENTS

- The unconscious patient will require all aspects of oral care to be provided on their behalf. They may have an Endo Tracheal Tube (ETT) in-situ, but this does not mean that toothbrushing cannot or should not be undertaken.

(Continued)

- If the patient has all their own teeth in place, approach the intervention with care and apply the same underlying principles as you would when brushing teeth for patients who require assistance.
- You may require support from a colleague to ensure you do not dislodge the ETT and to provide suction of excess toothpaste and secretions to avoid ingestion.
- Assessment of the oral cavity and condition of the teeth is vital for the fully dependent patient and oral care should be provided regularly, hourly if indicated.
- The condition of the patient may impact on the overall condition of the oral cavity and the lips, and therefore great care should be taken to avoid dryness, cracked lips, sores or infection.
- Document all findings in the nursing notes and report any changes to the nurse in charge.

DENTURE CARE

- If the patient is fully conscious, establish whether the patient has their own teeth or partial or full dentures.
- Ask the patient how they would like to proceed. Some patients will be happy to offer their dentures in a denture pot for cleaning at a basin, whilst others may prefer to keep dentures in-situ. It is important to discuss with the patient the need to regularly remove dentures for the purposes of cleaning, especially following mealtimes.
- It is also advisable to encourage patients to remove dentures overnight, placing them in a denture pot; this allows the mouth and delicate oral membranes to recover.
- It is essential that the denture pot is clearly and accurately labelled to ensure dentures are returned to the correct owner, and that water is changed daily. Some patients may feel self-conscious when their dentures are removed, and therefore it is crucial to offer privacy and uphold dignity throughout the process.
- Enable the patient to undertake this aspect of personal hygiene in the privacy of a bathroom or with the curtains drawn if they prefer.
- Ask the patient if they have their own toothbrush and toothpaste, some patients may not have been prepared for a hospital admission and therefore the equipment should be provided by the ward.
- When cleaning dentures, use a soft toothbrush and toothpaste, and be careful to avoid dropping into a basin as they can break.
- Clean the entire denture including the surface that fits the denture in place. Prior to reinserting, encourage the patient to gently brush the gum and oral cavity and rinse with cold water to aid the removal or prevention of plaque build up and tartar.

BRUSHING TEETH

- If the patient is unable to undertake their own tooth brushing, you will be required to undertake the process on their behalf.
- Prior to starting the process, clearly explain to the patient what you intend to do and ensure you have gained consent.
- Make sure the patient is in a comfortable position, and that you have all the necessary equipment to hand.
- Provide the patient with a towel to cover the chest area. If the patient has partial dentures, ask for consent to remove them for cleaning in the same way as full dentures.
- Apply a small amount of toothpaste to the brush (the same size as a pea is sufficient). Position yourself behind and slightly to the side of the patient supporting the patient's head and proceed

to brush the teeth without applying too much pressure. This will avoid causing any bleeding of the gums or oral cavity.

- Avoid applying too much pressure to loose teeth to avoid the risk of dislodging and potential swallowing or choking.

- Use small strokes at an angle of 45 degrees ensuring to brush all areas, top and bottom, inside and out including the tongue, palate, gums, and cheeks. Brushing should occur for 3-4 minutes. Ask the patient to rinse their mouth as vigorously as possible to remove any debris and tooth-paste and provide them with a small cloth or towel.

- Flossing or use of intra dental sticks should be encouraged to remove plaque and food from between the teeth. If the patient is used to doing this at home, ensure to maintain. If the patient consents, apply some soft paraffin or lip salve to avoid dry cracked lips, that can arise following use of a face mask or within a dry environment.

- Rinse and dry the toothpaste and store in a clean area or return to the patient's toiletry bag or a toothbrush holder.

- Do not store wet or damp to avoid possible infection.

- Safely discard disposable equipment in line with local policy and document the care pro-vided, noting any changes or new findings that have resulted as part of your overall oral assessment.

ACTIVITY: HAVE A GO

Ask permission from a friend or family member to brush their teeth then ask them to do the same for you. How does it feel to be the recipient of such a process? How did you feel undertaking the process? Does experiencing a similar procedure enhance your empathy?

Shaving

Assisting or enabling a patient to shave is an integral aspect of personal hygiene and provides the nurse with an opportunity to develop relationships and can also be undertaken at any point throughout the day, either during the process of washing and bathing or as a separate activity. As with all aspects of hygiene, the starting point is to establish how much the patient can do for themselves, encouraging and enabling the individual to participate partially or fully. Encourage the patient to utilise their own and pre-ferred toiletries and provide them with appropriate space and enough time that they do not feel rushed.

Be mindful of differences in cultural and religious preferences and ensure that you do not offend by offering to support a patient to shave when not advocated within their religion.

SHAVING: STEP BY STEP

EQUIPMENT

- Towel to place across the patient's chest area
- Basin of warm water if not in a bathroom at a basin

(Continued)

- Patient's own face cloth or disposable wipes
- Shaving foam/soap/gel
- Shaving brush (if not available, use hands to generate foam)
- Patient's own razor or new razor provided by the ward (dispose of this following use) – ensure that razors both manual and electric are not shared between patients to avoid cross infection and ensure safe disposal of sharps in line with local policies and procedures

or

- Electric shaver

PROCEDURE

- If you are shaving the patient, ensure they are sitting comfortably either on a chair or in the bed at working height that is suitable and safe.
- Prior to starting, ensure you have gathered all the equipment required. Check before shaving if the patient is taking any prescribed medication such as Warfarin or has any underlying conditions that may affect blood clotting such as Haemophilia. A cut or nick in the skin during the shaving process will need monitoring.
- When you have gained informed consent from the patient, you should check the overall condition of the skin, looking for blemishes, lesions or any signs of infection or trauma. This should be done whether you are undertaking a wet shave with shaving gel and razor or a dry shave using an electric shaver (Ette and Gretton, 2019).
- When undertaking a wet shave, ensure the water is warm enough to open the hair follicles and generate a foam either using gel or shaving foam.
- Apply to the face and then using short strokes, shaving in the direction of the hair growth.
- You should hold the skin taught to maintain purchase and avoid discomfort. Achieving a clean shave will reduce the possibility of the patient developing any skin abrasions and will add to the general feeling of wellbeing.
- Ensure that excess soap or foam is removed regularly and rinse the blade to avoid clogging with hair and foam. These actions should be repeated until the whole area has been shaved and then rinsed with warm water and dried thoroughly.
- The patient may want to use aftershave or a soothing balm, in which case enable the patient to apply themselves or apply on their behalf.
- Whilst it is predominantly men who require assistance with shaving, it is not exclusively the case. You may be required to assist female patients with the removal of facial hair.
- Excess facial hair might be a side effect of medication or underlying conditions such as Polycystic Ovary Syndrome (PCOS). This situation should be approached with respect and sensitivity and the principles of facial hair removal applied. Great sensitivity is also required when working with transgender patients who may seek support to manage hair growth. Adopting a non-judgemental approach and maintaining privacy and dignity is always an important aspect of all interactions with all patients.

Eye care

Eye care as an aspect of personal hygiene can also serve as an opportunity to assess the overall condition of the eye and the surrounding area. General eye care, eye cleansing and application of prescribed treatment can prevent eye infections, support treatment of infections or conditions, and relieve symptoms of underlying conditions or eye trauma, and help prevent damage to the eye when the patient is unconscious and unable to blink (Dougherty and Lister, 2015).

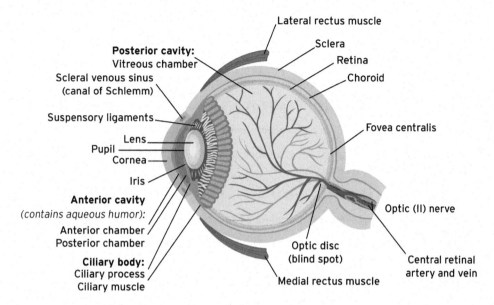

Figure 6.4   The eye

As with all aspects of personal care and hygiene, eye care should be underpinned by the concepts of good communication, patient dignity, infection control and prevention and patient advocacy and self-determination. Some patients who have underlying eye conditions including reduced vision and blindness may find it difficult to undertake their own eye care within a new environment, and as such you should help (Gwenhure and Shepperd, 2019). Eye infections can result in pain and discomfort and even long-term damage, and therefore care whilst cleansing the eye area should be applied. It may be not be possible for contact lens wearers to continue wearing contact lenses in hospital. This is because extra care is required to ensure contact lenses are taken out at night and that lens solution is available. If a patient is unwell, they may not be able to do this and therefore may need to wear glasses instead. Furthermore, sometimes patients are asked to remove contact lenses, for example when about to undergo surgery.

WATCH THE VIDEO

EYE CARE

Watch along as you read through this step by step procedure by scanning the QR code with your smartphone camera or via https://study.sagepub.com/rowberry.

EYE CARE: STEP BY STEP

- Gather all the necessary equipment prior to starting the process. This will avoid disruption of the process.

- Explain clearly what the procedure will involve and allow the patient to ask any questions they may have relating to the process.

- Gain informed consent from the patient prior to starting the procedure.

- Ensure the patient is in a comfortable position and uphold their privacy and dignity throughout.

- Wash your hands thoroughly and don appropriate PPE to reduce the risk of cross infection.

- On a clean tray or trolley, prepare all the equipment including sterile procedure pack, cleaning solution and lint free gauze swabs.

- Place a paper towel on the patient's chest and neck area.

- Ask the patient to keep their eyes closed whilst you clean the eyelids.

- Clean the eyelid from the inner aspect, near the lacrimal apparatus, towards the outer aspect. Use each swab only once prior to discarding.

- This should be repeated until such a point that all discharge has been removed.

- Ask the patient to open their eyes, and repeat the above process on the lower eyelid, again using swabs only once to avoid potential cross infection.

- Each eye should be regarded as a separate procedure and therefore two packs should be utilised.

- Infected eyes should be treated last to prevent the possibility of cross infection.

- Continue until all discharge has been removed.

- Ensure you do not touch the cornea with the gauze swab as this could be painful and could cause an abrasion.

- Dry the lids carefully, making sure the area is not left moist.

- Communicate with the patient throughout reducing anxiety and promoting dignity.

- On completion, discard all disposable equipment and PPE according to local policy.

- Ensure the patient is comfortable before documenting any findings.

Nail, hand, and foot care

Hands and feet are often overlooked as a fundamental aspect of personal hygiene and general care. However, for many reasons, including prevention and control of infection, they are central to maintaining personal hygiene.

NAIL, HAND, AND FOOT CARE: STEP BY STEP

- Familiarise yourself with local policy in respect of who can cut finger and toe nails. Some Health Boards/Trusts will not support the intervention being carried out by nurses, and as such alternative solutions must be found, including referrals to chiropodists or specifically trained staff. Remember, with the correct equipment, some patients can undertake their own nail care effectively.

- Encourage patients to wash their hands regularly, especially following use of the toilet and prior to mealtimes.

- If it is not possible for the patient to access a basin with water and soap, consider providing the patient with a wet/damp cloth and towel to wash their hands at the bedside.

- If they prefer, offer use of an alcohol-based hand gel, however, this should not be regarded as a substitute to handwashing with soap and water, but as a short-term alternative.

- Preventing infection underpins the nurse's role, and as such, maintaining good handwashing is important for the patient as well as staff.

- After the patient has washed their hands, they should be dried thoroughly, especially in between the digits/fingers. These areas if not thoroughly dried can remain moist and become a source of fungal infection. They should be offered the choice to apply hand cream. This will moisturise and help avoid dry and cracked skin. Ensure you have checked that the patient is not allergic to any ingredients and encourage them to use their own cream if they have access to it.

- Fingernails can harbour microorganisms and can be a source of infection. Patients should be encouraged to keep nails short, cut straight across to the level of the finger with nail clippers or scissors, and any rough or jagged areas filed smooth. Any residual dirt is best removed following immersion in a bowl of warm soapy water or during a bath or shower. Gently rub away any matter that the patient is unable to remove for themselves.

- Like the hands, the feet also require care of the skin and nails. When bathing or showering, do not overlook the feet. Care should be taken to wash and thoroughly dry the areas in between the toes, as like the hand digits, these areas if left moist can harbour fungal infections and become cracked and sore.

- Some patients will already be receiving treatment for various foot infections and conditions, and therefore it is vital that any treatment is accurately prescribed and administered appropriately.

- Toenails should be kept short, cut with clippers or scissors straight across. They should not be cut at the corners as this can lead to ingrowing toenails. There are some underlying conditions that will render this process difficult to manage including diabetes that can result in reduced sensation and circulation. Toenails can be tough and hard and some patients may also have underlying medical conditions that require specialist intervention from a foot care specialist such as a chiropodist.

- Conditions such as those that have an impact on peripheral sensation and circulation should be considered as part of an assessment to determine the most appropriate approach.

Hair care

For many patients, hair type and style are integral parts of individual identity and as such all effort should be made to approach hair care with respect towards individual practice and preference. Many patients will undertake the brushing or combing of their hair independently, provided they have brushes or combs to hand. However, for the dependent patient, assistance will be required, for example, to prevent their hair from knotting and becoming tangled. As with all aspects of care, you should approach this process with care and be careful not to apply too much pressure as this may be uncomfortable or painful for the patient. You also risk damaging the scalp if the skin condition is delicate and affected by any scalp conditions.

As with all interventions, prior to brushing or combing ensure you have gained consent and assess the general condition of the head and scalp, noting any abnormalities, lesions, trauma or cuts and bruises. Brushing and combing of the hair can result in general feelings of wellbeing and reflects the overall care and attention paid by the individual and/or staff to how the patient feels and appears.

In addition to brushing and combing, hair washing can have the same impact. Unwashed hair can feel dirty and as part of general personal hygiene the opportunity to wash hair as part of an independent bathing/showering should be made available. Hair washing can support a general feeling of wellbeing for patients. Washing hair stimulates the circulation of the scalp, whilst shampooing removes dirt, bacteria, microorganisms and oils. Aspects of hair care include daily brushing and combing, head bath to maintain cleanliness and treatment of hair including lice infestation.

Patients who are unable to leave the bed to wash their hair in a bathroom setting should nevertheless be helped to wash their hair. For the unconscious and conscious patient, there is equipment that can be utilised to facilitate hair washing whilst lying in bed. This equipment can range from an inflatable bowl to a rigid plastic tray (Lawton, 2019). In the absence of such equipment, a bowl can be utilised and placed beneath the patient's head. Do not attempt to move the patient or undertake hair washing until you have completed an assessment. This procedure may not be suitable for a patient who has a neck or spinal injury.

HAIR CARE: STEP BY STEP

- Gather all the required equipment including staff apron and gloves if deemed necessary, towels, waterproof sheeting, shampoo/conditioner, brush/comb, water tray or inflatable hair washing bowl and jug.
- Gain informed consent from the patient and ensure you communicate throughout the procedure, maintaining eye contact and providing reassurance, upholding patient dignity throughout.
- Remove the head of the bed and place towels or waterproof sheeting around the patient's neck and shoulder areas making sure the patient feels warm and comfortable.
- Place the tray or inflatable bowl under the patient's head.
- Apply water to the hair prior to applying shampoo. Ensure you have checked that the patient is not allergic to any contents and that it is suitable for their hair type. Ask the patient if they have their own and use it if that is what they prefer.
- After shampooing, rinse the hair thoroughly and dry with a towel making sure you dry the ears and folds in the neck.
- Some ward areas may have a hairdryer, if so, dry using the drier but be careful not to apply too much heat as to cause discomfort or pain.
- Change the bed linen and clothing as necessary.

- Discard all disposable equipment according to local policy and decontaminate any reusable equipment.
- Remove your apron and gloves if worn and wash your hands before recording the procedure appropriately.

ASSESSING, PREVENTING, AND MANAGING COMMON COMPROMISES TO SKIN INTEGRITY: DISCUSSION

Types of wounds

A wound can be defined as an injury to the skin and/or underlying tissues because of trauma, surgery, or underlying disease processes such as cancer. They can be categorised as acute, where healing occurs within an expected time frame, which is quantified differently within the literature, sometimes as four weeks, other times as six ; and as chronic. A chronic wound is a wound which does not heal within the above expected time frame, and delayed healing is often attributed to underlying conditions, pharmaceutical regimes, and infection. With the reasons for delayed healing varying between individuals, this highlights the importance of an individualised holistic assessment. Nurses tend to direct their focus towards the choice of dressing, but in fact the primary considerations should be of the underlying aetiology, that is what variables are causing this delay. The focus should be on solving the underlying problem.

Within this chapter, there is not scope to discuss the full principles of wound assessment, and further reading should be undertaken to complement the wound assessment looking at physiological factors such as disease and medications, psychological and social factors which may impact upon the wound. Locally, there should be a full assessment of the wound bed and quite often the TIME assessment is utilised as a framework for this.

Major categories of wounds, their underlying causes and generalised management plans are contained within the table below:

Table 6.1 **Major categories of wounds, their underlying causes and generalised management plans**

Wound type	Causes	Treatment
Pressure ulcers	Pressure, shear and friction. Risk elevated by underlying conditions, medications, continence status, nutritional status, age, mobility status.	Reduction of the pressure. Repositioning and offloading. Using specialist equipment, general wound management.
Moisture lesions	Urine and faeces, perspiration, exudate.	Full continence assessment, correct selection of continence products. Correct washing and drying of the skin using neutral pH cleansers. Use of barrier protection. Reducing the pressure.
Venous leg ulcers	Venous disease. Characterised by brown staining of the limbs, champagne bottle shape, swelling, varicose veins, eczema. Venous leg ulcers are shallow, tend to be limited to the gaiter area, irregular edged. However, there can be arterial disease occurring at the same time which may alter the appearance of the ulcers.	Gold standard treatment is graduated compression bandaging. Caution should be taken and full arterial assessment must be performed by a competent individual in order to commence therapy.

(Continued)

Table 6.1   (Continued)

Wound type	Causes	Treatment
Arterial leg ulcers	Peripheral arterial disease. Caused by narrowing or blockage of the arteries in the lower limb. Higher incidence in those who have diabetes, history of other arteriopathies such as coronary artery disease, CVA and smokers. Appearance of arterial ulcers tends to be more punched out, deeper, have necrosis.	Full arterial assessment is needed. Quite often requires surgical intervention – arterial bypass, grafts or angioplasty.
Diabetic foot ulceration	Ulceration on the foot. May be ischaemic, neuropathic or a combination of both. Healing is compromised because of a lack of blood supply and neuropathy. Very high risk of infection and osteomyelitis.	Debridement, infection prevention and management. Offloading of the pressure from the affected area using specialist foams or footwear. Revascularisation. Local wound care.
Malignant wounds and fungating tumours	Skin lesions because of primary or secondary tumours.	Some cancers can be surgically removed. For those that cannot, then treatment becomes palliative with management of exudate, pain, colonisation, and itching.
Burns	Wounds made by thermal, electrical, or electromagnetic energy.	Multifactorial approach from conservative management with cooling and dressings to surgical debridement with skin grafting.
Surgical wounds	Incisions made for the purpose of surgery.	Generally, heal by primary intention, with closure using sutures, clips or glue. Sometimes, wounds are left to heal by secondary or tertiary intention.

Negative pressure therapy

Vacuum assisted closure, sometimes referred to as negative pressure wound therapy, has revolutionised wound care over the last 15 years. It is a mode of therapy used to encourage wound healing. It is used both as a primary treatment of chronic and complex wounds and as an adjunct for temporary closure and wound bed preparation prior to surgical procedures such as flap surgery and skin grafts (Shintler, 2012).

KEY TERMS

Topical Negative Pressure (TNP) therapy: the application of local sub atmospheric pressure across the wound bed, which has a central role in the management of acute wounds.

Wounds suitable for treatment with topical negative pressure include:

- Acute trauma (upper/lower limb)
- Burns
- Chronic pressure sores
- Leg ulcers

- Diabetic ulcers
- Wound dehiscence
- Wound infection
- Necrotising fasciitis
- Postoperative sternal infections
- Skin grafts and flap surgery
- Wound bed preparation

NEGATIVE PRESSURE THERAPY: STEP BY STEP

- The equipment required consists of foam, an adhesive dressing, tubing, and the negative pressure vacuum assisted device/machine.

- The foam is cut to size, to fit the wound cavity exactly. Different colour foam pads are available; some are more pliable whereas others are less so and will require greater levels of pressure to achieve the required effect. The choice of foam is normally decided by the clinician.

- This is covered by a film dressing or silicone overlay to achieve a complete seal. The adhesive dressing also creates a closed environment for moist healing.

- A small incision is made in the film to insert a drainage tube, however when using gauze-based dressings, a fenestrated tube is used with no incision required.

- The tube is connected to the vacuum assisted closure device/machine. This enables excess fluid to be removed into a cannister. There can be some adhesion with the foams to the granulation tissue which can cause trauma on removal. It is worth placing a wound contact layer in between, such as a silicone-based dressing.

- The seal around the insertion point must be leak free to achieve the required suction.

- Once in position the dressing provides a stable environment over the wound surface. This also enables the wound to heal even in the mobile patient.

- Monitor for any shear stresses as this can affect the wound and in turn damage the fragile newly formed tissue.

- Pressures achieved are monitored by the machine. Negative pressure therapy is usually applied at a sub-atmospheric pressure of 125 mm Hg using PU (black) foam – that is, 125 mm Hg below atmospheric pressure to achieve the desired outcome, although evidence to support optimal pressures is limited (Jones et al., 2005). This decision however is normally made by the clinician.

- Pressure can be applied on a constant or intermittent basis, controlled by device functions on the device/machine. It is, however, often stated by patients that the intermittent mode is less tolerable due to the fluctuations in pressures applied, therefore caution is advised. Listen to the patient feedback and perspective in order to maximise positive patient experience and outcomes.

- Dressings should be changed every 48–56 hours except in exceptional circumstances (for example, over a skin graft).

- Dressings left for longer periods of time over the recommended 56 hours can lead to increased discomfort during dressing changes. This occurs as a result of granulating tissue adhering to the foam dressing.

- Wounds need to be regularly inspected to ensure the wound healing is achieved (Banwell and Musgrave, 2004).

GO FURTHER

For more information, read the following journal article on the vacuum assisted closure technique:

Yadav, S., Rawal, G. and Baxi, M. (2017) 'Vacuum assisted closure technique: A short review', *The Pan African Medical Journal*, 28: Article #246. doi.org/ 10.11604/pamj.2017.28.246.9606

Skin assessment: Pressure damage

The true incidence of pressure damage in the UK is unknown. Prevalence audits in England demonstrated an average of 9.04% of inpatients had a pressure ulcer (Gov.uk, 2022), with Wales' most recent national inpatient audit demonstrating a similar point prevalence of 8.9% (Clark et al., 2017). This has an estimated cost of £1.74 billion per year: the Department of Health and Social Care (2020) productivity calculator estimates the cost of a grade 4 pressure ulcer as £14,000. Besides the cost to the NHS, there is a significant cost to the person physically, psychologically, financially, occupationally, socially, and a significant impact on the quality of life. Figures vary, but several sources state that 50–95% of pressure ulcers are preventable, with simple interventions such as effective risk assessment, repositioning, adjunct equipment to reduce pressure and patient carer education. It is the responsibility of the entire healthcare team to prevent pressure ulcers; the remit normally falls on nursing staff and prevention is fundamental to effective and safe patient care.

A pressure ulcer is defined as 'localised injury to the skin and/or underlying tissue, usually over a bony prominence, as a result of pressure, or pressure in combination with shear. Several contributing or confounding factors are also associated with pressure ulcers; the significance of these factors is yet to be elucidated' (European Pressure Ulcer Advisory Panel, 2016). The sacrum is the most common area for development of pressure ulcers followed by the heels (Moore et al., 2019), however they can occur over any bony prominence, over the cartilage of the ears and nose and anywhere where a device has contact with the body.

WATCH THE VIDEO

SKIN ASSESSMENT

Watch along as you read through this step by step procedure by scanning the QR code with your smartphone camera or via https://study.sagepub.com/rowberry.

INITIAL SKIN ASSESSMENT: STEP BY STEP

As with all nursing interventions, it is essential that you gain informed consent from the patient prior to assessment. Privacy and dignity must be maintained throughout the procedure, and you must ensure that the patient is comfortable, i.e. their pain is managed, room temperature is adequate, and take into consideration the patient's current condition (breathing etc.).

- Ensure that communication is maintained with the patient, that dignity and respect are maintained, and the patient is comfortable.
- Only expose the parts of the body that are being checked at the time, keep all other parts covered. It is essential that all areas of the body are checked, with particular attention to bony prominences, ears and nose and areas in which there are devices. Check catheters, under anti-embolic stockings, under spectacles, oxygen delivery devices.
- Assess the bony prominences for any signs of erythema. If erythema is noted, apply pressure for a few seconds to assess whether it is blanching. Tissue that is blanching will return to its usual colour within 2 seconds. Blanching may not be visible in darkly pigmented skin, but colour of early pressure damage can be different to the surrounding skin therefore should be assessed for. Check for areas of skin loss and blistering. For patients with lighter skin tones, check for areas of dark discolouration or devitalised tissue, which is yellow, brown, or black in colour. For patients with darker skin tones, palpating areas over the bony prominences is recommended, any signs of the area being cooler or warmer to the touch or feeling softer or firmer than the surrounding tissue may be an indication of pressure damage. If these changes are noticed, then pressure should be offloaded from the area. Otherwise, unexplained pain over a bony prominence should also be taken note of and pressure offloaded with close observation. Suspected deep tissue injuries can also be difficult to detect on darker skin. It is extremely important that thorough assessment and management is undertaken in those with darkly pigmented skin as damage can quickly deteriorate into a deeper level ulcer without appropriate action.
- Ensure that the pressure is offloaded from any areas of concern immediately. This may be achieved by repositioning, or use of devices or pillows to offload pressure. There are silicone pads which can reduce the pressure in awkward areas.
- Consider the use of supplementary equipment to reduce the pressure, in line with local contracts. This may be static air filled devices or dynamic devices for the bed and chair.
- Patient and carer education is important, in encouraging movement, skin checks using a mirror if possible and reporting any areas of unusual pain.
- Document on a bedside communication chart, within the nursing notes and on a body map as per local protocol. Report any adverse incidents in line with local procedure.

Hygiene and skin integrity: Discussion

Pressure damage occurs because of sustained pressure, where the tissues are compressed between the surface and the bone. The pressure occludes the capillary bed and reduces the blood supply and oxygen supply to the tissues; thus, it begins to die. This can be alleviated by repositioning and offloading the pressure loads. The risk can be compounded by shearing forces, the act of the underlying structures such as bone and more superficial tissues moving in opposite directions to each other; this again can cause ischaemia, a disruption in blood supply to the area. These forces can be reduced by correct moving and handling techniques and positioning the patient, so they are not likely to slip down in the bed or chair and be subject to shearing. Friction is also considered simultaneously with shear, damage can occur because of friction with the surface such as dragging across the bedsheets, friction against a chair, shoes, or medical devices.

There are many factors which increase the risk of pressure damage including but not limited to age, sex, underlying medical conditions, medication use, continence status, mobility status and nutritional status. Risk is elevated by a lack of mobility and lack of sensation. However, we should assume that pressure damage can happen to anyone. It is important not to be complacent, do not assume that just because someone is independently mobile or self-caring that they are risk free. They can still develop pressure ulcers; indeed, they may sometimes be more of a risk than those who are not, because staff can assume that they are not at risk. Pressure ulcers can develop in children and young people, labouring mothers and those who score as 'low risk' in assessment as a result of short-term illness, undergoing surgery or interventions which affect mobility and sensation such as temporary sedatives, nerve blocks and epidurals.

Pressure damage is categorised into six grades, numbered one to four and two additional categories of unstageable and suspected deep tissue injury, however not all pressure ulcers look like the photographs you may see and will vary in size, shape, and tissue types, and some find it easier to categorise the damage according to descriptors.

GO FURTHER

It is important to be mindful that pressure damage appears differently on different skin tones. To learn more read the following article:

Black, J. and Simende, A. (2020) 'Ten top tips: Assessing darkly pigmented skin', *Wounds International*, 11 (3). https://www.woundsme.com/uploads/resources/d34b6a6f02b2659b00636c49b453046c.pdf (accessed October 13, 2022)

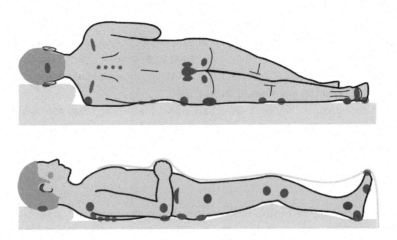

Figure 6.5   Body map with pressure points

Source: Wikimedia Commons/Jmarchn (CC BY-SA 3.0)

Table 6.2 Pressure ulcer grades and simple recognition

Grade of damage	Explanation
The red mark	This is not yet pressure damage, but an initial inflammatory response in an area which is highly susceptible to pressure damage. If there is an area of erythema over a bony prominence, ears or nose or underneath a device then firm pressure should be applied for a few seconds. When the pressure is released, check whether the area has blanched, that is turned white and then refilled. Even if the area is blanching, then the patient is still at high risk of pressure damage in this area and action must be taken to reposition off the area. Act on the red mark by offloading pressure.
Grade one	When pressure is applied to an area of erythema (redness), there is no blanching seen. That is, it does not turn white. This is grade one pressure damage. Skin tones vary in their response to this.
Grade two	Grade two pressure damage is superficial damage to the epidermis at the epidermal-dermal junction. This will appear as either a clear fluid filled blister or superficial skin loss in which the wound bed is pink.
Grade three	Grade three pressure damage is full thickness skin loss, that is loss of epidermis and dermis. There will be subcutaneous tissue visible as all of the skin layers are lost.
Grade four	Grade four pressure damage is down to the muscle, tendon, or bone. There may be some slough or necrosis, but the structures must be visible in order to classify it as grade four.
Suspected deep tissue injury	This will be either a blood-filled blister, or dark discolouration beneath intact skin. Sometimes, if the patient has had a fall, this can be confused with bruising. However, if the origin of the dark discolouration is uncertain, then treat it as if it were pressure related and remove the pressure.
Unstageable	An unstageable pressure ulcer is one in which the wound bed is obscured by slough or necrosis, where you are unable to visualise the wound bed. Until debridement of the devitalised tissue has been undertaken, you cannot see its true depth. Due to the level of tissue damage when slough or necrosis is present, it will always be a grade three or grade four post-debridement.

With darker skin tones, signs of erythema are not always as evident, therefore relying on this as an indicator of pressure damage is difficult. It may be useful to look for differences in skin tone, by comparing one affected limb to the other or areas surrounding. Some subtle signs include shiny skin as a result of swelling which pulls the skin tight. The area may be more painful for the patient, it may be firmer or softer, warmer or cooler compared to other skin areas. Identifying possible early pressure damage such as the red mark or grade one damage becomes more difficult.

At best, pressure damage causes pain and discomfort for the sufferer. In extreme circumstances, pressure damage can lead to sepsis, loss of limbs and even loss of life. It is the responsibility of all members of the healthcare team to prevent pressure ulcers. Up to 95% of pressure ulcers are avoidable, thus it is largely preventable harm.

Risk assessment

All patients should have a pressure ulcer risk assessment undertaken and the policy and guidelines for this will differ locally. It is essential that you familiarise yourself with the policies of the health board, trust or private provider that you are working with. There are a variety of different tools that may be used to assess risk of pressure damage, which will vary between healthcare providers, and you should use the standardised tool for the area in which you are working. Clinical judgement should also be exercised, as tools are just an aid to assessment and individualised planning is essential.

Each provider may have different frequencies at which to repeat risk assessments, with most often daily assessments undertaken or on each visit in community. It is essential that these risk assessments are repeated from scratch, as an assumed assessment copying the data from the previous assessment is as useful as no assessment at all. There will be various factors which increase the risk of pressure damage such as age, gender, underlying conditions, previous pressure damage, medications, and conditions which cause a lack of mobility or lack of sensation. Poorly managed continence and nutrition can also increase the risk of pressure damage, so it is vital that adjunct assessments of nutrition, mobility and continence are undertaken.

Documentation is extremely important in the prevention, assessment, and management of pressure ulcers. Risk assessment documentation allows for effective communication amongst the team and recognition of risk, effective care planning and safer care. There should also be sufficient documentation of skin assessment and repositioning of the patient. The age-old phrase 'if it wasn't documented, then it wasn't done', is applicable. Bedside records of care, most frequently the SKIN bundle (Gibbs et al., 2006) allows for documentation of skin assessment, repositioning, continence care and nutritional care. This documentation will be relied upon in investigations, which must be undertaken for all levels of pressure damage sustained. In addition to the SKIN bundle documentation at the bedside, there should be written entries documenting any changes within the nursing notes and documentation on a body map to accurately identify the position and nature of any wounds, as well as the date of discovery.

Local reporting systems should be used to report pressure ulcers and an investigation, root cause analysis and action plan should be undertaken to ensure learning from incidents and to improve practice. The serious incident reporting system in Wales and England mandates that all pressure ulcers of grade three, grade four and unstageable developed in NHS funded care must be reported to government and there must be a higher level of investigation. The presence of thorough documentation assists investigation. The documentation is essential to demonstrate that effective care was given and to demonstrate whether a pressure ulcer was avoidable or unavoidable. Care plans should always be put in place for patients who are at risk of pressure damage, which outline the frequency of repositioning and skin assessment, the equipment required to reduce the risk etc. It is imperative that care plans are formulated, individualised, and evaluated on a regular basis. A one-size-fits-all approach should not be taken in regard to repositioning; this should always be based on an individualised assessment. It is dependent on a variety of different factors, and clinical judgement should be considered, with thorough documentation of the rationale for decisions taken. Some patient's skin may tolerate not being repositioned for 6 hours, and issues such as waking them unnecessarily should be factored in. Other patients may be showing early signs of pressure damage in as little as an hour; these patients obviously require more frequent repositioning.

Adjunct equipment

Equipment can be used as an adjunct to, but never a replacement for, reducing pressure. Despite pressure-reducing equipment being used, the patient still needs to be repositioned to offload pressure regularly. Equipment is also prone to failure, so should be regularly checked to ensure that it is in good working order. For example, a deflated dynamic mattress is as useful as the patient just lying on the metal frame of the bed and can be more of a risk than using standard pressure reducing foam if left unchecked. However, dynamic mattresses are not suitable for use with patients suspected of having or with unstable spinal fractures as they can aggravate the injury. Patients with spinal fractures which have not yet been stabilised must be nursed in the supine position, thus offloading is far more difficult. The protection of the spine is more important at this stage, up until the fracture has been stabilised.

Instead, frequent log rolling and skin assessment are essential, as well as adjustment of skin loading using recognised techniques.

Most profiling beds in the inpatient setting will have a high specification foam mattress with castellations to reduce pressure. The same designs often come in cushions. These products are often marketed for patients who are at high risk of pressure damage, however this should not be relied upon solely and regular assessments should take place to ensure that the pressure reduction is sufficient.

The risk profile of the patient should be considered when deciding if higher specification equipment is required. There are non-powered static air-filled pressure redistributing mattress overlays, cushions, and heel offloading devices, which are made of thermoplastic polyurethane where movements redistribute pressure across the entire cell.

There are also mattresses on the market which are hybrid, that is, can be used as a standard foam castellated pressure reducing mattress or cushion. These products have alternating air cells which can be activated when a power box is attached. They have the benefit of being able to step up or step down the pressure relieving properties of the mattress without moving the patient. They can also be altered as condition dictates.

There is higher specification equipment in the form of entirely alternating dynamic pressure mattresses and cushions, which have cells which are filled with air in which alternating cells inflate and deflate to continually redistribute pressure. Again, it is key that the patient is still repositioned on this equipment as it reduces, but does not eliminate pressure ulcer risk.

Device related pressure damage

Any patient who must use a medical device for a period is potentially at risk of device-related pressure ulcers, thus it is important that thorough assessment of the skin underneath the device takes place. There should always be an assessment as to whether medical devices such as oxygen and catheters should be ongoing, not just for reasons of need, safety, and infection risks, but for their risk of pressure damage. This requires an individualised patient assessment to arrive at a solution for the individual patient; clinical judgement and the current evidence base should be consulted when arriving at a plan.

Oxygen delivery devices such as facemasks and nasal cannulas should be fitted to ensure correct positioning, but not overly tight to apply increased pressure to the tissues. Non-invasive ventilation devices which provide Continuous Positive Airways Pressure (CPAP) must have a tight seal over the nose and mouth to be effective; this can cause pressure damage particularly over the bridge of the nose. If pressure damage is occurring, alternatives such as a full-face CPAP facemask or nasal prongs can be considered. Alternative methods, such as utilising pressure reducing silicone strips across the bridge of the nose, can help to redistribute pressure without compromising the seal. These are not suitable for use on top of broken skin, but a primary wound contact layer could be tried beneath.

Anti-embolic stockings can cause pressure damage. Patients should be correctly measured following manufacturers guidelines. This should also be checked regularly as the size of the patient's legs can alter with oedema or reduction of oedema. The stockings should be removed at least once daily to monitor the skin condition beneath. A thorough holistic assessment should always be undertaken prior to both prescription and application of anti-embolic stockings; patients with compromised arterial status can be at high risk of tissue necrosis should they be applied. Patient education in relation to wearing these products must be given and follow manufacturer instructions.

Plaster casts are also a source of potential pressure damage. Application of casts should be undertaken by an appropriately trained professional and following correct techniques to minimise the risk of pressure damage. Due to the opacity of the casts, the patient should be questioned about any unusual pain beneath the cast, and this should be escalated for review. Patients should be advised or assisted to change position of the casted limb regularly, not to rest on the heel and to use a pillow under the cast.

Bedsheets can cause pressure damage if they are positioned too tightly, particularly on the toes. Top sheets should be left loose and not tucked under the mattress to reduce the risk. Too tight positioning of the bottom sheets on the bed can also cause a hammocking effect and reduce the pressure-reducing properties of the mattress. The layers between the patient and the mattress should also be minimised to sustain the pressure-reducing properties.

Caution should be taken with nasogastric tubes and endotracheal airways as they can cause pressure damage to both the skin and mucosa. These devices are often secured tightly to prevent movement, thus increasing the pressure on the tissues. Repositioning of these devices should occur regularly along with assessment of the tissues to ensure that there are no signs of damage.

Catheter tubing should be assessed for position when the patient is moved in bed or in the chair to ensure that it is not kinked nor underneath the patient. A catheter which is not properly positioned may not drain effectively, may cause a tugging effect and cause trauma to the urethra or neck of the bladder and can cause pressure damage to the skin or mucosa on which there is increased pressure. Spectacles can also be a source of pressure damage over the bridge of the nose and ear cartilage. Care should be taken to encourage or assist in repositioning spectacles and over the ear hearing aids regularly, as well as to ensure that the patient does not fall asleep wearing them.

Repositioning is the single most important concept in reducing pressure damage. We know that pressure ulcers are caused by pressure, so it makes sense that offloading this pressure lessens the chances of development. NICE recommend repositioning six-hourly for those at risk and four-hourly for those who are high risk. However, it is essential that reassessment of skin occurs, as there are some patients who could develop pressure damage in less than four hours. Some patients in conditions of high pressure and low sensation and movement can develop pressure damage in an hour or less. Imagine the patient collapsed unconscious on the floor; a hard surface coupled with the inability to sense the pain occurring in pressure damage and inability to move will mean that pressure damage will happen quickly. An individualised assessment should be undertaken to assess for the red mark; if a red mark is present after the scheduled time for turning, then it must be recognised that repositioning needs to happen more frequently.

When repositioning patients in the bed, ideally a new position should be chosen each time, however this will be dependent on their condition and tolerance. Repositioning does not always have to be assisted, and encouragement can be given to the patient to remind them to change their position. NICE guidelines do not mention a specific method of repositioning, and as always this will be patient dependent. Some patients cannot be positioned in a lateral position due to their condition. It is important to avoid positioning the patient on to an area of erythema. Appropriate manual handling aids should always be used, to avoid unnecessary shearing and friction.

There are times when helping the patient into a new position completely is not possible. For example, when a patient has respiratory disease or cardiac failure it becomes difficult to breathe when supine or lying on their side. It is common for these patients to want to be sat in an upright position for this reason, and some even sleep in the chair overnight. These are patients who are at higher risk of pressure damage anyway because of reduced oxygenation of the tissues and oedema. In this case, breathing would take priority. However, this does not mean that regular turns and assessment cannot occur, and the distribution of pressure will be ever so slightly different when returned to the position. These patients would require the higher specification equipment, consideration of the use of silicone redistributing devices over the bony prominences and education to keep moving as is practical.

When in the chair, people are more at risk of pressure damage. In bed, body weight is distributed over a larger surface area at the points that the body is in contact with the mattress. In the chair, 70% of the body weight is borne by the ischial tuberosities. So, a large amount of weight over a smaller surface area, which increases the pressure. It is for this reason that patients who have limited mobility and are largely sitting in a chair should be repositioned and have a skin assessment hourly.

Patients should be assisted to sit upright, on a chair which is neither too high nor too low. Chairs that are too high for the patient mean that they do not have a stable base and are at risk of slipping in the chair which increases the risk of falls and of shearing forces on the buttocks or sacrum. Being too low a chair will equal more weight being taken down through the ischial tuberosities. There should be consideration as to whether the patient requires a surface of higher-pressure reduction in the chair, that is a pressure-reducing cushion. Patients should not have hoist slings left underneath them when in the chair. It may be a task to fit the hoist sling in the seating position, but the seams of the sling can subject the person to unnecessary pressure, and it is also undignified.

Offloading of heel pressure is essential to minimise the risk of heel pressure ulcers developing. For example, those who have undergone surgery, patients who have experienced a stroke or those who have diabetic neuropathy. There are devices available specifically for offloading heel pressure, such as inflatable boots with cut outs in which the heel sits and inflatable wedges which allow heels to be suspended enough above the surface. These should not be draped with pillowcases or sheets as this defeats the purpose and creates again a hammocking effect. In the absence of specialist equipment, a pillow placed under the calf will suffice. Take care that the heel is not in contact with the pillow, as the pressure will remain; rather it should be suspended over the edge. The heels do not have to be elevated excessively, as this can cause discomfort for the patient. A general rule of thumb is that if you can slide a piece of paper between the heel and the surface, then the pressure is sufficiently offloaded. It is important to note that foam dressings designed for heels DO NOT reduce pressure in any way, so should not be used for this purpose.

Important consideration: we have discussed the fact that there is more pressure going down through the ischial tuberosities. Consider the patient who has difficulty maintaining balance while in the chair, possibly due to a stroke or muscle weaknesses. Those patients may tend to lean towards one side, thus putting even more weight and pressure through the one ischium. Coupled with a reduced sensation and ability to feel the pressure, this can be a great risk. It must never be assumed that if a patient is independently mobile and caring for their own needs, that they are not at risk.

When a pressure ulcer has already occurred

When a pressure ulcer has already occurred, then the aim becomes to heal the wound and prevent further damage. As pressure is the underlying cause of the wound, it stands to reason that further pressure will cause further deterioration or a delay in healing. The principles for avoidance of further damage remain the same as those for prevention. It is not possible to give an exact description of how to manage a pressure ulcer healing, because each pressure ulcer will have different characteristics (tissue types, inflammation, moisture, edges) and the individual patient factors which impact upon wound healing will be different. Each pressure ulcer needs a full holistic wound assessment and an appropriate management plan developed using the current evidence base and local wound care policy.

Assessment, prevention, and management of moisture lesions

Moisture lesions are damage to the skin caused by faeces, urine, perspiration or exudate. They can cause extreme pain and discomfort, and in some cases lead to the patient avoiding having an adequate fluid intake to avoid as frequent incontinence, which has its own consequences. As with pressure damage, many moisture lesions are preventable with effective care.

An adequate continence assessment should always be undertaken in line with local policy, and the correct continence aids chosen for the patient considering their own preferences. Devices such as a sheath for males can completely avoid urine encountering the skin. If continence pads are used, then the correct absorbency should be chosen. Too low an absorbency, and more urine comes into contact with the skin. Too high an absorbency for the patient's needs can also be detrimental; pads are designed to absorb moisture. They can draw moisture from the skin and skin damage can ensue.

Catheterisation comes with its own risk of infection and should only be used as a last resort to manage incontinence and clinical judgement used. Sometimes, if there is extreme pain, infected moisture lesions or lack of healing, catheterisation could be considered as part of a balanced risk assessment.

Consideration should also be given to correct cleansing and drying of the skin. Soap based products can have a high pH and dry out the skin; it is best to use neutral cleansers to wash the skin after episodes of incontinence. Skin should be thoroughly dried after washing, paying special attention to skin folds.

Barrier creams and sprays can provide a layer of protection on the skin against damage from urine and faeces. It is important that manufacturer guidance is followed when applying barrier creams and sprays as many are not designed to be applied regularly, but rather every 24–72 hours. There is some evidence to suggest that emollients can both moisturise and protect the skin from damage from incontinence of urine and faeces. Be mindful that some barrier protection products can clog the pores of the continence aids and reduce the absorbency, if applied too generously. You should only use products to manage continence which are licenced for use for the purpose. Procedure pads (square sheets often marketed as bed protectors) should not be used for this purpose. They are not designed to absorb urine and will keep it against the skin. Additionally, they can cause pressure damage as they crease underneath the patient. They should just be used for the purpose of undertaking procedures (wound dressings, enemas, catheterisation etc.) and then removed immediately after use).

Moisture lesions are normally reportable as a clinical incident, as they are preventable harm. Ensure that you follow local policy in terms of reporting moisture lesions. It is important to differentiate between moisture damage and pressure damage for the purposes of care planning and treatment. Moisture damage can increase the risk of subsequently developing pressure damage.

Differentiating between moisture damage and pressure damage

1   Is the area of skin damage over a bony prominence?

Unless caused by a medical device, which usually has an obvious diagnosis, if the skin damage is not over a bony prominence, then it will not be pressure damage. Moisture damage can of course occur in the region of bony prominences, but damage which is over the fleshy part of the buttocks can generally rule out pressure.

2   What shape is the damage?

Linear areas of skin loss in the natal cleft will be due to moisture damage. Similarly, areas of linear skin loss in the groin, under the abdominal apron, under the breasts or axilla will not be pressure. A patient does not have to be incontinent for moisture damage to occur, it can occur as a result of perspiration, exudate or lymphorrhoea.

Pressure ulcers will generally be the shape of the bone and regularly shaped if the damage was caused when the patient was static. They generally tend to be rounded in shape over the ischium, trochanter, elbows, ankles and heels, the shape of the sacral bone in sacral pressure ulcers. However, they can be more irregularly shaped if shearing forces were involved. Moisture damage will most definitely be irregular in shape, sometimes creating a mirrored effect.

3   How many areas of skin loss are there?

Pressure damage is usually limited to one area. Multiple areas of skin loss over the buttocks is indicative of moisture damage.

4   What is the depth of the skin loss and what tissue types are present?

Pressure damage can be of any depth down to bone. There may be necrosis in pressure damage. Moisture damage will generally be superficial skin loss, unless infected. There will be no necrosis in a moisture lesion.

5   What are the edges like?

Pressure damage will generally have distinct edges. The edges are more diffuse in moisture damage.

   It is important to note that although differentiation between the two types of skin damage is necessary, that there can be combination lesions in which there is moisture damage and pressure damage.

Treatment of wounds

Wounds come in varying presentations, and with many underlying aetiologies, thus it is important to undertake a full holistic assessment before proceeding to a dressing. As part of the holistic assessment, there should be consideration not just of the local characteristics of the wound such as tissue types, inflammation, exudate levels and surrounding skin but of the wider factors at play. There should be consideration of the underlying medical conditions that the patient experiences. Conditions such as cardiac failure, diabetes, arterial and venous disease, and chronic obstructive pulmonary disease can impact upon the rate of wound healing. Quite often, the underlying cause must be addressed in non-healing wounds, alongside local wound management. Medications that the patient takes can also have an impact upon wound healing. Corticosteroids, chemotherapeutics, anticoagulants, and non-steroidal anti-inflammatory drugs are known to impact wound healing.

   After holistic assessment, an individualised care plan should be formulated, the TIME principle can again be useful in this. Consider if the wound requires cleansing. Preparation of the wound bed through debridement of devitalised tissue should be considered through sharp, mechanical, larval, or autolytic debridement methods. Consideration of the characteristics of the wound bed is important, including consideration of whether there is infection, in which case a topical antimicrobial is advised. The exudate levels of the wound should be considered. There is a requirement for a moist wound healing environment, however excess exudate can be detrimental and should be absorbed with an appropriate secondary dressing. There may be issues with further skin damage, malodour, pain and leakage if exudate is not properly managed, which can have an impact upon the person physically, psychologically and socially. Compression bandaging can help to reduce high levels of leakage in the limbs, with caution to suitability. Also, consideration of the underlying cause of exudate is important: infective causes, venous, lymphatic, or cardiac causes should be also treated. Surrounding skin should also be managed by cleansing and use of barrier protection or emollients.

Clean or sterile technique in wound care?

There is quite frequently debate within the literature as to whether wound dressing requires an aseptic technique or simply a clean technique. Chronic wounds tend to be routinely colonised with bacteria, which quite often causes no harm until the critical colonisation stage. It is quite often advised to wash leg ulcers in a lined bucket in the patient's home, and for patients with burns to shower to clean the wounds. Quite often patients with leg ulcerations experience concurrent dermatological complaints such as varicose eczema, the dead skin can harbour bacteria and it is thought that washing the legs in this way reduces the risk of infection and does not increase it. Wounds in the perineal area are high risk and good attention to hygiene is required. This has benefits for the patient psychologically and socially.

There is no correlation between using tap water and rates of wound infection. In chronic wounds, the area can be washed with a suitable cleanser with a neutral pH, such as an emollient.

Does it need cleaning at all?

It should be assessed whether the wound requires cleaning at all. Irrigating with fluid, particularly room temperature saline, can reduce the temperature of the wound and in doing so delay healing. A moist, clean wound bed can be left without cleaning. There is a tendency for nurses to use gauze to rub the wound bed to ensure that it is clean, this can sometimes do more harm than good, disrupting new granulation tissue that is forming in the wound bed. Irrigation is preferable to cleaning using gauze swabs. Wound cleansing should be limited to those that have visible contamination (such as incontinence, road rash), infection or slough. There is rarely any requirement to use antiseptic solutions in wound care.

Sterile gloves debate

(See Chapter 11) Non-sterile clean gloves can be used for undertaking a wound dressing. When the procedure is being undertaken, the parts of the dressing which will contact the wound bed should not be touched by the clinician. Should the dressing need to be touched, for instance when packing a wound, then sterile gloves should be used in a hospital/care home environment. In the patient's own home, this is not considered necessary.

Despite the debates that have arisen above, there is still a requirement to maintain asepsis when undertaking a wound dressing so as not to increase the risk of transmission of pathogenic microorganisms from hands, equipment and from one body part to another. Therefore, the aseptic non-touch technique should be used. ANTT is discussed in more depth in Chapter 11. However, this becomes somewhat of an oxymoron when we are advising that legs be washed in a bucket in community, as it becomes impossible to avoid transfer of microorganisms, so this is where a clean technique would apply. There is still a requirement to have a dressing pack with a sterile field, aprons, gloves, and an aseptic approach to dressing application. In hospital settings, it is advised that strict aseptic non-touch technique is used for the procedure due to the higher risk of cross contamination.

In aseptic non-touch technique, we are used to hearing of key sites and key parts. Key sites are entry points for invasive devices or open wounds. In this case, the open wound. The key parts would be the wound dressing, forceps, scalpel etc. anything which comes into direct contact with the wound.

WATCH THE VIDEO

Watch along as you read through this step by step procedure by scanning the QR code with your smartphone camera or via https://study.sagepub.com/rowberry.

DRESSING A WOUND: STEP BY STEP

- Introduce yourself to the patient and explain the procedure.
- Carefully read the wound management plan in place for the patient.
- Gather the equipment that is required for the procedure, e.g. dressing trolley, dressing pack, cleansing solution, gauze, primary and secondary dressings.
- Clean the dressing trolley according to local policy with recommended cleaning solution or wipes.
- Store your equipment on the bottom shelf of the trolley.
- Ensure thorough handwashing using soap and water.
- Open the dressing pack using a minimal touch technique to maintain the sterile field.
- Open packs and dispense the gloves, dressings and any other required key parts, ensuring that they are dropped into the sterile field, and you do not touch it.
- Clean hands using alcohol gel providing hands are not visibly soiled.
- Don apron and then gloves.
- Remove old dressing.
- Remove gloves and clean hands. Don a clean pair of gloves.
- Clean the wound if deemed necessary (consult guidance on whether it is necessary and the technique to be used). Keep a 'clean' hand which picks up items from the sterile field and 'dirty' hand for the wound care.
- Apply dressing using non-touch technique.

The practice of maintaining asepsis and using a non-touch technique applies to other aspects of wound care also, such as the management of wound drainage systems and removal of sutures and clips. It is important to minimise or eliminate the transmission of microorganisms wherever there is a breach in the skin.

CHAPTER SUMMARY

In summary, this chapter has highlighted some of the fundamentals of skin hygiene and integrity. Skin integrity and wound management is a wide field, and you are advised to read further on topics such as wound assessment and management. There are a diverse range of treatments and dressings which could not be covered within this chapter.

Personal hygiene and maintaining skin integrity are fundamentals in nursing and play an important part in patient safety and comfort. Some conditions are not preventable, but it is important that nurses focus on prevention, as it is far more favourable to cure. Breaches to the skin integrity and subsequent pain, infection, odour and discomfort can have a significant impact on a person's quality of life.

ACE YOUR ASSESSMENT

Q1   How many square meters does the skin cover (approx.)?

   a   1.67 square meters

   b   1.59 square meters

   c   2.00 square meters

Q2   How many sweat glands does a square inch of skin contain (approx.)?

   a   900

   b   650

   c   720

Q3   Identify the correct functions of the skin.

   a   Protection, keep warm, stop foreign bodies.

   b   Protective barrier, stop foreign bodies, regulates vitamin A.

   c   Protective barrier, thermoregulation, provides vitamin D.

Q4   Identify the correct causes of pressure damage.

   a   Shear/friction, medications, mobility.

   b   Medications, increased mobility, clothing.

   c   Mobility, medications, trauma.

Q5   What can cause device related pressure damage?

   a   Oxygen masks, slippers, wet clothes.

   b   Anti-embolism stockings, plaster casts, trauma.

   c   Oxygen masks, non-invasive equipment (CPAP), plaster casts.

Answers

1   A

2   B

3   C

4   A

5   C

GO FURTHER

National Pressure Injury Advisory Panel (NPIAP) guidelines: https://npiap.com/page/Guidelines (accessed October 13, 2022).

REFERENCES

Banwell, P.E. and Musgrave, M. (2004) 'Topical negative pressure therapy: Mechanisms and indications', *International Wound Journal*, 1: 95–106.

Clark, M., Semple, M.J., Ivins, N., Mahoney, K., Harding, K. (2017) 'National audit of pressure ulcers and incontinence-associated dermatitis in hospitals across Wales: A cross-sectional study', *BMJ Open*, 21 (8): e015616.

Department of Health and Social Care (2020) 'Pressure ulcers: Productivity calculator'. https://www.gov.uk/government/publications/pressure-ulcers-productivity-calculator (accessed December 2022).

Dougherty, L. and Lister, S. (2015) *The Royal Marsden Hospital Manual of Clinical Nursing Procedures.* Chichester: Wiley-Blackwell.

EPUAP (2022) *Pressure Ulcer Prevention.* https://www.epuap.org/wp-content/uploads/2016/10/final_quick_prevention.pdf (accessed December 2022).

Ette, L. and Gretton, M. (2019) 'The significance of facial shaving as fundamental nursing care', *Nursing Times*, 115 (1): 40–2.

Gov.uk, (2022) 'Pressure ulcers, applying all our health'. https://www.gov.uk/government/publications/pressure-ulcers-applying-all-our-health/pressure-ulcers-applying-all-our-health (accessed December 2022).

Gwenhure, T. and Shepherd, E. (2019) 'Principles and procedures for eye assessment and cleaning', *Nursing Times*, 115 (12): 18–20.

Jones, S.M., Banwell, P.E. and Shakespeare, P.E. (2005) 'Advances in wound healing: Topical negative pressure therapy', *Postgraduate Medical Journal*, 8: 353–7.

Kolarsick, P., Kolarsick, M.A. and Goodwin, C. (2011) 'Anatomy and physiology of the skin', *Journal of the Dermatology Nurses' Association*, 3 (4): 203–13.

Lawton, S. (2019) 'Skin 1: The structure and functions of the skin', *Nursing Times*, 115 (12): 30–3.

McLafferty, E., Hendry, C. and Alistair, F. (2012) 'The integumentary system: Anatomy, physiology and function of skin', *Nursing Standard*, 27 (3): 35–42.

Moore, Z., Avsar, P., Conaty, L., Moore, D.H., Patton, D. and O'Connor, T. (2019) 'The prevalence of pressure ulcers in Europe, what does the European data tell us: A systematic review', *Journal of Wound Care*, 28 (11). doi.org/10.12968/jowc.2019.28.11.710

Rassool, G.H. (2015) 'Cultural competence in nursing Muslim patients', *Nursing Times*, 111 (14): 12–15.

Shintler, M.V. (2012) 'Negative pressure therapy: Theory and practice', *Diabetes Metabolism Research & Reviews*, 28 (1): 72–7.

Thompson, D. (2005) 'An evaluation of the Waterlow pressure ulcer risk-assessment tool', *British Journal of Nursing*, 14 (8): 455–9. doi: 10.12968/bjon.2005.14.8.17930. PMID: 15924028.

Yousef, H., Alhaji, M. and Sharma, S. (2022) 'Anatomy, Skin (Integument), Epidermis', *StatPearls*, November 14. https://www.ncbi.nlm.nih.gov/books/NBK470464/ (accessed January 30, 2023).

NUTRITION AND HYDRATION

7

HELEN BECKETT AND LOVELY SAJAN

NMC STANDARDS COVERED IN THIS CHAPTER

ANNEXE B NURSING PROCEDURES

2.6   Accurately measure weight and height, calculate body mass index, and recognise healthy range and clinical significance of low/high readings.
5.1   Observe, assess, and optimise nutrition and hydration status and determine the need for intervention and support.
5.2   Use contemporary nutritional assessment tools.
5.3   Assist with feeding and drinking and use appropriate feeding and drinking aids.
5.4   Record fluid intake and output and identify, respond to, and manage dehydration or fluid retention.
5.5   Identify, respond to, and manage nausea and vomiting.
5.6   Insert, manage and remove oral/nasal/gastric tubes.
5.7   Manage artificial nutrition and hydration using oral, enteral, and parenteral routes.
5.8   Manage the administration of IV fluids.
5.9   Manage fluid and nutritional infusion pumps and devices.

LEARNING OBJECTIVES

After reading this chapter, you should be able to:

- Understand the Anatomy and Physiology (A&P) related to the digestive tract
- Identify and understand the factors affecting the nutrition and hydration status
- Understand the nurse's role and responsibility in assessing nutritional needs using nutritional assessment tools and respond to those needs
- Understanding the practical skills needed to optimise nutrition and hydration status

STUDENT VOICE

I had no idea how complex this area of nursing was. Ensuring patients receive nutrition and hydration is about more than just mealtimes. You need to understand many key areas around the topic to ensure we do what's right for the patient.

Cleo, 2nd year, Adult Health

When caring for an infant or child who may be at risk of dehydration, it is really important to work in partnership with their parents or carers, in a family-centred care approach, as they know their child best.

Sian, 1st year, Child Health

INTRODUCTION

We take eating and drinking for granted every day, but we only need to be dealing with a common cold lasting a few days to know it can be more difficult to take diet and fluids when we are unwell. The importance of good nutrition starts from birth, and breast milk, where available and safe, provides the ideal nutrition for infants. It is extremely important to note that breastfeeding is not always possible, and that empathy and respect is paramount at these times. Having the right balance of vitamins, minerals, protein, and carbohydrates is key to a balanced diet, throughout a person's life. However, it is also important to note that the nutritional and hydration needs of patients will adapt, change and be different across their lifespan.

In this chapter we will look at some of the more complex aspects of ensuring patients receive adequate nutrition and hydration when they are unwell. This is a vital aspect of nursing care for all fields of nursing. The chapter will cover evidence-based practice and best practice in relation to the care and support of nutrition and hydration needs of patients.

Healthcare professionals are responsible for patient nutrition and hydration needs when they are unwell, and this requires a person-centred/family-centred approach to care that may involve a multi-disciplinary, and inter-disciplinary team, to improve the effectiveness of patient care. Person-centred care is an approach which includes dignity, respect, sharing of information, patient/family participation and individual/institutional collaboration (Baas, 2012). However, with this said, much of the responsibility does fall to nursing staff due of the amount of time and face-to-face contact spent with patients. Whilst a doctor may assess a patient to be malnourished and a dietician may outline a nutrition plan, they may not be able to action the plan the same way a nurse can. Maintaining nutrition and hydration for patients you care for will be a large part of your role regardless of the area or field of nursing you work in. Nursing students particularly need an in-depth knowledge of all aspects relating to this area of care. Your knowledge will develop and expand over the duration of your programme.

A 'balanced diet and adequate fluid intake' means different things to different people; this could be influenced by their cultural and social beliefs and values and may become incredibly complex when people suffer ill health, when their need and ability to take on diet and fluids may change considerably: there is no 'one-size-fits-all'. A sound underpinning knowledge of nutritional science, assessment skills, Anatomy and Physiology (A&P) and clinical skills will be important for your ongoing learning and clinical practice.

ANATOMY AND PHYSIOLOGY RECAP

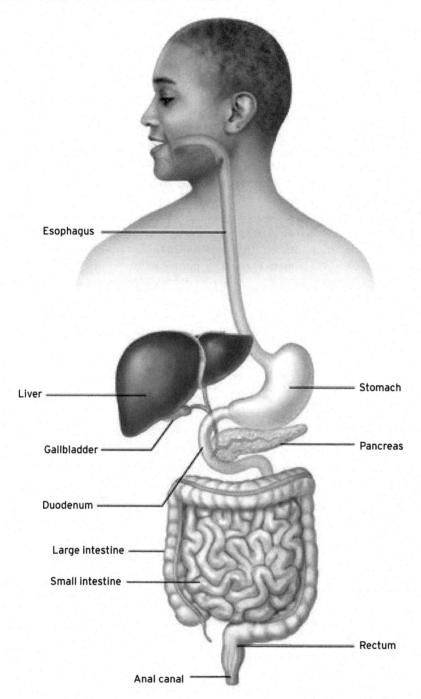

Esophagus

Liver

Gallbladder

Duodenum

Large intestine

Small intestine

Anal canal

Stomach

Pancreas

Rectum

Figure 7.1 The digestive system

Nutrition and hydration cross many A&P areas and body systems, further adding to the importance of this area. This section will firstly recap the A&P of nutrition and secondly consider fluids and hydration. See the Go Further section at the end of the chapter for more information and help with your learning.

Nutrition

The digestive system has multiple functions. For the purpose of this chapter, the A&P recap will focus on ingestion, digestion and absorption; other functions will be covered in further chapters. To help with your understanding recap your knowledge by making a list of the organs in the digestive system. Digestion of nutrients plays a key role in maintaining a person's health. Ingested nutrients, usually from food, are processed and broken down by mechanical and chemical means. Key structures within the digestive system such as the pancreas, liver and gallbladder play important roles in the digestion of nutrients. Large and small intestines each have jobs in facilitating macronutrients – proteins, fats and carbohydrates – and their absorption.

As you can see, the system is complex and comprises many anatomical structures and organs to be naturally effective (commonly described as 'in good working order' – see Figure 7.1). When patients have any disruption, illness, or trauma to any of these structures it will have a detrimental impact on their ability to take on adequate nutrition and hydration. Without the normal activity in this system, cell function and growth is at risk and can further lead to ill health in patients. Many patients must overcome these nutritional challenges after surgery for the rest of their lives. A patient may not be able to adequately absorb fat soluble vitamins, vital for normal body function, if they had resection of their terminal ileum. This means that nutritional support cannot be universal and must be tailored to the individual needs of a patient.

KEY TERMS

Absorption: the end products leave the digestive system and enter the blood supply to be distributed where they are needed.

BMI - Body Mass Index: this is a measurement used by healthcare professionals to assess if a person's weight is healthy. The calculation used is weight in kilos divided by height in metres. This is then compared on a BMI chart.

Digestion: the process of food breakdown. This can be via mechanical method (chewing and swallowing) or chemical method where the food mixes and reacts with enzymes as it moves through the GI tract.

Ingestion: the process of taking food into the digestive system.

Peristalsis: is a series of wave like movements that transport food through the digestive tract.

Fluids

Cellular fluid compartments can be categorised into intracellular and extracellular. Intracellular Fluid (ICF) relates to the fluid that sits in the intracellular compartment, the space inside a cell, and the Extracellular Fluid (ECF) sits outside the extracellular compartment, the space outside the cell. The ICF comprises predominantly potassium, proteins and organic anion solution and is controlled by cell membranes and cell metabolism. The ECF is a predominantly sodium and sodium bicarbonate solution. The ECF are further subdivided into interstitial fluid and intravascular fluid separated by a capillary membrane. Fluid movement between the compartments is controlled by hydrostatic pressure – this is pressure exerted by the fluid – and osmotic pressure – this is pressure exerted on a fluid to stop water passing across a permeable membrane. Any changes in the fluid's concentration or in the fluid volume will influence its movement between compartments. Both pressures can be affected when the body experiences ill health and disease, for example loss of fluid through burns or dehydration.

Considering the effects of dehydration on the osmotic pressure, if the water loss is higher than the electrolyte loss, the osmotic pressure of the ECF becomes higher than the cellular osmotic pressure. This change in osmotic pressure results in water movement from the cells causing reduction in osmotic pressure and gradual increase in ECF volume. This causes dehydration of the cells accompanied by the person feeling the symptom of thirst. Dehydration, depriving the body of water, is a great deal more serious than the body being deprived of food and is usually a result of failure to drink liquids, water loss to excess or a combination of both. Water loss can be further subdivided into sensible and insensible losses. Sensible water loss can be measured and arises from excretion of urine. Insensible water loss is not easily measured and is the fluid lost from the lungs during respiration or from the skin. Severe dehydration can result in shock and even death within hours.

Water within the body is also important in many digestive system functions, particularly in the process of hydrolysis, which is the process whereby enzymes act on food molecules when diet is taken. Adequate hydration is also important for maintenance of health for the renal system, respiratory system, and skin functions. There is a variation of body fluid content as we age, with infants having a higher concentration of water (approx. 70%); by childhood this will have reduced to approx. 65%, and in adulthood this further reduces to 60% (Koyfman, 2018).

Nutritional needs across the lifespan/cultures

From the first moments of life through to end of life care, the nutritional and hydration needs of the individual should be carefully and effectively assessed and supported throughout a person's lifespan, adapting and reacting to changes that they may experience. In this section some of the key aspects that impact an individual's nutritional and hydration needs will be discussed as they venture through their nutritional journey.

Infancy: Breastfeeding

According to the United Nations (1989) 'Convention on the Rights of the Child' every infant and child has the right to good nutrition, and this must begin at the very start of life. Breast milk provides the best nutritional support and protection to the newborn and infant. Colostrum, which is produced in the first few days of breastfeeding, can help build immunity and resist infections (Carneiro-Sampaio, 2016). The WHO and UNICEF both recommend that breastfeeding is initiated within the first hour of life and continues exclusively for the first six months of a child's life. As nurses it is important to support parents in their choice to breastfeed, and every opportunity should be taken by healthcare professionals to offer reassurance and evidence-based information regarding the benefits of breastfeeding. Parents who cannot breastfeed their child or who choose not to must be respected for their choice, they should be at the centre of their own care and as with other areas of maternity care, midwives and maternity support workers should promote informed choice.

Infancy: Weaning

As an infant grows and develops it is from around the age of six months that it is time to consider adding 'solids' to their diet, although breast milk can still provide nutrients up until the age of two. Weaning can be described as the introduction of solid foods into an infant's diet, and progressive reduction of breastfeeding; the WHO recommends that this starts when an infant is six months old (WHO, 2021). Weaning can be a challenging but crucial part of a child's development, as actions at this age can impact their food preferences, dietary and eating behaviours.

Childhood

During this age group there is rapid growth and development, physically, socially, and psychologically. School-aged children are often willing to eat a wider variety of foods and will further move towards making their own decisions about what they want to eat. Children at this stage will have growth spurts and increased physical activity, meaning that their nutrient and energy needs are often greater than those for adults.

Adolescence

Adolescents need a balanced diet rich in nutrients, this is particularly important at this stage as they are going through a period of rapid growth as they reach puberty. Puberty and adolescent age ranges vary significantly dependent on the source used and it is key to remember that there can be variations on actual age ranges. Person-centred care is vital in meeting individuals' needs. During this time young adults may feel stressed, anxious or may have concerns around body image. This may lead to wanting to control how much or what they eat, which in turn could impact their nutritional status. As nurses it is important to recognise the signs of an eating problem and offer the right support and guidance to these young adults.

Adulthood

Through adulthood the nutritional needs of individuals do not change greatly, however nutritional requirements continue to vary depending on sex, age, level of physical activity and for those who are pregnant or breastfeeding. Awareness of cultural and religious beliefs and practices in relation to diet must also be considered when caring for an individual. Eating a healthy balanced diet, keeping physically active and maintaining a healthy weight can all help to reduce the risk of developing chronic conditions such as cardiovascular disease, type 2 diabetes, and some cancers (WHO, 2020).

Older age

According to the British Nutrition Foundation (2016), in the UK, around 16% of the population is over 65 years old. Whilst the nutritional requirements remain largely the same for elderly individuals, their energy requirements can diminish, through decreased metabolic rate and physical activity. Many factors can impact the nutritional status of the older adult; this may include ill health and chronic conditions, medication interactions, and reduced mobility. Hydration status can also be impacted at this stage of life. The older adult may be vulnerable to dehydration due to physiological changes, and frailty both physically and mentally can increase the risk of dehydration in this age group.

Cultural and religious factors

Diet may vary based on various cultures and religious beliefs. It is important for nurses to have an understanding about these varying dietary preferences and provide meal options where possible by utilising correct options from the menus supplied by hospital catering facilities.

CLINICAL SKILLS RELATED TO NUTRITION AND HYDRATION

As outlined in the introduction, the topic of nutrition and hydration is vast. Water and nutrients are essential for sustaining life and maintaining health and it is important that people have the correct amount in accordance with their needs at various life points. Both nutrition and hydration have key roles in keeping body organs in optimum health. Failure to maintain these areas can lead to deterioration of conditions already diagnosed or new periods of ill health. Diet and fluids are responsible for tissue growth and repair; immunity; muscle strength as well as keeping organs such as the kidneys, skin and GI tract healthy (review A&P recap for further information). Failure to meet a patient's dietary and fluid requirements can result in detrimental effects such as weight loss, physical and mental health issues, fatigue, dehydration, dental decay, anaemia and obesity amongst others.

The clinical skills covered below are essential in developing and expanding your knowledge and practice in this area and are skills you should aim to develop throughout the full duration of your programme of study. Fundamental skills learnt in year one will be expanded upon in years two and three and even beyond into your early years of registration. The focus may differ slightly dependent on your clinical placement areas or areas you ultimately choose to work in.

Contemporary nutritional assessments: Discussion

Assessment is an essential part of any nurse's role. Nutritional assessment relates to the process of gathering and interpreting data with a view to making clinical decisions about the cause or nature of nutrition-related ill health (BDA, 2012). Effective nutritional assessment relies on keen nursing observations of the patient as well as effective communication skills. It also requires knowledge of systems of the body, what problems can occur when systems go wrong and of appropriate pharmacology. All these factors will help guide your assessment and develop the appropriate questions when performing the skill.

Any assessment is comprised of multiple data gathering routes; you will gather objective clinical data such as weight and height as well as subjective data regarding the patient's religious, cultural, spiritual and lifestyle needs as well as their thoughts and feelings, opinions, and anxieties for instance. In gathering this data, several contemporary nutritional assessment and screening tools are available to use, and you will come across many throughout your programme. For example, one of the most commonly used tools in healthcare settings is the Malnutrition Universal Screening Tool (MUST), which is explored in the activity below. A patient's BMI is an important data point on nutritional assessment tools, but it is important to know that several authors have in recent years criticised the BMI and its effectiveness (Rothman, 2008; Nuttall, 2015). For example, a young athlete may present with a BMI that would place them in the overweight category but in reality, their muscle increases their weight. Similarly, an older person with heart failure may be fluid overloaded and thus be classed as obese based on their BMI when in reality they may be severely malnourished. Despite this, the BMI remains extremely useful and effective when considered as part of a holistic, in-depth, and person-centred nutritional assessment, adding to the overall picture of the patient.

ACTIVITY: PAUSE AND REFLECT

Make your own list of other contemporary nutritional assessment tools that you have encountered in your practice settings to help build your knowledge. Have these tools been effective in identifying patients at risk of malnutrition?

Familiarise yourself with the Malnutrition Universal Screening Tool (MUST): https://www.bapen.org.uk/pdfs/must/must_full.pdf (accessed October 14, 2022).

How might this tool be better than others you have already used?

CONTEMPORARY NUTRITIONAL ASSESSMENT: STEP BY STEP

- Every patient should have a nutritional screen/assessment within 24 hours of admission.

- Introduce yourself to the patient, explain what you aim to do and gain consent. For some individuals such as those with a learning disability, you may want to ensure that a familiar person for them is available whilst the assessment is carried out – to assist with communication, and provide reassurance to the individual.

- Gather the equipment, you will need the following: gloves; apron; nutritional assessment tool; pen torch (for assessing oral cavity); tongue depressor.

- Ensure the patient and environment is as comfortable as possible. Does the patient want the curtains drawn, or move to another room if appropriate? Continuously ensure the patient is comfortable throughout the process. You can also be guided by a chaperone if this is required for the individual.

- Wash and dry hands thoroughly as per local infection prevention and control policy.

- Don Personal Protective Equipment (PPE) as per local policy.

- Gather objective data in the following areas: dietary history; social history; physical abilities/factors (neurological considerations); socio-economic factors; any current illnesses; psycho-social factors; GI symptoms/complications; weight/height/calculate BMI; medication history (prescribed and non-prescribed; oral health; physical appearance; recent weight loss/gain; biochemical profile. (See Chapter 2, The Importance of Assessment.)

- Gather subjective data in the following areas: how does the patient communicate with you; what body language do you observe; any anxieties displayed; does the person require assistance to communicate?

- Offer ongoing reassurance and rationale for your questions and points, you may need to provide a break from the assessment process if the person becomes overly anxious.

- Document your findings accurately and fully complete the nutritional assessment tool in line with local policy.

- Ensure the patient is still comfortable when you conclude.

- Escalate information appropriately to key persons (for example doctor, dietician), and make referrals if needed.

Assisting patients with eating and drinking: Discussion

Reviewing the A&P section above will allow you to consolidate your understanding of the GI tract and digestive system (see Figure 7.1). You will now have fundamental knowledge of problems that may arise if any structures encounter damage or disease. These issues can cause a variety of problems for patients trying to take on board adequate diet and fluids.

You will care for patients in a variety of settings who may require assistance to eat and drink. Malnutrition costs the healthcare industries significant sums of money and affects one in three inpatients (Elia, 2015). When patients become unwell, they are unlikely to want to take diet and fluids in the same way or in the same amounts they would when they are well, and this can cause challenges for nursing care. Malnutrition and dehydration can lead to or exacerbate complications such as skin breakdown, greater risk of infections, sepsis and poor or delayed wound healing, and this can cause additional distress and suffering to patients.

Many patients will be independent when taking diet and fluids and this must be encouraged and fostered, however some patients will need assistance from staff or families. Performing an effective nutritional assessment, as discussed previously, will help you understand if and how a patient needs help in this area. Some medical conditions will mean patients need assistance also, as outlined below.

Conditions that often require eating and drinking assistance

- **Post-surgery** – pain following surgical procedures can mean patients find eating and drinking more difficult.
- **Dementia** – many patients living with dementia in the community may not have the cognitive or physical ability to maintain adequate nutrition and this is a challenge in itself. The reasons for this may be multifactorial and complex. Examples include the inability to simply obtain food from a shop, inability to cook food or not experiencing the feeling of hunger. Up to half of older adults and half of patients living with neurological problems may have swallowing problems (Clavé and Shaker, 2015). This is then further compounded by an admission to a hospital, making nutritional support both challenging and even more important.
- **Cancer** – patients with cancer can experience distressing nausea and vomiting, pain or structural difficulties, meaning they are unable to remain independent with nutrition and hydration.
- **Swallowing difficulties** – these can be caused by a variety of conditions (e.g. patients who have had a stroke (CVA), some individuals with a learning disability) and mean there are additional safety concerns when patients are taking diet and fluids.

ACTIVITY: PAUSE AND REFLECT

From your experience or your learning, what other conditions may give rise to difficulties in eating and drinking? Have you cared for any patients where their cultural beliefs and values impact their dietary choices?

Assistance with feeding and drinking could come in the form of helping patients make appropriate choices when choosing meals. It could mean facilitating protected mealtimes to create a conducive environment. It could include utilising measures that highlight patients who are at risk in clinical areas (i.e., red lids), as well as adapted cutlery and utensils that allow patients to remain as independent as possible with this activity. Assisting patients takes time and must not be rushed – ensuring an optimum and safe position is always essential as well as responding to the needs of the individual and maintaining safety.

It is always necessary to continuously assess patients for their nutritional support. For example, when assisting in hydration a patient may be given a straw, yet not have the ability to draw on the straw to drink. A patient may be given a spouted beaker to drink from, yet not have the dexterity to stop the flow of fluid or cognitive ability to realise to drink from the spout. Assessment is key.

As a nurse there are a lot of things you can do to support a patient with their eating and drinking. Find out what food and drinks they like or do not like. Care you provide should always be person-centred, individual choices and preferences should always be listened to and acted upon. It is also important to note that patients should be offered a drink periodically to aid digestion and continuously assess safety to do so. Offer oral care pre- and post-meal; if the patient experiences nausea ensure anti-emetics are administered prior to this procedure – if this skill is delegated, ensure the person possesses the knowledge and skills to carry out the skill.

ASSISTING PATIENTS WITH EATING AND DRINKING: STEP BY STEP

- Levels of assistance needed will vary; promote the patient's independence as much as possible regardless of the time it takes.
- From completion of the nutritional assessment, ascertain the level of assistance the patient may require.
- Assist the patient to the dining area where available. You could consider using objects of reference such as the individual's plate or cutlery to ensure they recognise what you are offering/ prompt that it is a mealtime.
- If it is not possible to sit the patient in the dining area, they should be comfortably seated in a chair. Where this is not appropriate, the patient should be comfortably sat up in bed, supported with pillows if/when needed.
- Low level assistance may be in the form of opening packets, removing lids or cutting food.
- Always and continuously ensure the patient can reach everything.
- Prepare the area. Ensure the table is clean and free from clutter. Allow the patient to wash their hands. Consider: does the patient have aids (hearing aids/glasses/dentures)? Does the patient have a meal option that they have chosen and that meets their individual needs?
- Explain the process fully and gain consent to assist.
- Wash your hands and don PPE as per local policy.
- Sit near the patient at eye level, do not stand over the patient.
- Offer the patient small amounts of food or fluids. If the patient has sight impairments, explain what you are offering and when.
- Continuously assess safety needs/coughing.
- Encourage the patient to do what they can for themselves throughout the process.
- You may have to ask or encourage the patient to open their mouth.
- If the patient is sight impaired, consider placing their hand on yours on the utensil as a guide, always talking through what you are doing, prior to any actions.
- Do not rush the patient.
- When the patient has decided they are finished, dispose of any waste and wash your hands.
- Enable the patient to wash their hands.
- Accurately document what and how much the patient has eaten/drunk.

CASE STUDY

Sarah

Sarah Jones is a 78-year-old woman who was diagnosed with Parkinson's disease five years ago. Sarah currently lives alone at home and has home carers that visit twice daily. Lately she has been experiencing coughing and drooling when eating.

Questions

Think about how you would assess Sarah. What tools might be useful and what recommendations would you make to support her?

Certain groups of patients may require extra support with eating and drinking by artificial methods using nasogastric, naso-jejunal or percutaneous endoscopic gastrostomy tubes (described further in the section below).

WATCH THE VIDEO

INSERTING AND REMOVING NASOGASTRIC TUBES

Watch along as you read through this step by step procedure by scanning the QR code with your smartphone camera or via https://study.sagepub.com/rowberry.

Nasogastric feeding tube insertion – adult, infant and child: Discussion

Adults may require artificial feeding due to need for supplementary oral intake, altered level of consciousness and if they are deemed unsafe to swallow for example, in end stage Parkinson's disorder, stroke, advanced dementia and some patients with learning disability. A nasogastric tube can be inserted at the bedside by a competent healthcare professional or using endoscopic technique in patients with oesophageal obstruction, basal skull fracture and facial injury.

The National Patient Safety Agency, NPSA (2011) has advocated that patients who require a nasogastric tube insertion should be assessed and identified as appropriate for nasogastric feeding and the same should be documented in the medical notes. Nasogastric tubes used for feeding should have visual length markings and should be radio opaque to ensure visibility on the X ray. Following insertion, a small amount of gastric fluid is aspirated gently using a syringe to check the pH on a pH indicator strip, which is used to confirm the position of the nasogastric tube in the stomach. Until the position of the nasogastric tube is confirmed to be in the stomach by pH test or Xray, no liquid should be introduced into the tube. The safe range of pH to commence feeding is between 1 and 5.5. If no aspirate is obtained or pH test is inconclusive, x-ray is used to confirm the position of the nasogastric tube.

Infants and children who either are unable to take any or sufficient nutrition orally, but whom the gastrointestinal tract is functioning, may be fed by a Nasogastric (NG) tube, Nasojejunal (NJ) tube, or Percutaneous Endoscopic Gastrostomy (PEG) tube to meet their nutritional needs. Tube feeding may be considered in infants or children that have a medical condition which prevents them from taking in adequate nutrition orally. This could be for short-term conditions such as bronchiolitis or long-term conditions such as cerebral palsy. If a child requires long-term feeding via a NG tube, then a PEG tube may be considered. Other reasons why an infant or child may require a NG tube is if they are found to have an unsafe or immature swallow; this would be assessed by the Speech and Language Therapist (SALT). Premature infants may also require a short-term NG tube whilst they transition to full oral feeds.

Feeding devices

NG feeding tubes are inserted through the nose and extend through the oesophagus into the stomach. They can be:

- Poly Vinyl Chloride (PVC) tubes – recommended for short-term use and need to be changed weekly.
- Poly Urethane (PU) tubes – recommended for long-term use. 'Silk' tubes are more comfortable, they will have a guidewire throughout their length to aid the insertion process. The lifespan of these tubes is usually 6-8 weeks.

NJ tubes are like NG tubes, but they extend beyond the stomach and end at the second portion of the small intestine (jejunum). Tubes are placed under radiological guidance to ensure correct placement.

PEG tubes are inserted under general anaesthetic; a gastrostomy feeding tube or device is one which is inserted directly through the abdominal wall into the stomach. They are held in place inside the stomach by a plastic disc or flange.

In adult patients, consent should be obtained for the procedure and if a patient lacks capacity to consent, capacity assessment should be done as per Mental Capacity Act (2005). The patient's next of kin or advocate along with the multidisciplinary team should be involved in the process to take a decision in the best interest of the patient.

If a child or young person requires a feeding device to support their nutritional needs, an appropriate feeding regime should be considered. Decisions about the child or young person's care should always be in partnership with the family, and they may also have the support of a wider multidisciplinary team. This team may include a paediatric dietitian, community children's nursing team, consultant in charge of their care, SALT, school nurse and GP.

Feeding methods via NG/NJ/PEG

Bolus feeding: Gravity or feeding pump

- Feeds can be given via a 20ml or 60ml syringe, or a mobile pump.
- Times when a feed is administered can be flexible, particularly for children with long-term feeding devices. This can allow them to be sociable and mimic mealtimes.
- It is important to follow the accompanying prescription.

Continuous feeding: Pump only

- Using a continuous pump to administer feed allows an hourly rate to be set, this enables more accurate recording of feed administered.
- If a child has a PEG, then they can have overnight feeds. This is not recommended for children with a NG tube as it could become dislodged and there is risk of aspiration.
- For adult patients, feeding regime is provided by the dietician and care is taken that patients' sleep hours are not disturbed and sufficient rest time is provided between feeds.
- In clinical practice, follow the prescription.

As discussed previously in this section, some young infants may require a NG tube for a short period of time either as they transition to oral feeding if born prematurely or if they have an acute illness such as bronchiolitis, where supportive measures are used including nasogastric feeding. If an infant or child requires a NG tube, discussing and explaining this to the child (where possible) and their family is very important. Ensure they have all the appropriate information to give consent for the procedure to be undertaken. When passing a NG tube on an infant/child, it is important to have two people present, one to comfort and support the child and one to pass the tube. These should be healthcare professionals and not parents or carers, as they may become distressed witnessing the procedure. Prior to undertaking the tube insertion, it is important to gather all your equipment.

The equipment used for NG tube insertion in an adult is similar although size of the NG tube and syringe used for aspirating the gastric content varies as per the adult range of equipment. The expiry dates of the equipment used should be checked. Follow local policy and manufacturer guidelines in relation to use of equipment. Document the procedure and all relevant information clearly in patients' notes.

NASOGASTRIC (NG) FEEDING TUBE INSERTION AND REMOVAL – ADULT: STEP BY STEP

(Student nurses should only complete this task under the direct supervision of their practice supervisor)

EQUIPMENT

- Plastic apron
- Gloves
- Sterile pot
- pH paper indicating an acid range of pH 0-6
- Enteral syringe 20ml
- Nasogastric tube
- Tape to secure

PROCEDURE

- Gain consent from the patient.
- Discuss and agree a signal with the patient if the patient wants you to pause the procedure at any point.
- Assist the patient to sit in a semi upright position in the bed using pillows with head slightly flexed forwards.
- Wash hands and don PPE as per local policy.

(Continued)

- Check that the guidewire of the NG tube is engaged in tube.

- Assess the length of tube to be inserted, by obtaining the NEX (Nose-Earlobe-Xiphisternum) measurement. Measure the length from tip of the nose to the earlobe and from the earlobe to the xiphisternum. Keep a note of the marking on the tube at the level of the xiphisternum, the tube should be inserted up to that marking.

- Lubricate the tube as per manufacturer guidelines, check the nostril and gently insert the tube along the floor of the nose. If any obstruction is felt, rotate the tube and try to advance it in a slightly different direction. If obstruction is encountered still, use the other nostril. If it is not possible to pass the tube into the other nostril, stop the procedure and ask for assistance from another competent staff member.

- If appropriate, as you pass the tube down into the nasopharynx, ask the patient to sip some water or instruct the patient to try to swallow as swallowing closes the glottis enabling the tube to pass into the oesophagus. Reassure the patient continuously as the procedure is quite uncomfortable.

- Insert the tube to the correct length as per the NEX measurement. Ensure that the patient is not showing any signs of respiratory distress like coughing, rapid breathing, change in colour or feeling unwell.

- Securing the tube in the correct position, aspirate a small amount of gastric fluid gently using a 60ml syringe. Check the pH of the fluid using the pH indicator strip. If the pH is within the range of 1-5.5, this is acceptable.

- Document the pH level, time, date and length of insertion of the tube on a chart for future reference. This should be done every time the tube is accessed for aspiration, flushing or feeding.

- If no aspirate is obtained, try the following steps. Try to obtain aspirate after each step:
  o   Turn patient onto left side.
  o   Reposition the tube by advancing or withdrawing it by 10-20 cm.
  o   Try to obtain aspirate after 15-30 mins.
  o   Nil by mouth patients can be provided oral care to simulate gastric acid secretion.

- If no aspirate is obtained still or pH test is not conclusive, obtain an x-ray to confirm placement of tube in the stomach.

- Once the tube placement is confirmed by a competent practitioner, secure the tube to the nose and side of the cheek using the plaster provided with the nasogastric tube pack. The guidewire can be removed from the tube and water can be administered initially using a syringe following local policy. Follow the dietician's regime for feed administration.

- Dispose of used equipment as per local policy. Complete documentation in the patient's medical notes.

- When needing to remove the NG tube, remember that removal of the tube could be uncomfortable and may stimulate a gag reflex. Ensure that the patient is sitting in an upright position.

- Explain the procedure to the patient. Provide vomit bowl and some tissues in case the patient will need to use it.

- Gently remove the tape securing the NG tube in place. Pull the tube out quickly while reassuring the patient. Check that the patient is comfortable.

- Dispose of the used equipment as per local policy. Update the patient's medical notes.

NASOGASTRIC (NG) FEEDING TUBE INSERTION AND REMOVAL – INFANT/CHILD: STEP BY STEP

(Student nurses should only complete this task under the direct supervision of their practice supervisor)

EQUIPMENT

- Plastic apron
- Gloves
- Sterile pot
- pH paper indicating an acid range of pH 0–6
- Enteral syringe 20ml
- Nasogastric tube
- Tape to secure

PROCEDURE

- Wash and dry hands thoroughly as per local infection prevention policy.
- Cut a piece of tape long enough to cover two thirds of the child's cheek and place in easy reach.
- Depending on the age and development of the child, explain the procedure to them and their parents or carers (person with parental responsibility) and obtain verbal consent.
- Before starting the procedure, you must position the infant or child to ensure they are safe and secure.
  - o Infants under the age of 1 year should be wrapped securely in a blanket or sheet.
  - o Older children may sit in an upright position on an adult's knee or supported by pillows.
- If the tube is a replacement tube, use the alternative nostril to reduce the risk of mucosal erosion.
- Establish the correct length of the NGT by measuring the distance from the infant/child's tip of nose to earlobe to xiphisternum (NEX measurement), make note of the measurement as this must be recorded in the patient's notes following the procedure.
- In neonates measure from the tip of the nose to the ear lobe and then to the midpoint between the sternum and umbilicus (NEMU measurement).
- Check that the tube is intact. If the tube has a guidewire ensure that it moves freely within the tube and that it is not kinked or protruding from the end.
- Using the second person to hold the child's head, gently pass the tube into the child's nostril advancing it along the floor of the nasopharynx to the oropharynx until the measured mark is reached.
- If any obstruction or resistance is felt, you must withdraw the tube and try again or use the other nostril.
- If the infant/child shows any signs of distress, breathlessness, severe coughing, gasping or cyanosis – you must remove the tube immediately.
- You must not use the tube until the position has been confirmed, this is done by aspirating gastric content and testing on a pH strip. The pH must be below 5.0 to indicate correct tube placement (see evidence box for NPSA Guidelines).

(Continued)

- Once the correct position has been confirmed, if a guidewire is used, flush the lumen with sterile water and remove the guidewire using gentle traction.
- Secure the tube to the cheek using the pre-cut tape.
- Record in the child's notes the size and type of tube used, the length of the tube inserted, and that correct placement has been confirmed.

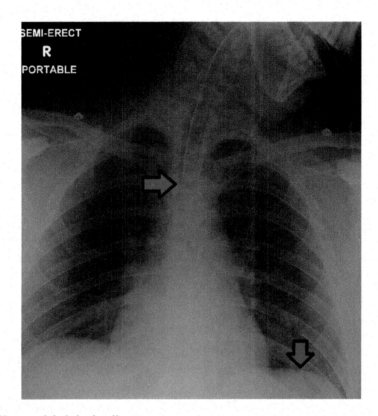

Figure 7.2   Nasogastric tube in-situ

Source: Wikimedia Commons/James Heilman, MD (CC BY-SA 4.0)

The NG tube can be seen on the above plain radiograph (also known as a chest x-ray). The upper-most arrow shows the tip of an endotracheal tube (or breathing tube) which is in the patient's trachea. Behind this tube you can see a prominent vertical line, which if you follow it downwards, you will see it travels below the level of the lung bases – this is the NG tube running down the oesophagus which lies directly behind the trachea. The lower arrow shows the tip of the NG tube sitting beneath the diaphragm in the stomach.

The first line for confirming the position of a NG tube is by testing the pH of the aspirate using CE marked pH indicator paper which has been manufactured to test human gastric aspirate. If the pH is 5.5 or less (5.0 in children and infants – although there are local variations in this) this reasonably indicates the NG is in the stomach and safe to be used. All pH results should be clearly documented with details of whether an aspirate was obtained, the pH value, who checked the pH, and when it was determined as safe to use (NPSA, 2011). Please be aware, your clinical area may have a differing policy, and this must be followed.

Risks associated with NG tube insertion

ACTIVITY: PAUSE AND REFLECT

What do you think are the potential risks around nasogastric tube insertion?

Misplacement of a nasogastric tube in the pleura or respiratory tract that is not detected could result in a pneumothorax, or if feeding has commenced aspiration of feed. Where there is suspicion of a base of skull fracture, NG tubes should be avoided as there is a risk of the NG tube perforating the base of the skull.

When an NG tube is used for an extended period of time, there is a risk of damage to the skin around the nostril and the skin can break down and create a pressure ulcer. To try and avoid this aim to use alternate nostrils when changing tubes and perform an assessment of the skin around the nostril to observe for any signs of redness or breakdown of skin.

Possible complications of NG tube insertion include:

- Pneumothorax
- Tube displacement
- Aspiration
- Nausea or vomiting
- Nasopharyngeal discomfort
- Rhinitis
- Sinusitis
- Nasal erosion/ulceration
- Otitis media
- Oesophageal perforation
- Reflux
- Fistula formation

ACTIVITY: COMMUNICATION SKILLS

How would you communicate and explain to the family/carer of a patient that they required a nasogastric feeding tube? Focus on your field of nursing. What other considerations might there be when communicating this information?

Feeding/medication via NG tube: Discussion

When accessing a NG tube to administer feed or medication there are several factors to consider prior to administration. The size of nasogastric tube, particularly in neonates and infants, can be very narrow and can easily become blocked by larger drug particles or viscous solutions. Fine bore nasogastric tubes in adults are also at risk of blockage due to feed or medications. Modified release medication should also not be administered through a NG tube.

Timing of feed and medication is also important as certain medications cannot be administered whilst feed is running or within a few hours of having a feed. Take Flucloxacillin as an example.

Absorption is decreased by the presence of feed, therefore feed should be stopped 1 hour prior to administration, and recommenced 2 hours after. You may also want to consider if the medication can be given by a different route, as this could preserve the life of the NG tube and prevent blockages.

MEDICATION VIA NG TUBE: STEP BY STEP

- Wash and dry hands thoroughly as per local infection prevention and control policy.
- Gather all equipment and medication needed, ensuring you have the most appropriately sized enteral syringe to safely administer the medication dose.
- Check local health board policy regarding NG medication administration.
- Explain the procedure to the patient, or if it is an infant or young child the parents, and obtain verbal consent. A best interests decision would be required here for any adult deemed to lack capacity to consent themselves.
- Check the patient's name, date of birth, hospital number and any allergies prior to commencing medication administration.
- Check and confirm the NG tube position; this is done by aspirating gastric content and testing on a pH strip. The pH must be below 5.5 (5.0 for children and infants) to indicate correct tube placement.
- Prior to medication administration flush the NG tube with 30ml of water using an enteral syringe.
- Using appropriately sized enteral syringes, prepare each medication separately as prescribed (please read Chapter 13 on medication management for more guidance on medication administration and safe practice). Never mix medications unless instructed by a pharmacist.
- For soluble or dispersible tablets:
  o   Remove the plunger from the syringe
  o   Place the tablet in the barrel and replace plunger
  o   Draw up 10ml of water
  o   Place a clean gloved finger over the tip of the syringe and shake gently
  o   Administer medication
- For liquids or suspension medication:
  o   Shake the bottle of medication well
  o   Draw the required dose of medication up into an appropriately sized syringe
  o   Administer medication
- If more than one drug is to be administered – flush between medications with at least 10ml of water to ensure that the medication is no longer in the tube.
- Once all medication has been administered, flush tube with 30ml of water.
- Document medication administered on medication chart and where appropriate on patient's fluid balance chart.

Responding to and managing dehydration and fluid retention: Discussion

Most commonly dehydration occurs when the body loses more fluid than it consumes. Dehydration can also occur due to loss of salt as well as water from the body. In the A&P section, we have discussed the various routes of water loss from the body. A person's fluid requirement and intake may vary due to various factors including their age, height, weight, activity and any associated health condition.

Recognising signs and symptoms of dehydration and responding to dehydration are vital responsibilities of a nurse. If dehydration is not treated on time and becomes worse, it could be a serious problem.

Table 7.1 shows the signs and symptoms of dehydration and factors contributing to dehydration.

Table 7.1 Signs and symptoms of dehydration and factors contributing to dehydration

Signs and symptoms of dehydration (RCN, 2019)

Thirst

Feeling dizzy/lightheaded

Sleepiness/tiredness

Dry, sticky mouth

Headache

Passing small amounts of dark, concentrated urine

Low blood pressure/hypotension

Rapid pulse/tachycardia

Factors contributing to dehydration (Shepherd, 2011)

Refusal to drink for fear of incontinence

Dementia, Alzheimer's disease or cognitive impairment

Reliance on health professionals to provide adequate fluids

Physical weakness or increased frailty

Pre-operative fasting

Medication, such as laxatives or diuretics

Illness causing physical and mental stress

Reduced sensation of thirst in older people

Fluid restriction for conditions such as heart failure or renal disorders

Diarrhoea and vomiting

Responding to dehydration

Managing dehydration may vary based on the severity of dehydration. There may not be any signs and symptoms during the initial phase of dehydration. Signs and symptoms develop as dehydration increases. As dehydration becomes severe, symptoms of hypovolaemic shock occur including diminished consciousness, lack of urine output, cool moist extremities, a rapid and feeble pulse (the radial pulse may be undetectable), low or undetectable blood pressure, and peripheral cyanosis (WHO, 2005: 4).

Dehydration can affect individuals of varying ages for various reasons. However, older adults are known to have greater risk of dehydration due to hampering of homeostasis related to metabolic changes in older age. For determining the hydration status of older persons, assessment and history taking is an important factor. Despite challenges associated with monitoring daily fluid intake and output in older persons, the assessment of daily fluid intake and output is considered as useful in the diagnosis of dehydration (Miller, 2015). This practical skill will be discussed later in this chapter.

Establishing dehydration in older adults can be done by use of diagnostic tests and screening methods. A test for dehydration due to water loss or insufficient fluid intake is serum osmolality which is the measurement of osmotic concentration of blood serum. The blood urea nitrogen/creatinine ratio is another test; however, this is not deemed as reliable as it may not distinguish between poor renal function and dehydration (Thomas et al., 2008). Some screening questions which could be of value when assessing dehydration are questioning about fatigue and whether they have missed drinks between meals (Hooper and Bunn, 2015). However, the early indication of dehydration in older persons includes confusion and alteration in mental status and memory.

Dehydration is common in children, and early intervention and treatment is required to prevent hypovolaemia and organ failure. Oral fluids and rehydration solutions are provided to manage initial phases of dehydration. As dehydration becomes severe, intravenous fluids are administered to replenish the fluid content. Considering an example of dehydration associated with diarrhoea in children, the table below gives further details on clinical assessment.

Table 7.2 Clinical assessment for degree of dehydration associated with diarrhoea in children

	A	B	C
General Appearance	well, alert	restless, irritable	lethargic or unconscious
Eyes	normal	sunken	sunken
Thirst	drinks normally, not thirsty	thirsty, drinks eagerly	drinks poorly, or not able to drink
Skin Turgor	goes back quickly	goes back slowly	goes back very slowly

Source: Adapted from WHO (2005)

Looking at Table 7.2, we can see that:

- if two or more of the signs in column C are present: the patient has 'severe dehydration'
- if two or more signs from column B (and C) are present: the patient has 'some dehydration'
- patients who fall under column A: 'no signs of dehydration'.

According to WHO (2005), the estimation of fluid deficit (and the requirement) in children with some dehydration or severe dehydration should be carried out by weighing them without clothing. (If weighing is not possible, a child's age may be used to estimate the weight.)

Table 7.3 Estimation of fluid deficit in children

Assessment	Fluid deficit as % of body weight	Fluid deficit in ml/kg body weight
no signs of dehydration	<5%	<50 ml/kg
some dehydration	5-10%	50-100 ml/kg
severe dehydration	>10%	>100 ml/kg

Source: Adapted from WHO (2012)

GO FURTHER

For details of treatment plans, read World Health Organization (WHO) (2005) *The Treatment of Diarrhoea: A Manual for Physicians and Other Senior Health Workers.* Geneva: WHO. https://apps. who.int/iris/bitstream/handle/10665/43209/9241593180.pdf (accessed October 14, 2020).

Managing the administration of IV fluids

Intravenous (IV) fluid therapy is administered by nurses very frequently in hospital settings in response to conditions including dehydration, diarrhoea, fluid loss and hypovolaemia. Sherratt (2014) highlighted the lack of nurses' training in relation to IV fluid therapy leading to them perceiving IV fluid therapy as being routine. It is important for healthcare professionals to understand the benefits and risks associated with IV therapy. The National Institute of Health and Care Excellence (NICE, 2017) has recommended the five Rs of fluid therapy prescription as: *resuscitation, routine maintenance, replacement, redistribution, and reassessment.* This guidance should be followed by healthcare practitioners when prescribing and administering IV fluids.

ACTIVITY: WHAT IS THE EVIDENCE?

Read the information on the following link and make notes as you read through each section.

- National Institute of Health and Care Excellence (2017) *Intravenous Fluid Therapy in Adults in Hospital* (CG174), nice.org.uk, May 5. https://www.nice.org.uk/guidance/CG174 (accessed October 14, 2022).
- National Institute of Health and Care Excellence (2015) *Intravenous Fluid Therapy in Children and Young People in Hospital* (NG 29), nice.org.uk, December 9. https://www.nice.org.uk/guidance/ng29/resources/intravenous-fluid-therapy-in-children-and-young-people-in-hospital-pdf-1837340295109 (accessed October 14, 2022).

Can you relate the assessment of patients requiring acute fluid resuscitation with any situation in your clinical area?

Have you identified any lack of training and education in IV fluid therapy in a CYP setting?

Intravenous fluids are usually prescribed by a doctor or healthcare professional with prescribing qualifications. The responsibility of administration of IV fluid and care of the venous access device (e.g., peripheral cannula) rests on the nurse or healthcare professional taking care of the patient. Therefore, the healthcare professional involved with the infusion therapy should possess all knowledge and skills and be competent in all areas of infusion care (RCN, 2016). There are various types of fluids used for fluid replacement therapy and for fluid resuscitation purposes.

Crystalloids

Crystalloids are aqueous fluids containing electrolytes which easily pass through the lining of blood vessels creating balance between the intravascular and extracellular space. Commonly used crystalloids are Normal Saline and Hartmann's solution (Lira and Pinsky, 2014). The properties of the fluids vary; they are used according to the type of fluid loss and patient's condition. Normal Saline (contains sodium and chloride) has an electrolyte concentration similar to plasma and is usually used to treat low extracellular fluid loss as in dehydration and for fluid challenge/resuscitation purposes. Hartmann's solution (which contains sodium, chloride, potassium, calcium and lactate) has balanced ionic composition more resembling the body's plasma levels and is usually given to patients who have fluid loss post-operatively (Cathala and Moorley, 2018).

Colloids

Colloids contain larger molecules which expand the volume of plasma and increase vascular pressure. Some examples of colloids are gelatins (prepared from collagen) and dextrans (synthesised from sucrose) (Lira and Pinsky, 2014). As all the intravenous fluids used for fluid replacement contain varying amounts of electrolytes, it is very important for the biochemical profile of the patient to be checked prior to administering intravenous fluids. As many colloid products are animal or human derived, it is imperative to obtain informed consent from patients who follow religions where use of animal products (or specific species) is a taboo.

Blood products

Blood products used for IV fluid therapy include red blood cells, fresh, frozen plasma, or platelets depending upon individual patient needs (Cathala and Moorley, 2018).

There is a lack of conclusive evidence over the choice of the type of IV fluid for fluid therapy (Philips et al., 2013). Nurses and healthcare professionals involved in administering IV fluid should refer to local protocols, policies, and NICE guidelines for IV fluid therapy. When considering the use of blood products, an individual's religious and cultural beliefs should be recognised and respected.

Total Parenteral Nutrition

Total Parenteral Nutrition (TPN) is an alternative method of nutrition when the feed is administered directly into the bloodstream intravenously. Indications for administering TPN include severe trauma, bowel obstruction, malabsorption, intestinal failure and non-functioning gut (Lawrence, 2017). Baseline assessment of the person requiring TPN should be done prior to commencing the nutritional therapy. This includes height and weight measurements, biochemical profile and fluid balance. The individual and family members of the person requiring TPN should be fully briefed on the therapy. The medical team, dietetic team and nutritional team are involved for the commencement of TPN. Based on the type of the feed, TPN is administered through a venous line centrally or peripherally using Aseptic Non-Touch Technique (ANTT). Healthcare professionals involved in administering the therapy should be qualified and proficient with the procedure and should report any issues related to the therapy to the medical or nutritional team as appropriate.

ACTIVITY: PAUSE AND REFLECT

In clinical practice, have you come across any patient who required intravenous fluid administration? What was the indication of IV fluid therapy? What type of IV fluid was used, considering the reasons for the fluid choice?

WATCH THE VIDEO

MANAGING THE ADMINISTRATION OF IV FLUIDS

Watch along as you read through this step by step procedure by scanning the QR code with your smartphone camera or via https://study.sagepub.com/rowberry.

ADMINISTRATION OF IV FLUIDS: STEP BY STEP

EQUIPMENT

- Medication Administration Record (MAR)
- IV fluid
- Administration set (gravity set, infusion pump set, blood infusion set, burette set)
- Infusion stand
- Plastic apron
- Gloves

PRIMING AND CONNECTING AN INFUSION SET

- Check the IV fluid prescription on the drug chart. Remember the 5 R's (right patient, right drug, right route, right time, and right dose) (Shepherd and Shepherd, 2020).
- Check the IV fluid expiry date and the bag for any leakage. If an outer covering is present, check that it is intact.
- Inspect the fluid for cloudiness, any change in colour and for presence of any particles/precipitates.
- Choose the correct administration set. IV sets vary based on the type of fluid administered and depending on how the fluid is administered, i.e. if using an infusion pump.

(Continued)

- Gather the required equipment and place it on a clean tray.
- Wash and dry hands thoroughly as per local infection prevention and control policy.
- Explain the procedure to the patient and obtain consent.
- Check the administration set for compatibility and expiry date.
- Ensure hands are cleansed as per local policy and wear disposable apron and gloves (RCN, 2016).
- Open the packaging of the set and check the tubing properly for any damage.
- Close the roller clamp on the tubing to prevent fluid and air bubbles from entering into the set when the bag is spiked.
- Using ANTT (2019) remove the protective covering from the inlet area of the infusion bag and the cap of the administration set spike.
- Employing ANTT, insert the spike firmly and fully into the inlet port of the infusion bag using a twisting motion.
- Hang the bag on the hook of the infusion stand while taking care that the end of the infusion set (with cover on) sits on the plastic tray.
- Squeeze and release the drip chamber of the infusion set to fill the chamber half with fluid. Avoid over filling the chamber as this would prevent visibility of drops dripping into the chamber.
- Check the drip chamber to ensure fluid flows into the tubing and close the roller clamp when fluid reaches the end of the tubing.
- Prior to connecting the infusion, check the patient's identity (Edward and Axe 2015) by verbal check, patient's notes, and check for allergies in the MAR and patient's records with consideration to factors preventing administration of certain fluid types.
- Clean and dry the needleless injection cap using 2% chlorhexidine and 70% alcohol (NICE, 2014).
- Using ANTT, remove the cap from the end of the infusion set and connect it to the needleless injection cap.
- Open the roller clamp and adjust the drop rate according to the prescription on the patient's drug chart.
- When administering IV fluids without use of an infusion pump calculating drops per minute, use the formula:

$$\frac{\text{Volume of fluid} \times \text{Drops per ml}}{\text{Time in hours} / 60} = \text{Drops per minute (RCN, 2019a)}$$

- When using an infusion pump, ensure the correct pump and the right administration set is used.
- Clamp the pump to an infusion stand. Perform the pump checks as per local policy.
- Remember that only healthcare professionals trained and assessed in using the infusion pump can administer intravenous fluids using the pump.
- Switch the pump on. Follow manufacturer instructions to feed the tube through the pump. Instructions for setting the pump may vary depending on the brand of the pump. This could again vary between hospital settings.
- Using the pump keys programme, set the pump to input the volume of fluid to be given and the time over which the fluid needs to be administered.
- Check the display screen on the pump to ensure that the data entered is correct.
- On pressing the start key, the infusion commences. Check that the pump is working, and the infusion has started. On checking the drip chamber of the tubing, drops flowing into the chamber

can be noted if the pump is working. Additionally, the display screen on the pump would show that the pump is infusing the fluid.

- Check that the patient is comfortable and there is no pain, discomfort or change in colour at the infusion site.
- Monitor the patient and the insertion site regularly following local policy.

Points to consider

- Check the infusion rate frequently, especially when fluids are administered using gravity set without use of an infusion pump.
- Observe the cannula (infusion site) regularly. Use scoring sheets to assess the site (Jackson, 1998). Remove the cannula if necessary. Adhere to the local policy.
- Check the administration set for any kinks or damage. Renew the administration set following local guidelines.
- Check the of infusion bag is at least 90cm higher than the patient. Monitor the position of the patient, e.g., flow rate can be affected by a bent arm if the cannula site is near or over the elbow joint.
- If the infusion does not flow correctly, flush the cannula with 0.9% Normal Saline as per local policy. Normal Saline flushed should be prescribed. If pain or swelling occurs upon flushing, the cannula should be removed. The cannula also needs to be removed if it is completely blocked and gentle aspiration of the cannula and flushing of the cannula were not successful.

ACTIVITY: COMMUNICATION SKILLS

Mr Thomas is a 38-year-old man, living in a deprived area of the city. He has difficulty in reading and writing. Consider how you would explain to the patient that they need IV fluid administration. Think about any issues in relation to consent.

Recording fluid intake and output: Discussion

Recording fluid intake and output is also referred to as 'recording fluid balance'. The terms refer to the balance of fluids needed to achieve metabolic function in the body (Welch, 2010). Over 50% of the body is made up of fluids which includes water and essential molecules. The body requires an electrolyte balance to function adequately. An imbalance of electrolytes can cause the body and systems to experience problems, some of which can be life threatening to the patient (cardiac arrythmias for instance). As with all sections to this point, an understanding of A&P – in particular fluid compartments, cells and electrolytes – is needed to make a successful assessment of the patient's fluid balance.

We take on fluids mainly from food and fluid in our diet and the predominant source of fluid loss is via urine output. However, we also lose fluid from the body via faecal matter, vomitus, sweating, respiration and via any drainage present (for example, post-surgery). When fluids in the body are depleted, it triggers our thirst response to take on more fluids. When osmotic concentration increases, the body can experience significant negative effects.

KEY TERMS

Negative fluid balance: deficit in overall volume within the body.

Positive fluid balance: the body's fluid intake is greater than its output.

Authors have debated in the literature whether the recording of fluid balance is a simple task, yet its recording has been criticised as inaccurate or inadequate (Vincent and Mehendrian, 2015). With that in mind, perhaps it is time to review the opinion that this is in fact a simple task. Certainly, the utmost care, attention and accuracy must be given when performing the skill, however the knowledge base needed to do this effectively is far from 'simple.' One key factor in improving in this area may be a greater understanding of the importance of it as well as the associated knowledge that is needed. Accurate record keeping is integral to quality nursing care (NMC, 2018a) and carries a responsibility. Reframing the importance and complexities of this task may go some way towards improving this skill, and in turn patient care in practice.

ACTIVITY: WHAT'S THE EVIDENCE?

More information about hydration is available on the RCN website, or via the link below. Make notes as you read through each section.

https://www.rcn.org.uk/clinical-topics/nutrition-and-hydration/hydration-essentials

---

The recommended daily fluid intake may be perceived to be simple; the reality is complex. There are variations in the amounts of fluid an adult should consume each day. These variations consider, age, gender, pre-existing conditions, external environment and any medications being taken. This could vary based on their requirement due to pregnancy, lactation or any illnesses.

Table 7.4 Recommended intake of fluids in adults (BDA, 2020)

Category	Fluid intake per day (from drinks)
Men	2000ml
Women	1600ml
Pregnant people	1900ml
Lactating people	2200-2300ml

For infants and children fluid requirements change depending on their age and range from 1L for under 3 years of age to 1.5L for older children. If a child is requiring intravenous fluids, then this is calculated depending on their weight.

Table 7.5   Daily fluid requirement for infants and children

Fluid requirement	Per day (ml/kg)
For the first 10kg	100ml/kg
For the second 10kg	50ml/kg
For each kg over 20kg	20ml/kg

Source: NICE.org, 2022

For example, for a child weighing 26kg, they would require 1000 + 500 + 120 = 1620ml/day.

Both sensible and insensible fluid losses differ between individuals based not only on their physiology, but also on their environment. This makes the reality of patient care difficult. A patient who is hyperventilating and receiving non-humidified oxygen may lose more fluid via their respiratory system. A patient with hyperthermia may have increased fluid losses linked to sweat production. If the country, nursing or residential home or ward is too warm, patients will be prone to more fluid loss. This makes fluid assessment more difficult, certainly beyond the scopes of recording an absolutely accurate input and output.

It is relatively simple to add together maintenance intravenous fluid therapy and subtract urine output. However reality is more complex: an example of this is how can you record fluid input from 'sips' of water? Should you record each and every sip, and how can you keep track of these during your other responsibilities? The range of fluid amount in a sip varies between 4 and 29 ml, with an average of 12.75ml (Halpern, 1985). Ten of these sips throughout the day may not seem a great deal, yet if a patient has a fluid restriction of 1L, these sips comprise over 10% of their daily intake.

ACTIVITY: PAUSE AND REFLECT

You are a second-year nursing student, caring for Mr Kubbitz who is 65 years old. He has no known chronic illness but has recently been feeling low in mood and his care and attention of himself has slipped. He lives alone. He occasionally misses meals as his appetite can be low due to lack of activity. Mr Kubbitz has had a recent hospital admission but is now at home and is under the care of the community nursing team. You have been asked to encourage Mr Kubbitz to maintain his oral intake. Based on your experience and knowledge, how would you encourage him to stay hydrated? What good practice have you seen?

When considering urine output, not all patients will have a catheter and certainly not all patients will be able to use a bed pan or urinary bottle. Some patients are incontinent of urine and faeces. The prevalence of urinary incontinence can be approximately 20% of hospitalised patients (Silva APM, 2005). This brings challenges towards measuring output. If a patient is incontinent of urine into a continence pad, a nurse may be able to measure the weight of the pad and consider this fluid volume. What if the patient is incontinent of both urine and faeces? How do we establish fluid loss from solid matter?

The reality of recording input and output is challenging but an understanding of all sources of intake and output as well as using and documenting accurate, quantifiable amounts of fluids is extremely important. Documentation should be in full and be legible, without symbols, abbreviations, approximations, or shorthand. Holistic patient care includes optimal hydration of patients. Understanding how vital water and hydration is to our wellbeing is extremely important.

Many additional patient complications can be avoided by accurately assessing and documenting fluid balance. Both dehydration and overhydration can have detrimental clinical consequences. Significant abnormalities in fluid balance should be reported and communicated to the relevant members of the team.

RECORDING FLUID INTAKE AND OUTPUT: STEP BY STEP

- Explain to the person about the importance of maintaining the fluid balance chart. Involve the family/carers in recording the chart if appropriate.

- Obtain information regarding the capacity of the fluid jug, glass, cup, beaker, mug etc. Ask the person to keep a record of what they drank including the time if they are able to do so. For persons who require assistance with eating and drinking, healthcare professionals can keep the record of the intake when they assist the individual with drinks or administer feed and fluids.

- Measure any other enteral intake including artificial feeds, soups etc. Measure the amount of parenteral intake including intravenous fluids, medications, blood transfusions, parenteral nutrition and catheter irrigations. These entries should be done on the relevant sections on the chart.

- Record the fluid output on the chart as correctly as possible. Avoid abbreviations, symbols and shorthand when completing the chart and record accurately intake and output; 'sips' or 'PU' written on a fluid balance chart tells us very little about a patient's fluid balance status.

- Measure or weigh all output including urine, vomit, post-operative drainage. Incontinence pads and nappies should be weighed, and the weight deducted from the weight of dry incontinence pads or nappies for obtaining the accurate output.

- Fluid balance is calculated by obtaining the difference between the fluid intake and output. Positive and negative fluid balance should be reviewed by the nurse and the doctor daily.

- If you have any concerns regarding a patient's fluid balance or imbalance report to the nurse in charge and/or the medical team.

ACTIVITY: COMMUNICATION SKILLS

Consider what methods of communication you would use to explain why monitoring and documenting fluid intake is important for a patient such as Mr Kubbitz. How will these methods of communication change if he has difficulties understanding verbal information, e.g., due to a learning disability?

How can you educate and involve parents in recording fluid intake of their unwell babies?

CASE STUDY

James

James is a 6-month-old boy who has been admitted with bronchiolitis, which has resulted in reduced oral intake. He does not require oxygen therapy but does need observation of his oral intake. James's parents are very anxious about him being admitted to hospital.

Questions

1   How might bronchiolitis impact James's feeding?
2   How can you support James's parents, and what advice might you offer about feeding?
3   How would you explain to James's parents about documenting fluid intake?

Responding to fluid retention

Fluid retention is a challenging health issue and occurs when there is a problem with the body's mechanism of maintaining fluid levels. Fluid retention is also known as oedema and can affect any part of the body: limbs, brain, lungs and other vital organs. Causes of fluid retention include sodium retention (in heart failure, kidney failure and liver failure), long-term corticosteroid treatment and inappropriate IV fluid therapy (Herlihy and Anderson, 2017). Signs and symptoms of fluid retention include:

- Sudden weight gain
- Swelling of hands and feet
- Distended jugular (neck) veins
- Shortness of breath, high respiratory rate
- Cough, chest pain
- Ascites (swelling in abdominal area)
- Increase in urinary output
- High blood pressure, bounding pulse
- Headache, blurred vision

Management of fluid retention involves treatment of the underlying condition and associated symptoms. Some interventions which could help with reducing fluid retention and relieving symptoms are elevating swollen limbs, controlling fluid and salt intake, monitoring daily weight, keeping an accurate fluid balance chart and using diuretics.

CASE STUDY

Ms Khuala

Ms Khuala is 63 years old and currently being nursed on a general medical ward. She has been receiving IV fluid therapy for the past three days to treat fluid loss due to gastroenteritis. She has developed swelling to her feet (oedema) and shortness of breath in the past hour. She has a history of non-insulin dependent diabetes mellitus type II and congestive cardiac failure.

(Continued)

Nausea and vomiting: Discussion

Nausea is an unpleasant symptom in which the patient may feel the inclination to vomit. It is an extremely common occurrence and can be caused by a wide variety of reasons. Assessment of nausea and vomiting is extremely challenging because the symptoms the patient may describe are subjective and difficult to quantify. While some numerical scoring systems have been used in isolated trials within specialist areas (such as palliative care or obstetrics), they have not been widely adopted in clinical practice nor fully validated for wider use.

Vomiting is a reflex, thought to have developed as a protective mechanism throughout our evolution. It prevents the ingestion of harmful or poisonous substances. While small amounts of vomiting can be distressing for patients, it can often be a self-limiting symptom which resolves spontaneously. For vomiting which is prolonged or profuse, it can be a serious symptom of an insidious underlying pathological process (such as a gastric obstruction) or in itself life threatening.

Nausea and vomiting are in fact separate symptoms and whilst they can be seen in isolation, they are often present together. The feeling of nausea that patients experience can be incredibly distressing and unpleasant for them and can quickly impair their quality of life. It usually originates in the upper gastrointestinal tract or pharynx (throat) and can be associated with dizziness or retching. Retching is the involuntary process of unproductive vomiting, in which the contraction of diaphragmatic muscles contract against a closed mouth. Vomiting represents the final event within the reflex, in which coordination of gastric, abdominal, and respiratory muscle cause rapid expulsion of stomach contents.

Vomiting can deplete the body of nutrients and fluids and upset a multitude of delicately balanced metabolic pathways. It is entirely possible for a patient to vomit to such an extent that they can cause themselves to have a relative alkalaemia due to an excess of gastric acid loss.

As with all aspects of nursing care, nursing assessment is a vital component to effective identification of the cause as well as the commensal of appropriate treatment and management for the patient. While all patients at all ages are at risk of nausea and vomiting, the key is identifying those who are at the most risk of adverse consequences. As innocuous as a small volume of vomiting may be for a younger patient, for an older more vulnerable adult with comorbidities, the reflux of gastric contents into the mouth may be aspirated into the lungs and cause a pneumonia. Aspiration pneumonia, as it's termed, is associated with significant morbidity and mortality.

Table 7.6   Common causes of nausea and vomiting

Post-operative
Drug induced
Hyperemesis in pregnancy
Chemotherapy / radiotherapy
Motion sickness
Excessive and prolonged coughing
Anxiety

Fluid and electrolyte imbalance

Bulimia nervosa

GI obstructions / ascites

Raised ICP

ENT problems

Food toxins / food poisoning

GI viral infections

Include any predisposing conditions such as GORD, gastric ulcers or indigestion also.

Many medications can also cause nausea and vomiting as a side effect. Alongside A&P, pharmacology knowledge also adds to our effectiveness in this area.

Vomiting in babies and children

All babies and children vomit occasionally, in most cases, it will last no more than two days and is not necessarily anything to be concerned about. Babies can often vomit, if they have gastro-oesophageal reflux, or are over fed. The most common cause of vomiting in babies and children is gastroenteritis. This is an infection of the gut that is usually caused by a virus or bacterial infection, which can also cause diarrhoea. Although unpleasant, babies and children usually recover well from the illness after a few days with no adverse effects. However, persistent vomiting in babies and children can cause them to become dehydrated. Signs of dehydration in babies and children include:

- Dry mouth
- Crying without producing tears
- Drowsiness or lethargy
- Reduced urine output, parents may report fewer wet nappies
- Sunken fontanel

More serious conditions that may cause a baby to vomit are pyloric stenosis and intussusception, both of which would need urgent medical review. Pyloric stenosis is a condition present from birth where the passage from the stomach to the bowel has narrowed, food/milk is unable to pass through easily and this can cause projectile vomiting. If the condition is not recognised and treated babies will become dehydrated and not gain weight. Pyloric stenosis is resolved through laparoscopic surgery where the muscle in the narrow passage is cut to widen it. Post-surgery feeding is recommended and increased as tolerated.

Intussusception is where the bowel telescopes in on itself causing the bowel walls to press on one another and cause the bowel to become blocked. If a child presents with severe pain, vomiting, looking pale and lethargic then intussusception should be suspected; they may also have a history of a high temperature, and their stools may contain blood or mucous. An ultrasound scan will usually confirm the diagnosis.

Intussusception is resolved usually through laparoscopic surgery, where the telescopic bowel is gently squeezed to separate segments; the bowel will be inspected to ensure there is adequate blood supply and that the bowel is healthy. Where there is found to be bowel that has inadequate blood flow or the bowel has died, then this section would be removed, and the bowel resected.

Following surgery children would be unable to take oral intake initially to allow time for the bowel to recover, intravenous fluids would be administered, and the child would have a NG tube inserted to drain stomach contents. After a few days children can begin to take fluids orally, gradually building up intake as tolerated.

Post-operative nausea and vomiting

One of the few scoring systems for assessment of post-operative nausea and vomiting was developed by Apfel (1998) and is known as the Apfel Score. It uses four items to predict patients at increased risk, and over recent years, has been validated by a small number of clinical trials. A person's score is based on sex, smoking status, history of previous post-operative nausea and vomiting and use of opioids during the procedure. A score of 1 predicts a 10% likelihood of nausea and vomiting, while a score of 4 suggests an 80% likelihood.

How is vomiting controlled and treated?

Vomiting is coordinated by the 'vomiting centre', an ill-defined area within the medulla oblongata within the brain. While some textbooks argue about the specific anatomy, one thing which many sources agree on is the presence of an area called the Chemoreceptor Trigger Zone (CTZ) which is located within the 'floor' of the medulla. The CTZ receives blood and chemical signals from the systemic circulation, which means it has a rapid response to vomiting stimulus. This also means that any medications which could target and supress the signals received by the CTZ have a role in reducing nausea and vomiting. The CTZ has numerous receptors (Dopamine, Serotonin and 5-HT3 are some examples) and it is these exact receptors which are targeted by many anti-sickness drugs which are used in clinical practice.

Medications that can cause nausea and vomiting include:

- Antidepressants
- Antibiotics
- Antihypertensives
- Bronchodilators
- Cytotoxic drugs
- Corticosteroids
- Digoxin
- Iron preparations
- Levodopa
- NSAIDS
- Oral contraceptives
- Opioids

When assessing the patient, remember to include biochemical disturbances and blood results – there could be reasons here that the patient is experiencing nausea and vomiting.

There are a range of medications that can be prescribed to treat nausea and vomiting; ensure to also assess the route of administration if the patient is actively vomiting (see Chapter 13, Medication Administration). Ensure you accurately monitor and record the effects of any medications administered. Likewise, there are a range of non-pharmacological interventions that can be implemented. Improving the comfort of patients experiencing these symptoms can be achieved through effective treatment and appropriate pharmacological and non-pharmacological interventions. Paying great care to this area of care can offer significant positive outcomes for distressed patients.

ASSESSING NAUSEA AND VOMITING: STEP BY STEP

In-depth assessment should be completed to identify the cause and influence the treatment and management of nausea and vomiting.

ASSESSING VOMIT

- Gather equipment - non-sterile gloves and apron, disposable receiver.
- Wash and dry hands thoroughly as per local infection prevention and control policy and don PPE.
- Where possible, obtain a sample of vomit in a receiver.
- Note observations of the vomit: colour, consistency, amount, presence of blood or other particles. Appearance:
  - Bright red - haematemesis - this can indicate upper gastrointestinal bleed.
  - Yellow/green - bilious - could indicate bile presence due to an obstruction.
  - Coffee ground - this could indicate the presence of old blood.
  - Brown/black - often in large amounts and can indicate acute stomach dilation following surgery or diabetic keto acidosis.
  - Brown, offensive odour - an offensive faecal odour can indicate a late sign of small intestinal obstruction.
- Discard the contents in the clinical waste after making your observations.
- Wash and dry hands thoroughly as per local infection prevention and control policy, change gloves and PPE.
- Offer reassurance and mouthcare to the patient.
- Document and report your findings to appropriate team members.

Certain food, drinks and medications can influence the appearance of vomit. Be mindful and accurate when describing your findings when the vomit has a brown appearance. The inclination to describe all brown vomit as coffee grounds needs to be avoided when looking to do the right thing for the patient. Coffee grounds has a distinctive colour and consistency. Personal observation and inspection are valuable and important in this area.

Management of nausea and vomiting

The distressing experience of nausea and vomiting can have further associated complications for patients, such as the risk of aspiration; pain and local trauma; alteration of nutritional status; loss of fluid and electrolytes; exhaustion and fatigue. Effective management is an essential nursing skill – this is not necessarily done alone but as part of the wider team. Management can fall into two categories: pharmacological and non-pharmacological management.

Pharmacological management

Neurotransmitters such as dopamine, serotonin and histamine are involved and send stimuli to the emetic chemoreceptor and vomit centre located in the medulla. Pharmacological interventions target this process and the receptor sites. The drug groups used include:

- Anti-dopaminergics such as metoclopramide and domperidone
- Antihistamines such as cyclizine
- Anti-cholinergics such as hyoscine
- Serotonin receptor antagonists such as ondansetron

A combination of medications can be used but using two medications from the same group should be avoided. Ensure timely administration of medications via an appropriate route and monitor and record the effectiveness.

Non-pharmacological management

These can include:

- Allow the patient time when eating or drinking and avoiding large amounts of either – offer small amounts often.
- Avoid fatty foods, offer dry foods instead.
- Have patients drink fluids at least half an hour before a meal.
- Allow and encourage the patient to relax when eating or drinking.
- Ensure the patient is sitting upright and remains seated for a while after meals.
- Encourage deep breathing when the patient feels nauseated and avoid restrictive clothing.
- Perform regular oral care.

CASE STUDY

Kato

Kato Thompson is 47 years old. They have been admitted to the ward you are working on with persistent nausea and vomiting for 3 days. They live with their wife and two children aged 17 and 14 years old and work full time as a bank administrator.

Kato's past medical history includes hypertension (recently diagnosed), low iron levels and a recent chest infection. Medication history includes Ramipril 10mg once daily; Ferrous Fumarate 210mg twice daily; and a recent course of antibiotics to treat the chest infection. Kato also deals with anxiety daily. They have been admitted to the ward, and you observe that they have produced bright red vomit.

Blood samples have been taken and sent to the lab, but no results are back at this point. Kato reports they have noticed unintentional weight loss recently when you chat to them, but cannot state how much. They appear anxious and distressed.

Considering what has been covered in this chapter, make a list of the things you will need to consider in relation to the assessment of Kato. Use the below questions for guidance.

Questions

1   What information might you want to gather and what questions might you ask?
2   What clinical skills might you need to use to help them?
3   From the knowledge you have gained are there any potential causes of nausea and vomiting to consider?
4   What nursing care, interventions and management can be offered to Kato?

Note any other considerations or thought points you have.

CHAPTER SUMMARY

This chapter has highlighted some of the important points and complexities of nutrition and hydration in patients you will work with. Evidence-based and best practices have been considered and outlined in relation to this. The nursing skills needed to provide quality care have been identified. You will develop these skills and knowledge base over the duration of your course. Revision and recap of A&P and associated pharmacology will assist your understanding and depth of knowledge.

Accurate and effective assessment of patients is a key and vital area of nursing and needed before effective management can take place. This chapter has discussed nutrition and hydration assessment and some of the tools you will encounter. This chapter is not exhaustive, and a deeper understanding of the practices adopted in the areas you work will further advance your practice and knowledge base. You can gain more information in the Go Further section below.

ACE YOUR ASSESSMENT

Q1   Peristalsis is

    a   the process of food breakdown
    b   the process of taking food into the digestive system
    c   is a series of wave like movements that transport food through the digestive tract

Q2   Nasogastric tubes are inserted through the nose to the

    a   duodenum
    b   stomach
    c   jejunum

Q3   Which of the following is not a sign or symptom of dehydration?

    a   Tiredness
    b   Thirst
    c   Swollen feet

Q4   Colloids are

    a   composed of large molecules which expand the volume of plasma and increase vascular pressure
    b   aqueous fluids containing electrolytes which easily pass through the lining of blood vessels creating balance between the intravascular and extracellular space
    c   red blood cells, fresh frozen plasma or platelets

(Continued)

Q5   What is the fluid requirement of a child weighing 10kg?
     a   500ml
     b   1000ml
     c   750ml

Answers

1   C
2   B
3   C
4   B
5   B

GO FURTHER

For quick look at hydration monitoring and effects of dehydration visit:

Royal College of Nursing (RNC) (2019b) 'Hydration essentials'. https://www.rcn.org.uk/clinical-topics/nutrition-and-hydration/hydration-essentials (accessed January 30, 2023).

The following site covers principles and protocols for IV fluid therapy, assessment and monitoring of the person's likely fluid and electrolyte needs, IV fluid resuscitation, IV fluids for routine maintenance alone and training and education for all healthcare professionals involved in prescribing and delivering IV fluid therapy:

National Institute of Health and Care Excellence (NICE) (2017) *Intravenous Fluid Therapy in Adults in Hospital (CG174)*, nice.org.uk, May 5. https://www.nice.org.uk/guidance/CG174 (accessed October 14, 2022).

This site covers information on IV fluid therapy for healthcare professionals who care for children and young people who need IV fluid therapy, children and young people under 16 years who need IV fluid therapy, their families and carers and commissioners and providers of healthcare services:

National Institute of Health and Care Excellence (NICE) (2015) *Intravenous Fluid Therapy in Children and Young People in Hospital* (ng29), nice.org.uk, December 9. https://www.nice.org.uk/guidance/ng29/resources/intravenous-fluid-therapy-in-children-and-young-people-in-hospital-pdf-1837340295109 (accessed October 14, 2022).

For a quick look at the benefits of nutrition and hydration, use this video:

Oral Health Foundation (2019) 'Sixty second guide to nutrition and hydration' (YouTube video), March 18. https://youtu.be/HHqL_esI5aI (accessed October 14, 2022).

REFERENCES

Apfel, C.C., Kranke, P., Eberhart, L.H., Roos, A. and Roewer, N. (2002) 'Comparison of predictive models for postoperative nausea and vomiting', *British Journal of Anaesthesia*, 88 (2): 234–40.

Aseptic Non-Touch Technique (2019) 'The ANTT-Approach'. https://www.antt.org/resources.html (accessed January 30, 2023).

Baas, L.S. (2012) 'Patient- and family-centered care', *Heart & Lung*, 41: 534–5. www.heartandlung.org/article/S0147-9563(12)00309-3/fulltext (accessed October 14, 2022).

BAPEN (2022) *BDA Nutritional Assessment.* https://www.bapen.org.uk/nutrition-support/assessment-and-planning/nutritional-assessment?start=1 (accessed December 10, 2022).

British Dietetic Association (BDA) (2021) 'Fluid (water and drinks): Food Fact Sheet'. https://www.bda.uk.com/uploads/assets/337cfde9-13c5-4685-a484a38fbc3e187b/Fluidfood-fact-sheet.pdf (accessed October 14, 2022).

British Nutrition Foundation (2016) 'Older Adults'. https://archive.nutrition.org.uk/nutritionscience/life/older-adults.html (accessed October 14, 2022).

Cathala, X. and Moorley, C. (2018) 'Selecting IV fluids to manage fluid loss in critically ill patients', *Nursing Times*, 114 (12): 41–4.

Clavé, P., and Shaker, R. (2015) 'Dysphagia: Current reality and scope of the problem', *Nature Reviews Gastroenterology & Hepatology*, 12 (5): 259–70. doi.org/10.1038/nrgastro.2015.49

Edwards, S. and Axe, S. (2015) 'The ten 'R's of safe multidisciplinary drug administration', *Nurse Prescribing*, 13 (8): 352–60.

Elia, M. (2015) 'The cost of malnutrition in England and potential cost savings from nutritional interventions (short version)', National Institute of Health Research. https://www.bapen.org.uk/pdfs/economic-report-short.pdf (accessed October 14, 2022).

Halpern, B.P. (1985) 'Time as a factor in gustation: Temporal patterns of taste stimulation and response', in: D.W. Pfaff (ed.) *Decisions During Sipping: Taste, Olfaction, and the Central Nervous System.* New York: Rockefeller University Press, pp. 181–209.

Herlihy, E. and Anderson, D. (2017) 'Hydration and fluid balance', in T. Moore and S. Cunningham (eds) *Clinical Skills for Nursing Practice.* Abingdon: Routledge, pp. 545–79.

Hooper, L. and Bunn, D. (2015) 'Detecting dehydration in older people: Useful tests', *Nursing Times*, 111 (32/33): 12–16.

Jackson, A. (1998) 'Infection control: A battle in vein infusion phlebitis, *Nursing Times*, 94 (4): 68–71.

Koyfman, A. (2018) 'Paediatric dehydration', *Medscape*, November 12. https://emedicine.medscape.com/article/801012-overview#a5 (accessed October 14, 2022).

Lawrence, S.K (2017) 'Nutrition', in T. Moore and S. Cunningham (eds), *Clinical Skills for Nursing Practice.* Abingdon: Routledge, pp. 545–79.

Lira, A. and Pinsky, M.R. (2014) 'Choices in fluid type and volume during resuscitation: Impact on patient outcomes', *Annals of Intensive Care*, 4 (4): Article #38.

Miller, H.J. (2015) 'Dehydration in the older adult', *Journal of Gerontological Nursing*, 41 (9): 8–13. doi.org/10.3928/00989134-20150814-02

National Institute of Health and Care Excellence (NICE) (2014) *Infection Prevention and Control. Quality Standard 5: Vascular Access Devices* (QS61), nice.org.uk, April 17. https://www.nice.org.uk/guidance/qs61/chapter/quality-statement-5-vascular-access-devices (accessed October 14, 2022).

National Institute of Health and Care Excellence (NICE) (2017) *Intravenous Fluid Therapy in Adults in Hospital* (CG174), nice.org.uk, May 5. https://www.nice.org.uk/guidance/cg174 (accessed October 14, 2022).

NICE.org (2022) *Treatment Summaries, Fluids and Electrolytes.* https://bnfc.nice.org.uk/treatment-summaries/fluids-and-electrolytes/ (accessed December 2022).

Nuttall, F.Q. (2015) 'Body mass index: Obesity, BMI, and health: A critical review', *Nutrition Today*, 50 (3): 117–28. doi.org/10.1097/NT.0000000000000092

Palmeira, P. and Carneiro-Sampaio, M. (2016) 'Immunology of breast milk', *Revista da Associação Médica Brasileira*, 62 (6): 584–93. doi: 10.1590/1806-9282.62.06.584. PMID: 27849237.

Phillips, D.P., Murat Kaynar, A., Kellum, J.A. and Gomez, H. (2013) 'Crystalloids vs. colloids: KO at the twelfth round?', *Critical Care*, 17 (3): Article #319.

Rothman, K. (2008) 'BMI-related errors in the measurement of obesity', *International Journal of Obesity* 32: S56–S59. doi.org/10.1038/ijo.2008.87

Royal College of Nursing (RNC) (2016) 'Standards for infusion therapy'. https://www.rcn.org.uk/clinical-topics/infection-prevention-and-control/standards-for-infusion-therapy (accessed October 14, 2020).

Royal College of Nursing (2019a) 'Flow rate and IV drugs'. https://www.rcn.org.uk/clinical-topics/safety-in-numbers/flow-rate-and-iv-drugs (accessed October 14, 2020).

Royal College of Nursing (2019b) 'Hydration essentials'. https://www.rcn.org.uk/clinical-topics/nutrition-and-hydration/hydration-essentials (accessed October 14, 2020).

Shepherd, A. (2011) 'Measuring and managing fluid balance', *Nursing Times*, 107 (28). https://www.nursingtimes.net/clinical-archive/nutrition/measuring-and-managing-fluid-balance-15-07-2011/ (accessed October 14, 2020).

Shepherd, M. and Shepherd, E. (2020) 'Medicines administration 2: Procedure for administration of oral medicines', *Nursing Times*, 116 (7): 42–4.

Silva, V.A., Souza, K.L. and D'Elboux, M.J. (2011) 'Incontinência urinária e os critérios de fragilidade em idosos em atendimento ambulatorial [Urinary incontinence and the criteria of frailness among the elderly outpatients]', *Revista da Escola de Enfermagem da USP*, 45 (3): 672–8. PMID: 21710074.

Thomas, D.R., Cote, T.R., Lawhorne, L., Tangalos, E.G. and Morley, J.E. (2008) 'Understanding clinical dehydration and its treatment', *Journal of the American Medical Directors Association*, 9 (5): 292–301.

UK Government (2005) *Mental Capacity Act 2005*. https://www.legislation.gov.uk/ukpga/2005/9/contents (accessed October 14, 2022).

Vincent, M. and Mahendiran, T. (2015) 'Improvement of fluid balance monitoring through education and rationalisation', *BMJ Quality Improvement Reports*, 9 (1): u209885.w4087.

Welch, K. (2010) 'Fluid balance', *Learning Disability Practice*, 13 (6): 33–8.

World Health Organization (2005) *The Treatment of Diarrhoea: A Manual for Physicians and Other Senior Health Workers*. Geneva: WHO. https://apps.who.int/iris/bitstream/handle/10665/43209/9241593180.pdf (accessed October 14, 2020).

World Health Organization (2020) 'Healthy diet', WHO, April 29. https://www.who.int/news-room/fact-sheets/detail/healthy-diet (accessed October 14, 2022).

World Health Organization (2021) 'Infant and young child feeding', WHO, June 9. https://www.who.int/news-room/fact-sheets/detail/infant-and-young-child-feeding (accessed October 14, 2022).

BLADDER AND BOWEL HEALTH

8

JEMMA GUSTAFSON AND TRUDI PETERSEN

NMC STANDARDS COVERED IN THIS CHAPTER

ANNEXE B NURSING PROCEDURES

2.9   Collect and observe urine and stool specimens.

6.1   Observe and assess level of urinary and bowel continence to determine the need for support and intervention, assisting with toileting, maintaining dignity and privacy and managing the use of appropriate aids.

6.2   Select and use appropriate continence products; insert, manage and remove catheters for all genders; and assist with self-catheterisation when required.

6.3   Manage bladder drainage.

6.4   Assess bladder and bowel patterns to identify and respond to constipation, diarrhoea and urinary and faecal retention.

6.5   Administer enemas and suppositories and undertake rectal examination and manual evacuation when appropriate.

6.6   Undertake stoma care identifying and using appropriate products and approaches.

LEARNING OBJECTIVES

After reading this chapter, you should be able to:

- Understand anatomy and physiology related to bladder and bowel health
- Identify and understand factors affecting the body's elimination
- Understand the nurse's role and responsibility in bladder and bowel health
- Understand the technical skills needed to maintain bladder and bowel health
- Explain the assessment and care of a patient requiring bladder and bowel care

STUDENT VOICE

I have learnt that continence and incontinence are equally important.

Sarah Davies, 3rd year, Adult Nursing

INTRODUCTION

The bladder and bowel play essential roles in an individual's overall biopsychosocial health. Nursing skills in relation to this area include assessment and management of conditions, the monitoring of bladder and bowel health, technical and supportive interventions, appropriate referral and signposting, health education and preventative health promotion activity. Care must be risk assessed, holistically focused, and sensitively conducted (or delegated and observed as appropriate) by a trained, competent practitioner (NMC, 2018a).

Bladder and bowel problems are often considered to be issues primarily relating to older adults. They may, mistakenly, be seen as simply part of the ageing process, especially for women in relation to bladder continence. It is true that older adults feature significantly (NICE, 2019). However, assuming poor function to be the 'norm' for this demographic can create a degree of therapeutic nihilism whereby belief in the effectiveness of prevention, treatment or care results in symptom reactive responses, e.g., the routine use of incontinence pads, rather than proactive, for example pelvic floor strengthening exercises. Up to 80% of incontinence can be cured or improved. There is much that nurses can do to help individuals experiencing, or at risk of experiencing, problems (Riemsma et al., 2017).

There is more to bladder and bowel health than continence. It covers a range of populations and conditions as well as being a measure of more general health. This chapter includes recognising healthy bladder and bowel function, recognising and responding to common conditions, nursing procedures and skills, psychological and mental health aspects and effective communication. The ethos is that of holistic, person-centered care.

NURSE'S VOICE

Start thinking differently about continence in a broader context from the onset – make the difference!

Llinos Walters, Specialist Continence Nurse, 2021

BLADDER AND BOWEL HEALTH

Bladder and bowel health are relative terms. For many individuals this will centre on the maintenance of functioning via the body's usual elimination routes. The aim is to preserve normal function of the bladder and bowel whenever possible. Ideally bladder and bowel excretion should be regular, relatively effortless and conducted in such a way as to retain muscle control (Gulanick and Myers, 2022).

For some individuals bladder or bowel heath will be achieved within the parameters of restrictions, such as surgical changes, or through the use of continence equipment. An understanding of 'normal' bladder and bowel health enables the nurse to recognise when an individual is presenting outside of these acceptable parameters. Equally, it is important to understand what 'normal' is for the patients related to their habits and elimination patterns.

Helping an individual attain and maintain bladder or bowel health may be as simple as ensuring that hydration levels are adequate and that the individual is consuming a varied, healthy diet alongside the promotion of general healthy lifestyle choices (NMC, 2018b).

KEY TERMS

Continence and incontinence: to maintain, or the inability to maintain, bladder and bowel control

Defaecation: an elimination of faeces from the body

Diuresis: an excess elimination of urine

DRE: digital rectal examination

DRF: digital removal of faeces

Dysuria: refers to painful urination

Elimination: to eliminate or get rid of a bodily fluid or product

Enuresis: a condition whereby the person has the inability to control urine during the night ('bed wetting')

Micturition: to urinate (normally or abnormally)

Nocturia: like enuresis but with nocturia the person has control and wakes to urinate

Peristalsis: the involuntary constriction and dilation of the intestine which moves products in a wave like forward motion

Peristomal: the skin surrounding a stoma formation

Polyuria: passing excessive amounts of urine while (usually) maintaining a normal fluid intake

PPE: personal protective equipment

PR: per rectum

PU: passed urine

PVR: post void residual, meaning the amount of residual urine left in the bladder after elimination

Stoma: a surgically formed opening in the body

TWOC: trial without catheter

Urostomy: a stoma made to divert the urinary system

Voiding: a term primarily used to describe something draining away or eliminating/discharging

ANATOMY AND PHYSIOLOGY RECAP

Bowel health/system

The stomach

Attached to the oesophagus, the stomach is the main receptor for ingested food/fluid. It contains gastric fluids to assist food breakdown. Once completed, the stomach's muscles move the food into the small intestine.

The small intestine

The small intestine consists of three areas: the duodenum, jejunum, and ileum. The small intestine, specifically the ileum and jejunum, absorbs nutrients from food. The duodenum absorbs secretions and enzymes from the bile duct and pancreas to assist digestive flow.

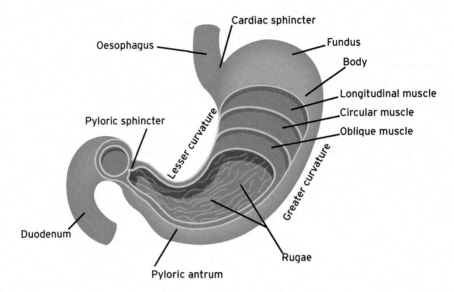

Figure 8.1 **Parts of the stomach**

The large intestine

The large intestine absorbs water from ingested products and produces mucus to assist digestive movement.

The liver and gall bladder

The body's biggest gland, the liver, detoxifies blood. It breaks down red blood cells, produces bile and stores glycogen from ingested carbohydrates. The gall bladder is a small sack that sits alongside the liver. It assists with the breakdown of ingested fat.

The pancreas

Another gland, the pancreas, works with the bile duct, carrying bile from the liver and excreting this into the small intestine, specifically the duodenum.

Bladder health

The kidneys

The kidneys filter waste products and extra water from the blood, excreting these as urine. They maintain the homeostasis and fluid balance of the body/blood.

The bladder

The bladder is the main receptor for waste and urine delivered from the kidneys via two tubes called ureters. Urine is eliminated from the bladder via another tube, the urethra. The urethra is longer in males.

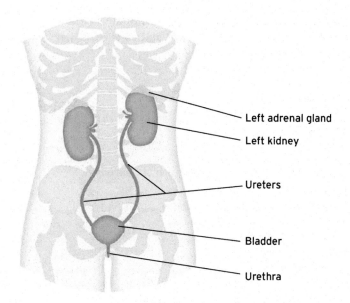

Figure 8.2 Outline of the renal system

The lymphatic system

The lymphatic system filters blood and products within the body. 'Leaking' fluids are mopped up by the lymphatic system and returned to the blood.

URINARY AND BOWEL CONTINENCE

'Normal' bladder elimination

Elimination refers to the voiding of waste from the body, via the bladder or bowel. Bladder elimination is referred to as micturition or, more commonly, urination. Continence means the person can control bladder and bowel movements. Generally, you would expect the elimination to be controlled and to occur from the urethra and anal canal. However, in patients who have had surgery or have certain underlying health issues this may not be possible.

Some patients require equipment aids, some may require surgery (an ostomy) to form a stoma. A stoma is an opening into the abdominal cavity that mimics what the natural biological elimination process of the body would be if fully functioning and not diverted.

Incontinence

Incontinence is a loss of elimination control. It may be voluntary or involuntary, temporary or permanent. Emotional and physical support is not the preserve of specialists. Continence nursing care is fundamental to the care of any patient. Incontinence may be temporary and acute. In some cases, it can be permanent and be the 'new normal' for the patient (Pizzol et al., 2021).

Patients lacking control of their bladder and bowel health can experience reduced self-esteem, confidence and quality of life. There are many factors and conditions that increase the likelihood of incontinence (see box below).

FACTORS INCREASING INCONTINENCE RISK

- Aging
- Certain mental health, cognitive and developmental conditions
- Muscle weakness
- Some medications
- Neurological dysfunction
- Surgery
- Immobility
- Faecal retention or impaction
- Childbirth
- Trauma
- Infection/inflammation

There are distinct types of incontinence. Differentiating between them affects the management and treatment provided:

- **Stress incontinence** – Due to weakened muscles, under pressure of exercising, impact or weight the pelvic floor muscles are not strong enough to control voiding.
- **Urge incontinence** – Occurs from the involuntary muscles of the bladder.
- **Overflow incontinence** – When there is a blockage or obstruction of the urethra, the bladder becomes too full and small amounts will leak out, and inconsistently 'dribble'. (Note: in the bowels faecal overflow incontinence can occur if the bowel is impacted.)
- **Neurogenic incontinence** – Dysfunction of the nervous system, can result in incontinence.
- **Mixed incontinence** – A combination of incontinence types.

(NHS, 2019; Pizzol, 2021)

ACTIVITY: PAUSE AND REFLECT

Consider the last practice area you worked in. How did incontinence and continence feature? Consider the clinical population, service provided and specialism, were there differences in approach?

Are there questions relating to this that you may want to explore further? How can you find out more?

Are you aware of how to signpost and seek specialist referral? Who can you ask, and how can you find out?

Can you further identify who you can discuss the above with? (e.g., practice assessor).

Bladder elimination

Normal bladder elimination (micturition/urination) should be functional, regular, without pain and forceless in effort. Any changes to the patient's norm require attention.

Based on an intake of the recommended 2L per day, an adult should pass 800–2000ml of urine (Moore and Cunningham, 2017).

A calculation, such as the one below, enables you to work out an average of how much a person should pass every hour, based on their weight. The urine to weight ratio (based on adult ratio) is calculated by ml/kg/hr (Cathala and Moorley, 2020; Gulanick and Myers, 2022).

The commonly expected outcome calculation is at least 0.5ml per kg (patient's weight) an hour (0.5ml/kg/hr)

The example is an acceptable range of urine output for a patient who is 60kg:

- Target urine output within 24 hours: 720–1008ml
- Target urine output within 12 hours: 360–504ml
- Target urine output within 6 hours: 180–252ml
- Target urine output within 1 hour: 30–42ml

Within any time range, action is required if urine output falls below or exceeds expected, acceptable parameters. Outside the ideal range output, at either end of the scale, are conditions which are defined by excess, or inadequate, urine production.

As highlighted above, the recommended fluid intake is 1.6L per day for women and 2L per day for men (this can vary, see Chapter 7). It is worth noting that too much oral intake may be as dangerous as dehydration. Drinking very excessive fluid, or not having a way to remove it, can cause overhydration. The body retains water consequently, losing/diluting valuable elements within the blood. Electrolyte imbalance can occur. Sodium (Na) balance may be compromised. Low sodium levels – hyponatremia – can result in disorientation, fatigue and confusion as well as more life-threatening symptoms including low blood pressure and potential cardiac arrest.

Consideration must be made to patients who are demonstrating other signs and symptoms or patients who are clinically deteriorating. Consider assessing the patient fluid input and output for an accurate fluid balance (see Chapter 7).

Anuria

In adults anuria is a severe condition where the patient has passed less than 500ml in 24 hours (<500ml/d). Reporting, assessing, and monitoring must commence if it is identified that the urine output is less than 0.5 ml/kg/hr (Gulanick and Myers, 2022).

Some conditions such as chronic/acute kidney problems, acute kidney injuries, cardiogenic shock, sepsis and hypovolemia can cause anuria. When urine is not passed, the kidneys struggle to eliminate waste products. This can be life threatening. Anuria is usually acute but people with chronic kidney conditions may live with anuria. Haemofiltration can be used to filtrate the waste from the blood to stabilise haemostatic balance as a form of management.

In such a case where anuria is acute, close monitoring of the patient will be required. This will mean following local guidance and policy while applying clinical judgement and tools to aid assessment. In a condition such as acute kidney injury where anuria occurs, the nurse will need to holistically assess, using an A–G assessment, monitor fluid balance (see Chapter 7), and monitor blood and urine samples to be collected and sent for sampling, measuring specifically the urea and electrolytes in the blood that will determine how the kidneys are functioning in filtering waste products. A build-up of the waste within the body will cause a variety of signs and symptoms that may need additional nursing interventions and medical attention.

Polyuria

Polyuria refers to excessive passing of urine. It is unlikely that the patient will become dehydrated because it is not a case of fluid imbalance. The body is making more urine for the body to pass. Polyuria may indicate an underlying medical condition requiring investigation. Polyuria may arise from a wide range of conditions including, but not limited to: endocrine dysfunction, e.g., diabetes mellitus; diabetes insipidus; pituitary adenoma; kidney dysfunction; and metabolic disorder, including hypocalcaemia and potassium depletion.

Lifestyle choices or habits, such as excessive fluid intake or caffeine intake, can cause polyuria. It can also arise iatrogenically via prescribed medication, for example diuretics or lithium. The patient may benefit from a medication review and titration where necessary (Baines et al., 2021). Polyuria may be accompanied by polydipsia and excessive fluid intake.

Bowel elimination

Prevention is usually better than cure. Ensure the patient eats a regular diet with adequate fibre, is well hydrated and active. Clinical factors and conditions can affect a patient's regular bowel habit, for example, obstruction, medication, chronic conditions such as diverticular disease, cancer, rectal prolapse and trauma. Untreated constipation, notably in older adults, can lead to a toxic confused state which may mimic or worsen dementia symptoms.

URINARY AND BOWEL ASSESSMENT

Bristol stool chart assessment tool

The quality and appearance of stools can indicate a range of conditions. Developed in 1997, the Bristol stool chart is a visual assessment tool that aids clinical judgement and forms part of initial and ongoing bowel function assessment. Examination can also be used pre- and post-operation, or treatment, to help identify adverse effects. The chart enables the nurse to assess bowel outputs using a standardised visual and descriptive tool thus minimising differences in perception or description between staff.

BRISTOL STOOL CHART

	Type 1	Separate hard lumps	Very constipated
	Type 2	Lumpy and sausage like	Slightly constipated
	Type 3	A sausage shape with cracks in the surface	Normal
	Type 4	Like a smooth, soft sausage or snake	Normal
	Type 5	Soft blobs with clear-cut edges	Lacking fibre
	Type 6	Mushy consistency with ragged edges	Inflammation
	Type 7	Liquid consistency with no solid pieces	Inflammation

Figure 8.3   Bristol stool chart

Source: Wikimedia Commons/Cabot Health, Bristol Stool Chart (CC BY-SA 3.0)

Stool quality indicates hydration/dehydration. The large intestine extracts water from stools and re-purposes this around the body, creating characteristic lumpiness of stool. This shows that the colon and large intestine are working effectively. The tool allows for identification of patterns, changes and frequency which guides intervention. For example, if the patient was having frequent type 2 stools, you might consider prompting and encouraging oral fluid intake (allowing for other relevant clinical factors) with the ideal goal of type 4 stool production.

The appearance of urine has long been recognised as a principal factor in assessment. Tools such as the one illustrated below were known to have been used by medieval apothecaries. However, unlike the Bristol stool chart, there is no one contemporary, standardised visual assessment tool for urine.

Whilst we do not taste urine anymore (yes, honestly, they used to!) visual assessment remains a vital element, providing insight into an individual's systemic state and changes and facilitating appropriate nursing and other treatment responses.

Visual assessment may prompt a urinalysis. It is important to recognise other sensory changes such as odour in the patient's urine to inform diagnosis of an illness, an acute problem or adverse reaction to treatment/medication, with considerations made to clinical conditions (Flamarion et al., 2021).

Urine colour: What can you see?

Generally speaking, urine in a fairly hydrated person should be a 'hay-coloured' or 'yellow tinged' clear fluid. The intensity of this colour may vary, dependent on the urobilin in the urine. Urobilinogen is a by-product of bilirubin. The breakdown of haemoglobin, when excreted, oxidises into urobilin. The visual presentation of urine can identify underlying affecting factors. These can include diet, hydration levels, clinical condition, and medication.

ACTIVITY: PAUSE AND REFLECT

Fatima is a 40-year-old Muslim woman. She was born in Sudan. She was recently admitted to your practice area. She has been asked to provide a urine sample. You notice the colour is dark brown.

1   What could you ask to identify the cause of the colouration?

Key considerations should include how much fluid she drinks (dehydration can cause dark urine), what symptoms she has (these may indicate an infection), whether she is taking any medication and what she has eaten in the last couple of days.

Fatima says that she is currently abstaining from food and drink in the day due to Ramadan. After sundown they eat. Her family's favourite is a traditional Sudanese dish which contains a large quantity of fava (broad) beans. Fava beans can turn urine brown. Abstaining from fluids could also result in her being somewhat dehydrated in the day so you may want to encourage her to drink fluids when she is able to.

2   Nurses should provide care in a culturally competent way. How could you improve your cultural competency?

Below are a few additional examples of medications/foods that can change the colour of urine.

(Continued)

- **Anticoagulants** – red, pink, blush colour: think bleeding?
- **Vitamin B-complex** – blue/green
- **Nitrofurantoin** – bright yellow
- **Levodopa** – brown
- **Amitriptyline** – green
- **Rhubarb** – pink
- **Asparagus** – bright yellow/green (odorous)
- **Beetroot** – pink

Other foods, infection, pH values and health conditions can also cause changes. Coloured urine can also be indicative of the kidneys doing their job as they should, excreting substances that are unable to be metabolised.

Table 8.1   Urine assessment: What to expect vs the unexpected

Urine colour	Description	Management
Clear-yellow	Normal urine could be described as 'straw-coloured'.	• Monitor vital signs. • Monitor fluid balance. If grossly positive, patient could be fluid overloaded and deplete of vital electrolytes such as sodium and potassium. • Blood test to measure urea and electrolyte balance (U&Es).
Amber-orange	Darker urine is typically 'concentrated' as it indicates reduced oral intake of water or excessive losses (such as diahorrea and vomiting).	• Monitor vital signs. • Encourage oral intake of fluids. • Monitor fluid balance. If grossly negative, patient may require intravenous fluids following a review by a responsible clinician. • Blood test to measure urea and electrolyte balance (U&Es). • Medications review may be required as diuretic medications (such as furosemide) may be causing excess fluid losses.
Pink or rust	Redness in urine is often a sign of blood within the urine. This can come from a number of causes, such as: • Menstruation • Infection • Trauma • Post-cystoscopy • Anticoagulation medication use • Coagulopathy • Malignancy	• Monitor vital signs. • Monitor fluid balance. • Conduct urinalysis. • Blood test to measure urea and electrolyte balance (U&Es) as well as haemoglobin levels and infection markers (FBC). • Medication review – anticoagulants/antiplatelet medication may need to be stopped. • Keep catheter in-situ. • Full A-G assessment.
Bright red blood	Often called 'frank haematuria', this demonstrates active bleeding from the urogenital system.	• This can often be extremely frightening for the patient, so remember to give reassurance! • Monitor vital signs. • Monitor fluid balance. • Escalate immediately to the patient's medical team. • Blood test to measure urea and electrolyte balance (U&Es) as well as haemoglobin levels and infection markers (FBC). • Medication review – anticoagulants/antiplatelet medication may need to be stopped. • Keep catheter in-situ. • Full A-G assessment.

This list is not exhaustive. There are other conditions that may influence the colour of the urine (Cathala and Moorley, 2020; Gulanick and Myers, 2022).

Consideration must be made in regard to patients who are demonstrating other signs and symptoms or patients who are clinically deteriorating.

Visual assessment

Clarity

Clarity refers to the visual presentation of the urine. Can you see through the urine? Is it clear? The urine may have a tint of colour but present as transparent with nothing occluding. Some normal urine may be a little cloudy even if the patient is well hydrated. Very clear urine may indicate over hydration. An abnormal visual can be described as cloudy, or turbid. Can you see any particles, crystallization, sediment or debris?

Odour

Fresh urine should have little or no smell. Odour may result from ingested medication, food or fluids. It can also indicate clinical conditions such as an infection, or the existence of excess waste products such as ketones.

Osmolarity

Osmolarity is the concentration of the urine. This may be determined by particles or sediment. This may give you an idea of kidney function and the need for further investigative tests.

Common bladder assessments

Urinalysis is a simple non-invasive procedure. It is a common diagnostic tool that can identify a range of elements including indicators of infection. The urine is tested with a small diagnostic reagent strip. It is commonly known as the 'dip stick' test.

What is tested:

- **Glucose** – Excretion of sugar in the urine. Excessive glucose may indicate diabetes. This should be as part of a broader diagnostic investigation.
- **Proteins** – The kidneys filter waste products, however the body needs protein. When protein is detected in the urine, this means the kidneys may not be functioning optimally, indicating a potential infection or an acute kidney injury (NICE, 2019).
- **PH** – The normal pH of the body is 7.35–7.45. Urinalysis can identify if urine is acidic or alkalotic. This may indicate kidney stones or other underlying kidney problems.
- **Leukocytes** – The primary function of leukocytes (white blood cells) is to fight infection. Their presence demonstrates that they are attacking bacteria, inflammation or an infection. Normally the kidneys would filter blood products from the urine. This may indicate a functioning discrepancy in the kidney/kidneys.
- **Nitrates** – A by-product, produced in the presence of bacteria, usually in the urinary tract, nitrates also indicate infection. Thus, a supportive diagnostic test for a Urinary Tract Infection (UTI).
- **Blood** – See above for the principles of kidney filtration. Unlike white blood cells, red blood cells may cause visible colour change. This is not always the case. Blood may be invisible to the eye but present and identifiable by the test.

- **Bilirubin** – Produced in the liver and formed from the breakdown of red blood cells. Bilirubin in the urine can identify gall bladder or liver conditions which will need further investigation. In order to get rid of excess bilirubin the body excretes and eliminates it via urination (Hoilat and Savio, 2021).
- **Ketones** – Produced by the liver to aid the fatty acid metabolism process. With a balanced diet ketones should be metabolised and should rarely be detectable in urine (or blood). However, if the body does not get enough glucose (sugar) the body will switch to using the stores of body fat and be unable to metabolise the ketones, resulting in ketones in the urine. This is significant when caring for a patient with diabetes. Diabetic ketoacidosis can be a life-threatening condition. Diabetic ketoacidosis can also result from illnesses such as chest infections, flu and UTIs. Ketones can also occur in individuals without diabetes who are not eating or drinking adequately (some popular, very limiting, diets promote this) or have severe diarrhoea and vomiting or certain other medical conditions.

Following a positive urinalysis test, the sample, or a further midstream specimen of urine, should be sent for further investigation for cultures and sensitivities. Urinalysis should not be a sole diagnostic tool. Consideration needs to be made to other signs and symptoms. When the additional specimen is sent for further investigation, signs and symptoms should be added to the request form under additional clinical information.

Some conditions that may cause changes in bladder and bowel health include:

- **Hyponatremia** – symptoms for hyponatremia (low calcium levels in the blood) include increased urine output
- **Hyperkalaemia** – high potassium levels in the blood. This can lead to urine abnormalities
- **Drug toxicity** – diarrhoea
- **Acute kidney injury** – decreased urine output
- **Diabetes** – increase and frequency in urination
- **Bladder/bowel dysfunctions/cancers**
- **Infection and inflammation**

(Gulanick and Myers, 2022)

ACTIVITY: PAUSE AND REFLECT

Jay visits you in General Practice setting. He has symptoms of burning when urinating and incomplete voiding. The doctor has asked you to test the urine using the 'dip stick' method. Jay is a first language English speaker but has a limited vocabulary and struggles to understand complex language.

1   How will you explain, in easy-to-understand language, the following to Jay: what the test is for, what the test consists of, why it is being done and what potential follow up there may be?
2   Are there terms you might be familiar with, but Jay may not be? How would you re-word these to ensure understanding?
3   How would you check that Jay understood what you told him?

CLINICAL SKILLS RELATED TO BLADDER AND BOWEL HEALTH

HOW TO TAKE A MIDSTREAM SPECIMEN OF URINE (MSU) AND URINALYSIS TEST: STEP BY STEP

- Hand hygiene performed as per local guidelines.

- Introduce yourself to the patient, check identity and allergies. Discuss signs and symptoms with the patient to obtain a holistic assessment and help diagnosis.

- Gain consent to undertake the procedure. Maintain dignity and privacy at all times.

- An explanation should be provided regarding the procedure. Explain to the patient that they will need to urinate in the specimen bottle. The patient will need to part the labia and clean the meatus with a little soap and water from front to back or cleanse the tip of the penis. Assistance can be provided as appropriate. Consider cultural sensitivity, any preferred helper gender and any requirement for a chaperone. Use an aseptic non-touch technique if assistance is given to the patient.

- Explain that the urine flow needs to be midstream, meaning the first bit of urine is passed before collecting the sample 'midstream'. Avoid bottle contamination and ensure the sample is enough. Complete elimination into the toilet.

- If the individual will struggle with a small pot, a larger collection vessel (i.e., a disposable bowl or urine bottle) may be used to collect, prior to decanting into a urine bottle.

- Dignity and privacy must be maintained at all times.

- Hand hygiene performed as per local guidelines.

- Check, prepare and clean the trolley. Use personal protective equipment.

- Check and prepare all equipment needed is in date and intact (unopened) and where necessary sterile.

- Hand the specimen bottle to the patient and allow them to carry out the procedure unless initial discussion indicates assistance or a different receptacle is needed.

- Once complete, conduct hand hygiene and don apron and clean gloves in a clean area.

- Dip the reagent strip into the urine, covering all coloured testing sites for no longer than a few seconds.

- Hold the strip alongside the guidance/visual categorising chart on the side of the container.

- Wait the required time before observing colour changes and reading the results (usually no more than 90 seconds, however manufacturer guidance may differ, so check).

- Note results and assess if a sample needs to be sent for culture and sensitivities.

- Dispose of waste appropriately as per disposal policy.

- Wash hands.

- Send a MSU sample if indicated.

- Provide health promotion advice as indicated.

- Inform the necessary involved health professionals of actions taken and results.

- Document results and additional actions.

Align the reagent strip in line with the parameters on the bottle. Below is an example of the strip alongside the parameters for ketones. You are able to see that you get a clear visible and logical result that the ketones are elevated within the urine above 16mol/L. Armed with this result and potentially other positive results and signs and symptoms, it would be advisable to send an MSU/CSU for further investigation and culture sensitivities.

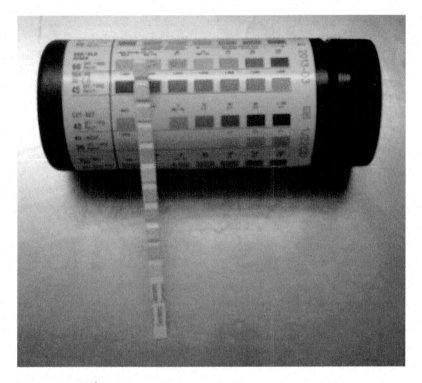

Figure 8.4 Reagent strip/result

Source: Wikimedia Commons/J3D3 (CC BY-SA 3.0)

ACTIVITY: WHAT IS THE EVIDENCE?

Detecting UTIs in adults over 65 years old and catheter users

It is general practice to perform a urinalysis test (dip stick) to detect a urine infection, however current evidence suggests this test should not be used to formally diagnose a UTI in adults aged 65 years or older (NICE, 2019), although the test can still be used in order to detect components in the urine that will give a practitioner an indication what is happening systemically, e.g. glucose, blood, bacteria and white blood cells.

A significant number of older adults, and patients with long term catheters, may have bacteriuria - bacteria present in the urine. Without any additional symptoms, this is normal. It is vital that patients are assessed holistically. You should assess for additional signs and symptoms suggesting infection is present. If symptoms are present, a midstream urine specimen or catheter specimen should be sent for culture.

To avoid antimicrobial resistance asymptomatic bacteriuria should not be treated with antibiotics. A high percentage of adults over 65 are regularly, and unnecessarily, prescribed antibiotics because of urinalysis. This adds to diagnostic overshadowing. Antibiotic treatment via IV access can increase the risk of infection, phlebitis, extravasation and adverse drug reactions (Gharbi et al., 2019).

Additionally, do not dip stick urine from a catheter from a patient using self-catheterisation. A catheter specimen of urine should be sent if clinical judgement supports this (meaning that the patient has signs and symptoms of a UTI).

CATHETERISATION AND URINARY DRAINAGE: DISCUSSION

All catheters used in the UK should have a UKCA mark to indicate they are fit for purpose and can be used clinically. The mark is indicative that the manufacturer has conformed to safety regulations and legislation in terms of medical equipment (UK Government, 2022). Ensure that a comprehensive assessment of the equipment is undertaken in order to assess size required and suitability. This will also assess sterility (where applicable), dates and safety.

A catheter is a general medical term used for a tube that breaches an aseptic site and is inserted into the body for medical use. This may be for acute intervention, for comfort and support, or chronic maintenance. Catheters are sometimes also called cannulas; some examples include vascular, arterial, drains and urethral. Catheters have different functions: some take fluid away from the body, and some can be used in order to insert medication, fluid or other treatment into the body. Urethral catheterisation is a common, invasive procedure.

A urethral catheter takes urine away and out of the body. Although a specialist task, medication can be given through the urethral catheter to target precise areas, such as directly into the bladder for disease management. In this instance the catheter may not be inserted to purely drain the urine but specifically to treat, for example chemotherapy into the bladder as treatment for bladder cancer following a trans urethral resection of a tumour (Anderson, 2018).

Some clinical indications for catheter use

- Surgical procedures that require urinary drainage (pre- or post-surgery)
- Acute deterioration
- Urinary retention
- Blocked urine flow
- Trauma
- Nerve damage to bladder
- Spinal injury or spinal cord compression
- Medication
- Bladder irrigation
- Accurate monitoring of fluid balance

ACTIVITY: PAUSE AND REFLECT

'Need' is the prime rationale for assessing if a patient requires a urethral catheter. Why do they need it? What for? The need for treatment? How long is it needed for?

Assessment determines the need. Does the patient have urine output below 500ml in 12 hours? If the patient is continuing to urinate, post void volume must be assessed, calculated and documented with ongoing monitoring. In the case of the patient going into complete urinary retention or oliguria, a bladder scan should be performed by a competent practitioner in order to assess if, and how much, urine is retained.

Scanning the bladder with ultrasound is a technique where sound waves are pulsed into the bladder, creating a series of vibrations. These vibrations create echoes within the body which are measured in order to build a black and white image of non-dense and dense tissue. An approximate measurement of urine present is produced giving an amount of residual quantity (Moore and Cunningham, 2022).

BLADDER SCANNING: STEP BY STEP

- Gain consent for the procedure.
- Prepare all equipment, ensure that it is all in date, maintenance checked and clean.
- Ensure the patient is ready and prepared for the procedure.
- Ensure privacy and dignity at all times.
- Locate the bladder anatomically (below navel, above pubic bone).
- Adjust the parameter on scanner and insert patient details.
- Place ultrasound gel on the patient and a spot on the ultrasound gun.
- Place ultrasound gun to abdominal area to locate bladder on the screen.
- Once the bladder is detected the scanner will indicate that it is measuring urine.
- Ensure this is recorded, and print report.
- Clean the patient, safely dispose of equipment, wash hands.
- Disinfect scanner and equipment.
- Document findings and inform the appropriate medical professional.

Bladder scans can be used if the patient is not in retention and is eliminating but you are unsure if they are fully emptying their bladder. This is a post-void scan.

Catheterisation should be a last resort procedure due to its invasive nature. It should not be used to 'treat' incontinence. Additional avenues should be explored to support the patient experiencing incontinence. Additional continence accessories should be used to support and protect the skin, whilst promoting independence. The following may encourage and support the patient:

- Convene catheters
- Continence diaries
- Intentional roundings
- Incontinence pads (only if necessary)
- Health promotion
- Good communication
- Supporting mobility to bathroom or commode

Catheters and bladder drainage

The need to catheterise a patient must have accurate clinical rationale in order to protect the patient from the risk of an invasive procedure. Risk could include infection, bleeding, medically restricted mobility and displacement. These can add further symptoms and deteriorating factors to a patient's already acute or frail clinical status. Improper assessment of need and management of urethral catheters can severely impact on clinical status and wellbeing, adding to morbidity and duration of hospital stay, resulting in meaning more time spent managing and caring for a patient with a catheter with time and money implications at organisational level (Centres for Disease Control 2015; Gilbert et al., 2018).

Once need and rationale for catheter insertion is identified, the procedure can be undertaken by a competent registered practitioner or suitably identified and supervised student nurse in line with local guidance and policies. It is important to recognise that there are different types of catheters and different sizes that enter the bladder. Both need and patient will affect the chosen type and size. Routine catheterisation should be avoided for reasons that cannot be evidenced, such as incontinence. Once inserted, a catheter passport is provided to the patient. The passport records treatment and care provided; this helps with communication and continuity and will alert service providers of products used, problems, dates and management. Local catheter types may differ. Catheter choice will be dependent on a holistic, person centred, multidisciplinary team assessment. Factors to consider:

- Lifestyle
- Comfort
- Patient wants and needs
- Local policy and formulary
- User-friendlyness
- Accessories and other features
- Reason for insertion

Intermittent Catheterisation: Discussion

A less invasive way to drain the bladder is by an intermittent catheter, self-administered by the patient. Considered the gold standard of catheterisation (NICE, 2018), 'self-catherisation', following education and training, enables the patient to drain the bladder as required. The catheter is only inserted long enough to drain the urine, then removed. The same technique as for an indwelling catheter is used but with self-management of bladder health, promoting independence, confidence and wellbeing. If the patient cannot manage this technique, it can be done by a competent practitioner in the interim.

The skill includes the patient inserting a catheter through the urethra and into the bladder in a time period just enough to drain the bladder (into a clean bowl, bag or toilet). It is then removed. The skill should be performed in a place that offers privacy, space and good lighting. The patient may choose to use a mirror to aid insertion. Patients undertaking this procedure should have an appropriately sized catheter. Learning should be over time at specific times throughout the day so that it fits into their lifestyles. Some may benefit from a continence diary.

Indwelling catheters

Indwelling catheters are often called 'long-term' catheters. However, their function may be short or long term dependent on need. This the main skill discussed in this chapter which includes a step by step procedural guide. An indwelling catheter has the same level of invasiveness as an intermittent catheter; however it stays in the bladder for a longer period of time. Once the catheter is inserted correctly into the bladder urine will appear in the tubing; this will show that you are in the right location. To retain the catheter a small balloon at the distal end is inflated with sterile water, usually supplied in a pre-drawn syringe (fluid quantity and pre-drawn syringe dependent on local manufacture guidelines). The catheter can stay in-situ for up to 12 weeks, and be replaced as needed, again guided by manufacturer guidelines. Ongoing assessment is needed. Regular flushing and maintenance may be needed in the interim.

Rationale for an indwelling catheter needs careful consideration. Insertion may be required for patients unable to urinate independently or who are in urine retention. Other rationales may include the need for accurate measurement of urine passed for fluid balance reasons, or if the patient is on a fluid restriction due to being overhydrated, secondary to a clinical condition, for example congestive cardiac failure where kidney damage may occur because of build-up of urine and where intervention is critical to maintain renal perfusion.

Documentation is key in the tracking, management and maintenance of the skill, and to continuously assess need and changes. Documentation includes the stickers present on catheters – one should be included in patient/nursing notes and one in the catheter care plan. Each medical device supporting the needs of the patient should be care planned. The care plan can identify trends, changes and clinical judgement. In terms of urethral catheterisation care planning, the care plan will support nursing care and intervention, enable practitioners to identify signs of infection, record maintenance of ANTT and the duration the device has been in-situ. This supports the efficacy and continuity of care provided by the nurse (NMC, 2018b).

Suprapubic catheters

This is where the catheter is inserted directly into the bladder through the abdominal wall. This may be more suitable for a catheter that is needed for a longer term as part of management for a chronic illness as it is less visible. This method avoids insertion in the genital area and thus may lessen the risk of infection as the abdominal area may be easier to keep clean. The patient may find it preferable if sexually active.

A suprapubic catheter may be more suitable for patients who have had surgery or illness affecting the urethra, genital area or bladder. Consideration must be made to risk of infection, frailty of the patient, skin and anatomy of the genital area, surgery or disease to bladder or urethra, patient's posture and positioning (Gibson et al., 2019).

Catheter sizes

Prior to catheterisation, ensure a thorough assessment has been done to ensure the products picked are appropriate to the patient's need. Always ensure that the smallest possible size for the patient is chosen to avoid trauma on insertion, urethral and bladder spasms and the risk of the urine bypassing the catheter.

Fr/Ch is the abbreviation used to describe the method used to measure the gauze (dimensions) of the catheter. Manufacturers differ in sizing methods used. Fr is the French Scale and Ch is Charrière (method).

Common measurements:

- Male: 12Fr,14Fr, 16Fr
- Female: 12Fr, 14Fr
- Suprapubic: 16Fr, 18Fr

WATCH THE VIDEO

CATHETERISATION

Watch along as you read through this step by step procedure by scanning the QR code with your smartphone camera or via **https://study.sagepub.com/rowberry**.

FEMALE CATHETERISATION: STEP BY STEP

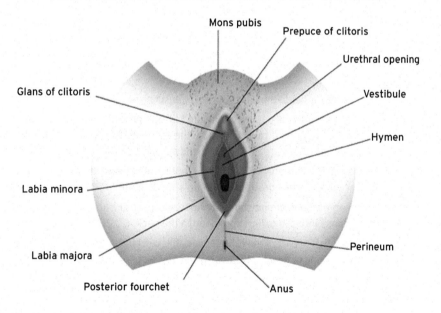

Figure 8.5 The external female genitalia

EQUIPMENT

- Catheter bag holders and hangers
- Urine drainage bag

(Continued)

- Leg bag
- Unistand floor stand
- Catheter pack
- Lubricant
- Catheters
- Abdominal strap
- Urine meter drainage bag

PROCEDURE

- Explain and discuss the procedure with the person, ensure privacy and obtain consent. Ensure you have underlying knowledge and theory to support the skill and are competent to undertake the skill. Inform the patient of the rationale and process. Ensure an assessment is carried out and that anatomical requirements, need and rationale are evident.
- Ensure the right equipment/products are picked.
- Check and prepare the equipment required. Ensure sterility (where applicable) and cleanliness of packaging and that all equipment is in date.
- Wash hands.
- Prepare the trolley/surface and equipment, ensuring ANTT is followed. Check all expiry dates and that sterility and packaging is intact.
- Take the trolley to the bedside, prepare patient. Ensure dignity and privacy is maintained.
- Wash hands.
- Open the catheter pack on to the top of the trolley, ensuring ANTT is maintained.
- Perform hand hygiene, then using the orange/yellow disposal bag as a 'sterile glove', move the items around the aseptic critical field.
- Fix the orange/yellow disposal bag to the side of the trolley, ensuring no contamination of the aseptic field.
- Hand hygiene. Open all additional equipment needed for the procedure and drop them into the aseptic critical field. Be careful not to contaminate the area with the outer packaging. Catheter and 2x pairs sterile gloves (these are additional to the pack as you will need to decide on sizing).
- Slide, or carefully drop, the catheter in the micro aseptic critical field. If 10ml of sterile water is part of the catheter pack and pre-drawn up this can also be placed on the aseptic field.
- Clean the top/opening of the cleaning solution and leave to air dry (usually 0.9% sodium chloride). Open and dispense into the gallipot provided in the pack.
- Open sterile anaesthetic gel (if part of the catheter pack this can be placed on the sterile field). If not, keep in packaging on the side of the aseptic field (the micro aseptic critical field). Prime the catheter.
- Open the catheter bag but leave in micro aseptic field.
- Prepare the patient and place the procedure/surgical sheet underneath the patient.
- Using the saline solution and gauze (or sterile cleansing swabs) part the labia and clean wearing gloves, use saline soaked gauze to clean the vaginal area and catheter. Part the labia, always using one swab action, away from the meatus/urethral opening.
- Prime and insert a little anaesthetic gel at the tip of the urethra, and following a little time insert the tip of the syringe and insert the remaining anaesthetic gel into the urethra (usually approx. 6ml remaining).
- Follow manufacturer guidance for the anaesthetic gel to take effect (usually 2–3 mins).

- Remove gloves, hand hygiene and don new pair of sterile gloves.
- Insert the tip of the catheter into the urethra and advance slowly in an upward motion. Advance approx. 5-6cm (dependent on manufacturer guidance).
- If resistance is felt, ask the patient to cough and relax. Do not advance if resistance is felt following this.
- Always observe the patient for any pain or discomfort.
- Once urine is seen in the sterile catheter packaging, advance a further 2-5cm.
- Inflate the distal balloon using the external port; using the prefilled syringe of sterile water ensure ANTT, and withdraw the catheter carefully to ensure internal security.
- Attach the chosen catheter bag.
- Remove all used PPE and wash hands, retain stickers and labels needed for documentation.
- Discard all used and contaminated equipment and PPE.
- Document procedure and stick labels in appropriate catheter care plan.
- Assess and monitor patient post-catheterisation for adverse reactions or systematic responses.

(Dougherty and Lister, 2015; Moore and Cunningham, 2017; RCN, 2021)

MALE CATHETERISATION: STEP BY STEP

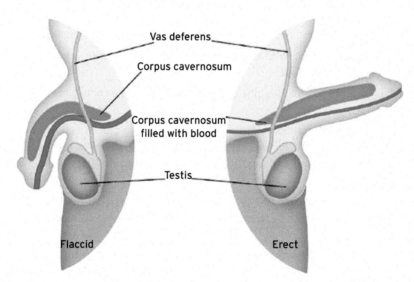

Figure 8.6 The flaccid and erect penis

EQUIPMENT

- Catheter bag holders and hangers
- Urine drainage bag
- Leg bag
- Unistand floor stand

(Continued)

- Catheter pack
- Lubricant
- Catheters
- Abdominal strap
- Urine meter drainage bag

PROCEDURE

- Explain and discuss the procedure with the person, ensure privacy and obtain consent. Ensure you have underlying knowledge and theory to support the skill and are competent to undertake the skill. Inform the patient of the rationale and process. Ensure an assessment is conducted and that anatomical requirements, need and rationale are evident.
- Ensure the right equipment/products are picked.
- Check and prepare the equipment required. Ensure sterility (where applicable) and cleanliness of packaging and that all equipment is in date.
- Wash hands.
- Prepare the trolley and equipment, ensuring ANTT is followed. Check all expiry dates and that sterility and packaging is intact.
- Take the trolley to the bedside, prepare patient. Ensure dignity and privacy is maintained.
- Wash hands.
- Open the catheter pack on to the top of the trolley, ensuring ANTT is maintained.
- Perform hand hygiene, then using the orange disposal bag as a 'sterile glove' move the items around the aseptic critical field.
- Fix the orange disposal bag to the side of the trolley, ensuring no contamination of the aseptic field.
- Hand hygiene. Open all additional equipment needed for the procedure and drop them into the aseptic critical field. Be careful not to contaminate the area with the outer packaging. Catheter and 2x pairs sterile gloves (these are additional to the pack as you will need to decide on sizing).
- Slide, or carefully drop, the catheter in the micro aseptic critical field. If 10ml of sterile water is part of the catheter pack and pre-drawn up this can also be placed on the aseptic field.
- Clean the top/opening of the cleaning solution and leave to air dry (usually 0.9% sodium chloride). Open and dispense into the gallipot provided in the pack.
- Open sterile anaesthetic gel (if part of the catheter pack this can be placed on the sterile field). If not, keep in packaging on the side of the aseptic field (the micro aseptic critical field). Prime the catheter.
- Open the catheter bag but leave in micro aseptic field.
- Prepare the patient and place the procedure/surgical sheet underneath the patient.
- Hand hygiene, and apply sterile gloves.
- Retract the foreskin if present.
- Clean the urethral meatus, ensuring ANTT and being careful not to touch the glans penis (also referred to as the head or tip of the penis).

- Position and extend the penis forward at a 90 degree angle in line with the patient's thigh.

- Prime the penis tip of the urethra, continue to insert the syringe into the urethral opening and slowly insert the remaining anaesthetic gel.

- Gently hold onto the penis, following manufacturer guidance for the anaesthetic gel to take effect (usually 2-3 mins).

- Remove gloves, hand hygiene and don new pair of sterile gloves.

- Hold penis at 90 degree angle and insert catheter tip into the opening of the urethra, advance 15cm-25cm (also dependent on manufacturer guidelines).

- If resistance is felt, ask the patient to cough and relax, but do not advance if resistance is felt following this.

- Always observe the patient for any pain or discomfort.

- Once urine is seen in the sterile catheter packaging, advance a further 2-5cm.

- Inflate the distal balloon using the external port; using the prefilled syringe of sterile water ensure ANTT, and withdraw the catheter carefully to ensure internal security.

- Attach the chosen catheter bag.

- Remove all used PPE and wash hands, retain stickers and labels needed for documentation.

- Discard all used and contaminated equipment and PPE.

- Document procedure and stick labels in appropriate catheter care plan.

- Assess and monitor patient post-catheterisation for adverse reactions or systematic responses.

ASSOCIATED SKILLS – CATHETER SAMPLE OF URINE (CSU)/ASSOCIATED THEORY: STEP BY STEP

- Explain and discuss the procedure with the person, ensure privacy and obtain consent. Ensure you have underlying knowledge and theory to support the skill and are competent to undertake the skill. Inform the patient of the rationale and process.

- Check and prepare the equipment required for the procedure. Ensure sterility (where applicable), cleanliness of packaging and that all equipment is in date.

- Review the catheter care plan/passport.

- Observe the patient's catheter. If no urine is visible in the tubing, wash hands, don apron and apply non-sterile gloves - proceed to manipulate the catheter tubing.

- Apply a non-traumatic clamp a few centimetres distal to the sampling port.

- Clean the sampling port with 2% chlorhexidine in 70% isopropyl alcohol and allow to air dry for 1 minute and 30 seconds. When visibly dry, continue to next step.

- There are two systems in which the urine can be removed from the catheter:
  o Needle and syringe (10ml): Using a sterile syringe and needle, insert the needle into the port at an angle of 45° using ANTT. Pull back on the syringe plunger to aspirate urine into the syringe. Withdraw the needle/syringe maintaining ANTT.
  o A needleless system (10ml syringe): Insert the key part of the syringe (without the needle) firmly into the middle of the sampling port. Using ANTT, pull back on the plunger of the

(Continued)

syringe and aspirate urine from the catheter. Once finished, remove syringe maintaining ANTT.

- Immediately transfer the urine from the syringe into a sterile urine sampling container.
- After transfer immediately discard the syringe into an appropriate sharps box.
- Back to the patient – clean the sampling port with an alcohol wipe and allow to air dry.
- REMEMBER: un-clamp and remove the clamp from the catheter.
- Dispose of all waste in appropriate bins.
- Remove apron, gloves and wash hands.
- Document procedure.

CARE PLANNING

Once a catheter is inserted, ongoing assessment and maintenance is required. To ensure consistency, a care plan or care bundle should be completed as part of nursing documentation (local policy applies). Such documentation helps maintain consistency of maintenance. The documentation can be an informative tool in troubleshooting problems. The catheter should be reviewed every shift, more routinely if there are identified or potential issues. Reviews enable early identification and intervention, prompting the clinician to remove at the earliest opportunity.

Cleaning of the meatal/genital areas daily with cleaning solution, and per requirement, is needed (local policy will apply). Catheter bags should be routinely emptied every 12 hours, and as necessary, to avoid over filling and to avoid infection. Visual assessment, fluid balance and clinical judgement should be ongoing. Monitor large gaps where urine is not apparent by assessing for blockages, kinks in tubing or crystallization/stone of urine in the tubing. Ensure the catheter is placed significantly lower than the patient (below bladder level) for the gravity system to work. Although the catheter drains urine from the bladder, there is no positive pressure that pulls it from the bladder. Intervention, if required, will be done following medical review. Maintenance medication may be prescribed to flush the catheter and clear blockages (see later in the chapter for procedural direction). Ensuring a closed system and maintaining a sterile clean environment, attach or detach leg bags or overnight bags when strictly necessary and clinically indicated to protect from infection. Always protect the patient by using standard precautions and ANTT in line with local policies.

Catheter drainage bags should be changed every 7 days. If still required after 28 days, the catheter and drainage will need to be replaced. If the catheter is no longer needed, remove. Daily assessment will determine if the catheter needs to be removed at any point in the 28 days.

Post-insertion

After inserting the catheter, the assessment and continuous management of the catheter and patient is vitally important. Immediately after insertion, careful observation is needed due to the phenomenon known commonly as a sepsis storm (formally cytokine storm) (Fajgenbaum and June, 2020), which is a life-threatening runaway inflammatory response of the body as a result in this instance of an invasive procedure or bacteria that has entered the body via catheterisation. The patient will present septic, and will likely have a pyretic post-procedural fever. Local sepsis protocols will need to be followed (The Sepsis Trust, 2018).

To avoid infection risk on insertion and pre-catheterisation, careful cleanliness and ANTT should be adhered to. Maintaining ANTT and cleaning is an integral part of any clinical procedure. Catheterisation is an invasive procedure you cannot achieve without breaching ANTT, therefore a surgical ANTT approach should be used.

ASSOCIATED SKILLS – REMOVAL OF URINARY CATHETER: STEP BY STEP

- Explain and gain consent for the procedure. Always maintain privacy and dignity.

- Hand hygiene and don appropriate personal protective equipment for the procedure.

- Wearing gloves, use saline soaked gauze to clean the vaginal area and catheter. Part the labia, always using one swab action, away from the meatus/urethral opening.

- For male patients, wearing gloves, use saline soaked gauze to clean the penis near the urethral entrance. Using circular motions around the shaft towards the head of the penis.

- Having reviewed the patient catheter documentation, use a syringe to remove the volume of water inserted into the balloon holding the catheter in-situ.

- Once the required amount of water is removed, and the balloon deflated, ask the person to take a deep breath in. On exhalation, gently retract and remove the catheter fully. You should NOT feel any restriction and the patient should not feel any pain. If you can feel restriction, stop and re-assess.

- Once the catheter is discarded, clean around the genitalia areas and make the patient comfortable.

- Discard and dispose of used equipment within infection control protocols.

- Clean hands and ensure the patient is comfortable. Encourage the patient to drink 1.6L-2L (variations apply) of fluid a day to maintain good bladder health.

- Post-removal, closely observe to ensure the patient passes urine. This is called post-catheter voiding.

(Bardsley, 2017)

Following removal of a catheter ensure the patient is closely monitored for the next 4 hours. It would be expected they would urinate during that time, if they have not then this must be escalated to the medical team. Timings may vary depending on other conditions the patient may have. If the patient experiences pain before this time this must be escalated immediately.

NURSE'S VOICE

You as a student nurse are ideally situated to challenge attitudes and move the focus of continence care from ritualised management to a structured proactive holistic approach.

Llinos Walters, Specialist Continence Nurse, 2021

Urostomy

Urinary drainage can occur mechanically with the support of surgery if the bladder has been removed due to trauma or bladder cancer. Urine can be diverted and drained through a stoma – an external abdominal opening that mimics what the natural elimination opening of the body would be doing. For urinary elimination, a urostomy may be used as a diversion. The urostomy is sited through the abdominal cavity. The surgeon uses a part of the small bowel called the ileum and joins both ureters (from the kidneys) as a diversion portal to drain urine into the exit stoma. Urine is passed through the stoma into a urostomy bag which collects the urine and is changed and emptied as required (Taylor et al., 2019).

CASE STUDY

Ryan

Ryan has recently started attending secondary school. He had an accident involving acute abdominal trauma. This resulted in an urostomy which it is hoped may be temporary, however there is no agreed plan on when it may be possible to reverse it. Ryan's mum, Rebecca, is a nurse in the local clinic. Despite being a nurse, she feels uninformed about urostomies, having never nursed anyone with one. Rebecca has noticed that Ryan has recently become a little withdrawn and is reluctant to go to school. Ryan has on a few occasions stated that he feels 'unwell', however he seems to improve once his mum says they can stay home. Ryan recently admitted that some of the other students in the class had been making jokes – they have been calling Ryan 'pee bag', this came from an overheard comment from the school nurse who asked Ryan in the corridor if the 'pee bag' was 'OK'. Rebecca is angry about this and approaches the school nurse.

Questions

1   What are your thoughts about how the school nurse spoke to Ryan? Could the nurse have done this differently? Did the nurse act in a professional way? What could the nurse have done differently? What interpersonal skills could they have employed?
2   How could Rebecca communicate worries most effectively with the school nurse?
3   Rebecca is both a nurse and Ryan's mother. What conflicts and similarities may arise in relation to holding both these roles and how could Rebecca be helped to manage these?

STOMA CARE: DISCUSSION

It is important the patient understands how to care for their stoma formation themselves. Support is usually provided by a specialist colorectal nurse who provides ostomy health promotion post-surgery. While this is specific post-surgical care, it is important that all nurses have a basic knowledge and understanding of ostomy procedure, assessment and care.

Different types of stoma formation

Stoma - faecal diversions

This surgical procedure brings a piece of the bowel through the abdominal wall to the outside of the abdomen. A stoma may be required because an individual has had surgery to remove parts of the bowel, because of bowel obstruction, because of damage to the bowel, incontinence, or if the patient has malformation of the bowel.

There are two types of faecal diversion stoma, formed from the colon (large bowel) and ileum (the small bowel). Known respectively as a colostomy (colon) and an ileostomy (ileum).

Commonly, an ileostomy is formed as a temporary loop ileostomy to divert for surgery repair or treatments given to the rectum. Full or total colectomy, meaning that the whole colon is removed, results in a permanent ileostomy.

Stoma sizing

Stoma sizing differs according to procedure and individual anatomy. Sizing of the equipment and ostomy bag/pouch is important. Patients may know the size that they require their pouches or bags to be. This information can be obtained from the medical notes or surgical report. Manual sizing can be done if this information is not readily available. Each adhesive ring has different printed sizes which can be manually compared to the size of the stoma for best fit (see stoma clinical skills section for further direction). Good fixation and skin adherence assists with the seal of the equipment. This protects the patient's privacy by preventing leakage and masking smell. Good adherence provides comfort, it also protects the skin. Compromised skin integrity to the peristomal skin increases the risk of pain, pressure damage, infection and, potentially, systemic complications such as sepsis.

CHANGING/EMPTYING COLOSTOMY BAG: STEP BY STEP (ONE PIECE SYSTEM)

EQUIPMENT

- The chosen ostomy bag/pouch - these can be pre-cut or will need to be cut to size. Pouches come in a range of inclusive skin colours and there is a choice of flushable accessories and bags. Patient preference should be sought
- Scissors - to cut open equipment or accessories
- Dressing/procedure pack - to maintain an aseptic/clean environment
- Cleaning solution - to cleanse the stoma and surrounding skin (patient's preference)
- Sizing chart - to correctly identify the size the adherent ring needs to be
- Gloves - ANTT
- Abdominal belt - a belt is used for extra support, providing comfort for the patient
- Adherent removal spray - to assist with removal of the old pouch
- Adhesive strips - for extra adhesion support if required
- Stoma guards - to protect the stoma bag from impact (patient preference if prescribed)
- Skin barrier cream (patient's preference if prescribed)

PROCEDURE

- Explain and discuss procedure with the person. Ensure privacy and consent is sought. Ensure you have the underlying knowledge and theory to support the skill and are competent to undertake

(Continued)

the skill. Ensure you are aware of, and inform the patient of, the rationale for the procedure. Ensure an assessment is carried out for need and that rationale is evident.

- Change the ostomy bag when the bowels are least active, when the patient is ready, and the time is suitable.
- Check and prepare the equipment required for the procedure. Ensure sterility (where applicable) and cleanliness of packaging and that all equipment is in date.
- Prior to the procedure, ensure that both anatomy and need have been assessed and the right equipment/products picked.
- Wash hands.
- Prepare trolley/surface and equipment, ensuring ANTT is followed. Check all expiry dates, sterility and that packaging is intact.
- Clean the top/opening of the cleaning solution and leave to air dry. Open and dispense into the gallipot provided in the pack. Drop any other equipment (if sterile) needed onto the aseptic field.
- Check the patient's care plan or speak to the patient about ostomy bag sizing.
- Size and cut the sized skin-adherent pad of the ostomy bag.
- Take trolley to the bedside, prepare patient and ensure dignity and privacy is maintained.
- Wash hands, don gloves.
- Prepare the patient. Protect privacy and dignity.
- Open the trolley dressing pack. Insert the procedural/surgical sheet underneath the ostomy bag for protection.
- Gently remove the adhesive pad from the patient's skin working from the top of the ostomy bag down (use adhesive remover where needed and if the patient prefers this).
- Once removed, discard into the appropriate clinical waste.
- Use the gauze soaked with the cleaning solution to clean around the stoma.
- Assess the peristomal skin (surrounding skin).
- Using dry gauze pat the area dry, ensuring the peristomal skin is dry for adherence.
- Discard gloves, hand hygiene.
- Don new set of gloves, measure the stoma with a measuring facility (if unsure and it is not documented).
- Cut the stoma adhesive skin pad to appropriate size.
- Cut around the sizing diameter, ensure the edges are smooth.
- Close the end of the bag (or clip, dependent on manufacturer).
- Remove the backing of the adhesive skin pad and insert over the stoma, smoothing to ensure adherence.
- Ensure the patient is comfortable.
- Remove and dispose of PPE.
- Document the procedure and the appliances or accessories used.

CASE STUDY

Ellie

Ellie, 26, is a non-binary person with Crohn's disease. Ellie was recently fitted with a stoma. This is not currently permanent. The stoma has had an impact on Ellie's body image and sense of self. Ellie uses a lot of social media; image is important to them. They previously did a lot of keep fit posts and jokes that Crohn's 'kept them thin'. They admit that they are worried that they will now put on weight. Ellie's mother is obese.

Ellie is in a relationship with Jack. They have been together for two years. They do not live together. Jack is in a flat at one end of town and Ellie has a flat at the other. Jack is aware that Ellie has a stoma and drove Ellie to hospital to have the operation. Jack is supportive and states that it makes no difference to the relationship. Ellie has insisted that Jack cannot see the stoma and has kept it covered. They have not been intimate since the operation.

Ellie is coping with stoma care at a practical level but finds it distressing. They can barely look at the stoma and thinks that it makes them look disgusting, they are concerned that it will leak in public. This has led to them going out less. Ellie works in a busy office and has not yet returned to work. Their work colleagues do not know about the stoma though they know Ellie has had an operation and that there were 'problems with their stomach.'

Ellie had one previous episode of depression, five years ago, following the death of their father. This was treated with antidepressants by the GP. They have started to feel low in mood again and are having difficulties going to sleep and some early morning waking. Ellie is tearful and says they have intrusive negative thoughts.

Jack has been trying to support Ellie by finding positive stories online, but they will not read them – 'I don't want to be known as the person with the bag'.

Questions

1   Ellie is non-binary. What would be important in meeting with them for the first time, when referring to them with colleagues and during your ongoing engagement?
2   How would you engage with Jack? (Assuming that Ellie is willing for this to happen.)
3   What would you need to be aware of in relation to risk and Ellie's mental health?
4   How could you gently challenge some of Ellie's negative thoughts?
5   How could you help Ellie come to terms with living with an ostomy?

Body image/peristomal skin conditions

Skin integrity is vitally important, and maintaining healthy skin is integral to the overall health and care of the individual. Prioritisation must be considered for patients suffering with bladder and bowel health issues. The peristomal skin area refers to the skin surrounding the stoma formation. Healthy peristomal skin should be maintained to reduce the occurrences of Peristomal Skin Conditions (PSCs). Risk factors include damage from accessories, tubing, straps and adhesive and skin breakdown from bodily fluids coming into contact with the skin more often. This may be because of the ostomy bag not being cut accurately, or the adhesive not adhering enough. Other factors such as age, body mass index, hydration and nutrition can have an impact. The main concern is leaking of faecal matter and discharge onto the skin.

It is estimated that patients with ileostomies are at greater risk of suffering from PSCs if pouches are not correctly attached. The pathophysiology of the ileum means looser stools are passed, allowing faeces to come into contact with the skin. More frequent pouch changes may create unnecessary erosion and stripping of the skin. Leaking appliances and PSCs are often the biggest concern of ostomates. Nurses must identify the right and most appropriate equipment and accessories to avoid incidences of PSCs. Specialist advice should be sourced from a colorectal nurse to avoid using incorrect accessories or processes.

Good recognition, knowledge, assessment and physical examinations in order to prevent and treat PSCs are significant in protecting patients from the stress and discomfort of PSCs, such as faecal induced erosion, maceration, contact dermatitis and erythema. Patient compliance must also be taken into consideration when PSCs are detected. A stoma formation can be challenging for a patient's body image and wellbeing. Patients may feel they need to change their ostomy bags or pouches more often to minimise odour or reduce any visual 'bump' under clothing. Speaking to the patient and understanding what is important to them will help shape their care and prioritise your nursing interventions and clinical decisions (Carter, 2019).

NURSE'S VOICE

What we think is important as nurses is not very often what is important for the patient living with a stoma formation.

Iris Williams, Colorectal Clinical Nurse Specialist, 2021

ADMINISTERING SUPPOSITORIES AND ENEMAS: DISCUSSION

Suppositories

Suppositories are solid pieces of medication inserted through the rectum into the lower bowel, with the intention of being expelled. They may have two functions:

- Evacuant: To stimulate bowel elimination and movement, suppositories are inserted in order to lubricate or stimulate faecal matter. When dissolved, they soften stools for ease of passing.
- Retention: To retain medication or treatment that cannot be given by any other route or where the rectal route offers necessary, faster absorption.

Enemas

An enema is a bolus of fluid that is flushed through the rectum into the lower bowel with the intention of it being expelled.

———————————— **WATCH THE VIDEO** ————————————

ADMINISTERING SUPPOSITORIES

Watch along as you read through this step by step procedure by scanning the QR code with your smartphone camera or via **https://study.sagepub.com/rowberry**.

ADMINISTERING ENEMAS AND SUPPOSITORIES: STEP BY STEP

EQUIPMENT

- Relevant medications to give rectally
- Documentation
- Disposable absorbent pad
- Lubricant
- Gloves and apron
- Wipes/cleaning products (POS procedure)
- Hand sanitizer

PROCEDURE

- Explain and discuss procedure with the person, ensure privacy and consent is sought. Carry out allergies and identity checks.
- Ensure you have the underlying knowledge and theory to support the skill and are competent to undertake the skill. Ensure you are aware of, and inform the patient of, the rationale for the procedure. Ensure an assessment is carried out for need and rationale is evident.
- Check and prepare the equipment required for the procedure. Ensure sterility (where applicable) and cleanliness of packaging and that all equipment is in date.
- Prior to the procedure, ensure anatomy and need have been assessed and the right equipment/products picked.
- Wash hands.
- Prepare patient, remove any clothing garments. Protect privacy and dignity as much as possible.
- Position the patient onto their left side. This position helps the medication move into the rectum. Ensure their knees are bent and the right knee is slightly further over.

(Continued)

- Tuck the absorbent pad under the hip and buttocks.
- Hand hygiene, don gloves and apron.
- Using the water-based lubricant, cover the suppository or enema and place some at the opening of the rectum.
- Communicate throughout the process.
- Using your non-dominant hand, push up on the right buttocks and separate them.
- Assess for any abnormalities, record and report if appropriate. Avoid giving the medication if there are any abnormalities or bleeding and seek medical advice.
- Ask the patient to take a deep breath. As they exhale out and the muscles relax, insert the tip of the enema into the anus and squeeze the bottle to dispense the medication into the rectum. If you are using a suppository, push the medication, using one finger, into the rectum.
- Gently remove enema or finger. Do not push or exert pressure. If you feel resistance, stop.
- Remove PPE and dispose of any contaminated equipment in the appropriate refuse. Wash hands.
- Re-position the patient. Inform the patient that the medication may act quickly and ask them to inform you when they need to use the bathroom if assistance is needed.
- Document.

Rectal examination and manual evacuation, when appropriate

- **DRF** – digital removal of faeces
- **DRE** – digital rectal examination
- **PR** – per rectum

There are many reasons why a nurse might perform a rectal examination. An assessment should be made pre- and post-medication administration to ensure safe and successful administration (NMC, 2018b; 2019; RCN, 2019). For example, placement of medication within the rectum is imperative to its action and successfulness. Evidence suggests that giving analgesic medication per rectum with significant stool formations remaining reduced the effectiveness by 32% (Hagen et al., 1991). This is startling evidence that suggests that your patient's pain management will be much less effective if they retain faeces. Therefore, being able to assess stool quantity and perform an evacuation will improve the absorption, metabolism, distribution and excretion of medication. (This is formally known as pharmacokinetics.) This awareness and assessment of pharmacokinetics can be applied to all principles of medication administration in all other sites. Understanding how the drugs work in the body is important, which ultimately maximises results, reduces adverse drug reactions and errors, and improves medication management (Mardani et al., 2020).

An examination of the rectum is a contribution to your A–G assessment. The exposure (E) part of the assessment can identify and guide diagnosis, treatment, investigation and management of the patient's care.

Some examples of occasions when and why a nurse can use DRE/DRF:

- Evacuating stool and faecal matter, if the patient's rectal tone is loose or patients are unable to defecate the remaining stool.

- Evacuating stool for accurate positioning of suppositories and enemas.
- To assess effects of medication.
- To directly stimulate recto-anal reflex to aid defecation for those who cannot, or conditions may stop them doing so either temporarily or permanently. In some cases, not doing this could be life threatening.
- To assess for abnormalities.
- To assess tone, sensation and contraction.

Below are some instances/examples where caution should be applied or DRE/DRF and manual evacuations might be avoided:

- Patients who have undergone surgery or experienced trauma of injury.
- Patients who have a history of abuse.
- The clinician or nurse is not trained, competent of experienced/supervised.
- Patients who suffer from Irritable Bowel Diseases (IBDs) such as Crohn's disease, ulcerative colitis.
- Anal pain.
- Infection.
- Fragile skin and tissue.
- Recent radiotherapy in pelvic/abdominal regions.
- Children, unless the nurse is specifically trained and experienced.
- Obvious signs of bleeding.
- An unstable patient.

This list is not exhaustive and will require further clinical judgement and guidance from local policy and specialism (Leeds Teaching Hospital NHS Trusts, 2021; NMC, 2018b; RCN, 2019).

—————————— WATCH THE VIDEO ——————————

RECTAL EXAMINATION

Watch this step by step procedure by scanning the QR code with your smartphone camera or via https://study.sagepub.com/rowberry.

PSYCHOLOGICAL FACTORS AND MENTAL HEALTH RELATED ISSUES

Bladder or bowel conditions can affect the psychological wellbeing of an individual in relation to both seeking help and coping. Contemporary reviews of the literature highlight several limiting factors including quality of life, social determinants of health, perceptions of physical 'norms' relevant to ageing, stigma and knowledge of treatment options. The intimate nature of conditions means that the person may have had little opportunity to discuss symptoms and 'normal' functioning informally with friends and family. Lack of routine continence questions in general consultations place the burden on the individual to raise it. This may be impacted by feelings of shame and a perception that it is not 'worth' raising as a concern if symptoms are not severe. Cultural aspects and gender differences between the health professional and patient may also impede openness (Mendes et al., 2017; Norton et al., 2017; Toye and Barker, 2020).

Living with a bladder or bowel condition can affect an individual's life on many levels, from practical considerations such as symptom management through to how living with the condition impacts emotionally on relationships and the self. Treatment, such as surgery, can be life changing in a positive way, but it can also mean having to come to terms with permanent changes. Ostaszkiewicz et al.'s (2021) narrative review suggests that the adjustment experiences of individuals living with other chronic conditions may have transferable relevance to those living with urinary incontinence.

For many people coping is something that develops over time and can be aided by supportive care that gradually reduces as the person's resiliency develops, however some people may go on to develop mental distress which may be both significant and long lasting.

Mental health, bladder and bowel health

As well as the impact of coping with a condition on the individual's mental health and wellbeing, psychological states can themselves affect bladder and bowel functioning. In this section we will explore some common mental health conditions that link with bladder and bowel.

Stress

Psychological or emotional stress is not the same as the stress referred to in stress incontinence. The latter refers to physical stress.

Glynn et al. (2021) point out that the impact of stressful life events on the symptoms of gastrointestinal disorders is well documented. Contemporary research increasingly highlights connections between the brain and the gut via the brain–gut axis (Ancona et al., 2021). This includes the central nervous system, the autonomic nervous system, the enteric nervous system and the hypothalamic pituitary pathway (Tsigos and Chrousos, 2002).

Individuals experiencing conditions such as irritable bowel disease or Crohn's disease may recognise, through experience, that stressful events can be linked to flare ups. The regular stressors connected with living with the condition can result in an individual not recognising their own stress levels. Whilst the individual may assert that they are fine, they may be in a state of unrecognised arousal much of the time.

Teaching the person to recognise stress is a first step to managing it. Symptoms of increased stress may include:

- Muscle tension
- Headaches
- Dizziness
- Upset stomach
- Rapid heartbeat
- Problems with concentration
- Forgetfulness

- Impaired decision-making and judgement
- Worrying
- Rumination – going over things in your mind repeatedly
- Irritability
- Sleep problems (too much or too little)
- Appetite changes (eating too much or too little)
- Increased unhealthy coping behaviour (smoking, drinking or drug use)
- Avoidance
- Feeling overwhelmed
- Sexual dysfunction

Practically, nurses are in a position to teach basic stress management skills. This may include simple relaxation and breathing exercises. Mindfulness has gained traction in recent years as a useful approach to stress management generally and in relation to gastrointestinal disorders (Ewais et al., 2019).

Depression

Increased rates of depression have been recorded in individuals with IBD (Mambro and York, 2021). Depression may be mild to moderate to severe. Signs of depression may include:

- Low mood that is continuous
- Poor self esteem
- Feeling hopeless
- Loss of motivation
- Feeling guilty
- Tearfulness
- Difficulty in thinking clearly and making decisions
- Irritability
- Thoughts of wanting to harm oneself or wanting to die

Physically, the individual may experience appetite changes, low energy, somatic symptoms – aches and pains – and a focus on physical symptoms. There may be evidence of weight loss (or occasionally gain). Sleep may be disturbed with early waking, difficulty falling asleep or night-time waking, libido may be decreased, and menstruation disturbed. The person may be physically slowed down in speech, thought and action. If anxiety is also present, the person may appear agitated.

Socially, the individual may isolate themselves, avoiding friends and family. There may be interpersonal difficulties at home and work. There may be a lack of interest in previous hobbies or activities. Severe depression can lead to psychosis (delusions and hallucinations) and neglect. This is considered an emergency situation requiring hospitalisation.

Depression itself can impact on bowel and bladder function. Extreme depression can slow gut movement. A loss of interest and enjoyment in food and drink may lead to poor nutritional input, resulting in constipation and dehydration. Amotivation may result in little physical activity and a sluggish system. Hygiene and self-care can deteriorate in severe depression and, in extreme cases, incontinence may result from this.

The National Institute for Health and Care Excellence (NICE, 2021) recommends that staff be alert to the potential for depression, particularly where there is a previous history and a chronic health condition with functional impairment. Two main questions can be asked to identify potential depression:

During the last month, have you often been bothered by:

1   feeling down, depressed or hopeless?
2   having little interest or pleasure in doing things?

Follow-up to a 'yes' response to either question depends upon the role and competence of the nurse as well as local procedure and practice. Only practitioners competent in mental health assessment should assess. Practitioners who are not competent in mental health assessment should refer to an appropriate professional. This may be the patient's GP or primary care service.

All staff should be aware of indicators of suicidality. Any statement or action that appears to be indicative of suicidal intent should be escalated and responded to as a potential emergency situation. IBD has been linked with higher than expected rates of suicide in adults (Gradus et al., 2010; Sánta et al., 2020). An extensive Danish and Finnish study of paediatric onset IBD and mortality over a 23-year period uncovered a fourfold increased risk of suicide, the majority of which occurred in individuals who had reached the age of 18 or more (Malham et al., 2019).

Anxiety

Anxiety can occur in conjunction with depression and as a standalone condition. Many of us experience worry and anxiety to a degree but when it becomes more extreme, persistent and interferes with daily living it may be considered problematic. Anxiety can present with a wide range of physical and psychological symptoms which can include distressing thoughts which may be out of proportion to the situation, constant tenseness, hypervigilance, and feelings of depersonalisation and derealisation. Panic attacks are a form of anxiety.

Somatic symptoms may include abdominal discomfort, bowel changes and aches and pains. These can confuse the overall physical health picture. A meta-analysis of the international literature, examining the relationship between urinary incontinence, anxiety, and depression, conducted by Cheng et al. (2020) concluded that patients with urinary incontinence had higher rates of both depression and anxiety than the general population, regardless of age, although they found a paucity of studies, quality concerns and small sample sizes. Both depression and anxiety have been linked with long-term urinary incontinence (Steers and Lee, 2001; Kwak et al., 2016).

Space precludes a fuller exploration. This is, however, an area with much to offer the interested reader who may want to consider carrying out further self-directed learning around psychological approaches to the management of bladder and bowel conditions, for example the potential for psychosocial interventions such as cognitive behavioural therapy and motivational interviewing in symptom management, coping and treatment concordance.

Working with individuals with learning disability

Keenan et al. (2018) point out that individuals with a learning or intellectual disability are at greater risk of developing incontinence, yet their needs are not always met in the most effective manner. Learning disability nurses require a good knowledge of bladder and bowel care. Nurses primarily skilled in other fields should liaise with learning disability colleagues and the multidisciplinary team, including continence specialists, with the aim of promoting continence in the most appropriate way, focusing on a person-centred, individual approach tailored to the individual's capacity, ability, personality and needs. Similarly, nurses should be aware of how someone with a learning disability may be challenged in relation to expressing themselves when in discomfort, distress or pain, and work with multidisciplinary colleagues to find the best way of managing this for the specific individual.

Working with other populations who may have challenges in understanding or expressing their needs

This may include individuals with neurological conditions, brain injury, sensory loss (vision/hearing), verbal limitations and dementia. Each situation and each individual are unique. What is most important is that bladder and bowel assessment, care and management are conducted in a way that reflects this, that dignity is valued, that independence is encouraged and that every effort is made to identify what works best for that person, informed by relevant others (professionals, carers, and family/friends) and by best practice and guidance.

CASE STUDY

Evelyne

Evelyne is 78 years old. Originally from the Caribbean, she has lived in the UK for the last 58 years. A nurse by background, Evelyne worked for years as a senior nurse in a county hospital. Widowed three years ago, Evelyne recently moved into a semi-supported care setting. Evelyne has Alzheimer's disease. Her short-term memory is affected, and she has demonstrable evidence of cognitive decline. Evelyne is currently still active and relatively independent. She has developed incontinence, something she finds distressing. The carers who call in daily have found soiled clothing pushed down the back of the sofa. Evelyne denies this. Her native language is French. She often has difficulty finding the right words in English and uses a French word instead. Evelyne has one son, who lives around three hours away by car, he visits once every few months.

Questions

1   How would you approach the issue of continence care with Evelyne?
2   Alzheimer's disease is a common, progressive cause of dementia. It can impact memory, thinking, reasoning, language or perception. How might this affect your communication around incontinence with Evelyne?
3   Learning disabilities and difficulties, neurological conditions, mental ill health and emotional distress can all impact on multiple areas, including communication and comprehension. In certain situations, with some individuals, this may also have implications in relation to capacity and consent for interventions. Would you know who to approach for additional or specialist information and support in your work setting? How could you find out?

Tips for continence promotion and management

- Use the right words and language – ask the right questions. Not everyone considers themselves incontinent. Someone with bladder or bowel frequency or urgency may manage their problem in their day-to-day life with no leaks or spills. It can still inconvenience them though – and this can be made worse with illness or a stay in hospital. The word 'incontinent' still has stigma attached to it, so some people may feel ashamed and try to deny or hide the problem. Simply asking whether their bladder or bowel causes any pain or problems should be enough to open up the conversation.
- A bladder/bowel diary is an effective investigation. You can get so much information from this simple piece of paper. It can help identify trends and patterns to assist with planning toileting routines. It can help identify incontinence type, which helps with care planning. It can monitor progress and can be used as a feedback tool.

- Pads might solve your problem but at your patient's expense – 'use it or lose it'. Individuals in cognitive decline can 'unlearn' continence if toileting is not maintained. Make sure that you've exhausted all other treatment options. Pads should be used on a short-term, temporary basis unless otherwise rationalised.
- Toileting can achieve more than just taking someone to the toilet, it can mean improving mobility, balance, and core stability, reduce the risk of pressure and moisture damage, and provide an opportunity to get to know the person.
- Initiate conversations regarding toileting, continence and incontinence.
- Do not take youth and fitness for granted. Interventions can impact temporarily on an individual's continence.
- Positioning can influence an individual's ability to void. Imagine using a bedpan or a hoist.
- Take advantage of the 30 minutes after eating when the gastrocolic reflex is strongest. Toileting at this time may help reduce constipation and faecal incontinence.
- Pelvic floor exercises are effective when done regularly.
- Often it is a number of small factors that we can assist with rather than one solitary intervention that makes the difference.
- Encourage your patients to always attempt to pass urine before and after sexual intercourse.

Llinos Walters, Continence Specialist Nurse, 2021

CHAPTER SUMMARY

The chapter has focused on nursing support in relation to bladder and bowel health. It includes essential knowledge and clinical skills for assessment, intervention and support, and encourages reflection on broader aspects.

There are numerous types of interventions nurses undertake to support bladder and bowel health.

- Assessment and identification of bladder or bowel changes is vital in identifying a patient's baseline and for diagnosis of conditions.
- Infection prevention and control policy and practice will help manage any identified infections.
- Recognition of how bladder and bowel health related conditions can affect patients' mental wellbeing, and appropriate interventions and signposting within the parameters of clinical competence.
- Health promotion, support, health literacy and education can support patients in understanding their conditions.

ACE YOUR ASSESSMENT

Q1   What factors can increase incontinence?

  a   Medications, trauma, aging
  b   Aging, heavy drinking, medications
  c   Drinking lots, cold weather, aging

Q2   What colour is healthy urine?

  a   Yellow/brown
  b   Yellow/green
  c   Clear/yellow

Q3 What does MSU stand for?

    a   Multistream specimen of urine

    b   Midstream specimen of urine

    c   Morningstream specimen of urine

Q4 Identify the correct indications for catheter use.

    a   Trauma, acute deterioration, surgical procedure

    b   Limited mobility, trauma, surgery

    c   Severe incontinence, surgery, acute deterioration

Q5 Identify the correct reasons a nurse may perform digital rectal examination.

    a   Faecal evacuation, constipation, assess tone

    b   Assess medication effects, assess tone, assess for abnormalities

    c   Constipation, assess abnormalities, assess tone

Answers

1   A

2   C

3   B

4   A

5   B

GO FURTHER

Current standards of care for patients and servicers suffering with gastrointestinal conditions:

- https://ibduk.org/ibd-standards
- https://www.crohnsandcolitis.org.uk/improving-care-services/ibd-standards

Signposting and support:

- https://www.bladderandbowel.org/bowel/bowel-treatments/maintaining-a-healthy-bowel/
- https://www.cancercare.org/diagnosis/colorectal_cancer
- "No Butts" campaign – 'No Butts: Get to know the symptoms of bowel cancer '. https://www.itv.com/lorraine/articles/no-butts

REFERENCES

Ancona, P., Petito, C., Iavarone, I., Petito, V., Galasso, L., Leonetti, A. [...] and Gasbarrini, A. (2021) 'The gut–brain axis in irritable bowel syndrome and inflammatory bowel disease', *Digestive and Liver Disease*, 53 (3): 298–305. https://doi.org/10.1016/j.dld.2020.11.026

Anderson, B. (2018) 'Bladder cancer: Overview and disease management. Part 1: Non-muscle-invasive bladder cancer', *British Journal of Nursing*, 29 (9): 27–37.

Baines, G., Da Silva, A.S., Cardozo, L., Bach, F., Parsons, M., Robinson, D. and Toozs-Hobson, P. (2021) 'Defining nocturnal polyuria in women', *United States Neuroulogy and Urodynamics*, 40 (1): 265–71.

Bardsley, A. (2017) 'How to remove an indwelling urinary catheter in female patients', *Nursing Standard*, 31 (19): 42–5.

Carter, C. (2019) *Critical Care Nursing in Resource Limited Environments*. Abingdon: Routledge.

Cathala, X. and Moorley, C. (2020) 'Skills for newly qualified nurses 1: Understanding and managing accountability', *Nursing Times*, 116, October 15. https://www.nursingtimes.net/roles/newly-qualified-nurses/skills-for-newly-qualified-nurses-1-understanding-and-managing-accountability-15-10-2020/ (accessed October 17, 2022).

Centers for Disease Control and Prevention (2015) 'Catheter-associated urinary tract infections (CAUTI)', cdc.gov. https://www.cdc.gov/hai/ca_uti/uti.html (accessed October 17, 2022).

Cheng, S., Lin, D., Hu, T., Cao, L., Liao, H., Mou, X., Zhang, Q., Liu, J. and Wu, T. (2020) 'Association of urinary incontinence and depression or anxiety: A meta-analysis', *Journal of International Medical Research*, 48 (6). doi.org/10.1177/0300060520931348

Clayton, J.L. (2017) 'Indwelling urinary catheters: A pathway to health care-associated infections', *AORN Journal*, 105 (5): 446–52. doi: 10.1016/j.aorn.2017.02.013

Dougherty, L. and Lister, S.E. (eds) (2015) *The Royal Marsden Manual of Clinical Nursing Procedures* (9th professional edition). Chichester: Wiley.

Ewais, T., Begun, J., Kenny, M., Rickett, K., Hay, K., Ajilchi, B. and Kisely, S. (2019) 'A systematic review and meta-analysis of mindfulness based interventions and yoga in inflammatory bowel disease', *Journal of Psychosomatic Research*, 116: 44–53. doi.org/10.1016/j.jpsychores.2018.11.010

Fajgenbaum, D.C. and June, C.H. (2020) 'Cytokine storm', *The New England Journal of Medicine*, 383 (23): 2255–73. doi.org/10.1056/NEJMra2026131

Flamarion, E., Reichert, C., Sayegh, C., de Saint Gilles, D., Bariseel, R., Arnoux, J.B. [...] and Penet, M.A. (2022) 'Orientation diagnostique devant une coloration anormale des urines: La roue à urines 2.0 [Abnormal urine color assessment: The urine wheel]', *La Revue de Médecine Interne*, 43 (1): 31–8 doi.org/10.1016/j.revmed.2021.02.009 (accessed October 17, 2022).

Gharbi, M., Drysdale, J.H., Lishman, H., Goudie, R., Molokhia, M., Johnson, A.P., Holmes, A.H. and Aylin, P. (2019) 'Antibiotic management of urinary tract infection in elderly patients in primary care and its association with bloodstream infections and all-cause mortality: Population based cohort study', *British Medical Journal*, 364: Article #1525. doi.org/10.1136/bmj.l525

Gibson, K.E., Neill, S., Tuma, E., Meddings, J. and Mody, L. (2019) 'Indwelling urethral versus suprapubic catheters in nursing home residents: Determining the safest option for long-term use', *Journal of Hospital Infection*, 102 (2): 219–25.

Gilbert, B., Naidoo, T.L. and Redwig, F. (2018) 'Ins and outs of urinary catheters', *Australian Journal of General Practice*, 47 (3). doi.org/10.31128/AFP-10-17-4362

Glynn, H., Möller, S.P., Wilding, H., Apputhurai, P., Moore, G. and Knowles, S.R. (2021) 'Prevalence and impact of post-traumatic stress disorder in gastrointestinal conditions: A systematic review', *Digestive Diseases and Sciences*, 66 (12): 4109–19. doi.org/10.1007/s10620-020-06798-y

Gradus, J.L., Qin, P., Lincoln, A.K., Miller, M., Lawler, E., Sørensen, H.T. and Lash, T.L. (2010) 'Inflammatory bowel disease and completed suicide in Danish adults', *Inflammatory Bowel Disease*, 16: 2158–61. doi.org/10.1002/ibd.21298

Gulanick, M. and Myers, J.L. (2022) *Nursing Care Plans: Diagnoses, Interventions, and Outcomes* (10th edition). St. Louis, MO: Elsevier.

Hagen, I.J., Haram, E.M. and Laake, K. (1991) 'Absorption of paracetamol from suppositories in geriatric patients with faecal accumulation in the rectum', *Aging Clinical and Experimental Research*, 3: 25–9.

Hoilat, G.J. and Savio, J. (2022) *Bilirubinuria*. https://www.ncbi.nlm.nih.gov/books/NBK557439/ (accessed January 30, 2023).

Keenan, P., Fleming, S., Horan P., Byrne, K., Burke, E., Cleary, M., Doyle, C. and Griffiths, C. (2018) 'Urinary continence promotion and people with an intellectual disability', *Learning Disability Practice*, 21 (3): 28–34. doi.org/10.7748/ldp.2018.e1878

Kwak, Y., Kwon, H. and Kim, Y. (2016) 'Health-related quality of life and mental health in older women with urinary incontinence', *Aging and Mental Health*, 220: 719–26. doi.org/10.1080/13607 863.2015.1033682

Leeds Teaching Hospital NHS Trusts (2021) 'Guidelines for digital rectal stimulation and manual evacuation of faeces in adults', Leeds: Trust Clinical Guidelines Group. www.lhp.leedsth.nhs.uk/ detail.aspx?id=1481 (accessed October 17, 2022).

Macmillan Cancer Support (2016) 'Urostomy support', macmillan.org.uk, February 29. https://www.macmillan.org.uk/cancer-information-and-support/impacts-of-cancer/urostomy (accessed October 17, 2022).

Malham, M., Jakobsen, C., Paerregaard, A., Virta, L.J., Kolho, K.-L. and Wewer, V. (2019) 'The incidence of cancer and mortality in paediatric onset inflammatory bowel disease in Denmark and Finland during a 23-year period: A population-based study', *Alimentary Pharmacology & Therapeutics*, 50: 33–9. doi.org/10.1111/apt.15258

Mambro, A.D. and York, S. (2021) 'Should mental health support and monitoring form part of regular IBD assessment and treatment?', *Gut, 70*: Article# A11.

Mardani, A., Griffiths, P. and Vaismoradi, M. (2020) 'The role of the nurse in the management of medicines during transitional care: A systematic review', *Journal of Multidisciplinary Healthcare*, 13: 1347–61. doi.org/10.2147/JMDH.S276061

Mendes, A., Hoga, L., Gonçalves, B., Silva, P. and Pereira, P. (2017) 'Women's experiences of urinary incontinence: A systematic review of qualitative evidence', *JBI Database of Systematic Reviews and Implementation Reports*, 15 (5): 1350–408. doi.org/10.11124/JBISRIR-2017-003389

Moore, T. and Cunningham, S. (2017) *Clinical Skills for Nursing Practice*. Abingdon: Routledge.

National Health Service (NHS) (2019) 'Urinary incontinence'. https://www.nhs.uk/conditions/ urinary-incontinence/ (accessed October 17, 2022).

National Health Service (NHS) (2022) *Urinary Catheters*. https://www.nhs.uk/conditions/urinary-catheters/ (accessed January 30 2023).

National Institute for Health and Care Excellence (NICE) (2018) 'Urinary tract infection (catheter-associated): Antimicrobial prescribing (NG113)'. London: NICE. https://www.nice.org.uk/ guidance/ng113 (accessed October 17, 2022).

National Institute for Health and Care Excellence (2019) 'Incontinence - urinary, in women', NICE, October. https://cks.nice.org.uk/topics/incontinence-urinary-in-women/ (accessed October 17, 2022).

National Institute for Health and Care Excellence (2021) 'Depression. All NICE products on depression. Includes any guidance, advice and quality standards' [portal page], nice.org.uk. https://pathways.nice.org.uk/pathways/depression (accessed October 17, 2022).

Norton, J.M., Dodson, J.L., Newman, D.K., Rogers, R.G., Fairman, A.D., Coons, H.L., Star, R.A. and Bavendam, T.J. (2017) 'Nonbiologic factors that impact management in women with urinary incontinence: Review of the literature and findings from a National Institute of Diabetes and Digestive and Kidney Diseases workshop', *International Urogynaecology Journal*, 28 (9): 1295–307. https://doi.org/10.1007/s00192-017-3400-x

Nursing and Midwifery Council (NMC) (2018a) *The Code: Professional Standards of Practice and Behaviour for Nurses, Midwives and Nursing Associates*. London: NMC. https://www.nmc.org.uk/globalassets/sitedocuments/nmc-publications/nmc-code.pdf (accessed October 17, 2022).

Nursing and Midwifery Council (2018b) *Future Nurse: Standards of Proficiency for Registered Nurses*. NMC, May 17. https://www.nmc.org.uk/standards/standards-for-nurses/standards-of-proficiency-for-registered-nurses/ (accessed October 17, 2022).

Ostaszkiewicz, J., Dunning, T. and Watt, E. (2021) 'Adjusting to urinary incontinence: Insights from a review of research into adjustment to chronic illness', *Australian and New Zealand Continence Journal*, 27 (3): 60–5.

Pizzol, D., Demurtas, J., Celotto, S., Maggi, S., Smith, L., Angiolelli, G., Trott, M., Yang, L. and Veronese, N. (2021) 'Urinary incontinence and quality of life: A systematic review and meta-analysis', *Aging Clinical and Expert Research*, 33: 25–35 https://doi.org/10.1007/s40520-020-01712-y

Riemsma, R., Hagen, S., Kirschner-Hermanns, R., Norton, C., Wijk, H., Andersson, K.-E. [...] and Milsom, I. (2017) 'Can incontinence be cured? A systematic review of cure rates', *BMC Medicine*, 15: Article# 63. https://doi.org/10.1186/s12916-017-0828-2

Royal College of Nursing (RCN) (2019) 'Bowel care: Management of lower bowel dysfunction, including digital rectal examination and digital removal of faeces', NMC. https://www.rcn.org.uk/Professional-Development/publications/pub-007522 (accessed October 17, 2022).

Royal College of Nursing (2021) 'Catheter care guidance for health care professionals', rcn.org.uk, July 27. https://www.rcn.org.uk/professional-development/publications/catheter-care-guidance-for-health-care-professionals-uk-pub-009-915 (accessed October 17, 2022).

Sánta, A., Szántó, K.J., Sarlós, P., Miheller, P., Farkas, K. and Molnár, T. (2020) 'Letter: Suicide risk among adult inflammatory bowel disease patients', *Alimentary Pharmacological Therapy*, 51: 1213–14. doi.org/10.1111/apt.15708

Steers, W.D. and Lee, K.S. (2001) 'Depression and incontinence', *World Journal of Urology*, 19: 351–7.

Taylor, C., Munro, J., Goodman, W., Beeken, R.J., Dames, N., Oliphant, R., Watson, A.J.M. and Hubbard, G. (2019) 'Experiences of wearing support garments by people living with a urostomy', *British Journal of Nursing*, 28 (22): S26–S33. https://doi.org/10.12968/bjon.2019.28.22.S26

The Sepsis Trust (2022) *The Yellow Manual*. Sepsis Trust. https://sepsistrust.org/wp-content/uploads/2022/06/Yellow-Manual-6th-Edition.pdf (accessed December 2022).

The United Kingdom Government (2022) 'Using the UKCA marking', Department for Business, Energy & Industrial Strategy. https://www.gov.uk/guidance/using-the-ukca-marking (accessed October 17, 2022).

Toye, F. and Barker, K.L. (2020) 'A meta-ethnography to understand the experience of living with urinary incontinence: "Is it just part and parcel of life?"' *BMC Urology*, 20 (1): Article#1. https://doi.org/10.1186/s12894-019-0555-4

Tsigos, C. and Chrousos, G.P. (2002) 'Hypothalamic-pituitary-adrenal axis, neuroendocrine factors and stress', *Journal of Psychosomatic Research*, 53: 865–71.

Tubbs, S.R. (2021) '"You must master human anatomy…"', *Clinical*, 34 (8): 1121. https://doi.org/10.1002/ca.23784

World Health Organization (WHO) (2021) 'Evidence of hand hygiene as the building block for infection prevention and control', WHO. https://www.who.int/publications/i/item/WHO-HIS-SDS-2017.7 (accessed January 30, 2023).

MOBILITY AND SAFETY

9

JAMIE WHEELER AND LOVELY SAJAN, WITH SARAH KINGDOM-MILLS (LEARNING DISABILITIES CONTRIBUTION)

NMC STANDARDS COVERED IN THIS CHAPTER

ANNEXE B NURSING PROCEDURES

7.1 Observe and use evidence-based risk assessment tools to determine need for support and intervention to optimise mobility and safety, and to identify and manage risk of falls using best practice risk assessment approaches
7.2 Use a range of contemporary moving and handling techniques
7.3 Use appropriate moving and handling equipment to support people with impaired mobility
7.4 Use appropriate safety techniques and devices

LEARNING OBJECTIVES

After reading this chapter, you should be able to:

- Discuss the principles of mobility
- Identify and understand the factors affecting the poor mobility and safety status of the patient
- Understand the nurse's role and responsibility in assessing mobility needs using mobility assessment tools, and respond to those needs
- Understand the technical and clinical skills needed to optimise handling and mobility techniques

STUDENT VOICE

It's easy to see manual handling as mandatory training as many of us have had this before starting the course, however it is extremely important to recognise the significance of this part of our education. Ensuring the patient, us and our colleagues are safe at all times is pertinent – whatever environment or field we work in.

Dan, 2nd year, Mental Health

INTRODUCTION

Being able to mobilise is vital to promoting a person's health and wellbeing. Mobility improves blood flow to limbs and all organs of the body. Our normal level of mobility (ability to move physically) can be affected due to periods of ill health affecting our muscle function, thereby preventing normal body activity. This can impact any sphere of a person's life including physical, psychological, and social aspects. In healthcare settings, nurses play an important role in encouraging early mobilisation thus preventing several complications associated with impaired mobility. This chapter will cover best practice and evidence-based approaches in optimising mobility and patient safety in healthcare settings.

The benefits of maintaining mobility are multifaceted and the advantages include and are not limited to the physical, mental, and psychosocial wellbeing of the patient. In order to help others understand the benefits coming from improving mobility, Arjo (2022) have formulated principles of the Positive Eight (see link below) which help patients obtain physical and physiological benefits while promoting independence and self-respect.

GO FURTHER

Visit https://www.arjo.com/int/knowledge/positive-eight/ to learn more about the Positive Eight philosophy.

The Positive Eight has eight key principles – mobility; improving vital functions; reduced consequences of immobility; quality of life; reduced need for support; reduced injuries and improved efficiency; reduced sick leave, turnover and compensation claims; and improved care and financial outcomes. The first four principles mainly focus on the patient. Stimulating and maintaining patients' mobility has a direct effect on optimising the functioning of the body organs like lungs, heart, circulation, bones and muscle structure. Risk to patients' physical and psychological ill health is also minimised, thereby reducing the cost of treatment related to health-related complications. Due to sustained independence, improved recovery times and confidence, the overall quality of the patient's life is also improved. The next four principles of the Positive Eight focus on the caregiver. As a result of improved independence level, the caregiver does not need to provide more assistance to patients, which reduces the risk of physical strain and injury, and frees up time for the caregiver. Hence the caregiver's health and wellbeing is maintained and there is a higher level of job satisfaction. This in turn promotes better quality of care and better financial outcomes for the care facility. When adopting these principles, it is also important to consider the limitations and abilities of the patient.

Healthcare professionals play an important part in promoting mobility and maintaining safety of the patients in hospital and domiciliary care. The Health and Social Care Act Regulations (UK Government, 2014) advocate that healthcare providers should risk assess the health and safety of patients receiving care, and staff taking care of the patients should be appropriately qualified, competent, equipped with skills and experienced to ensure safe delivery of care. An integral element in ensuring safety involves appropriate care planning of moving and handling. All patients coming into a healthcare facility should have a moving and handling plan. Nursing students can also engage in formulating the moving and handling plan under the supervision of practice area staff. While simple moving and handling tasks can be assessed by nurses, the more complex care requires referral to the physiotherapist. The joint assessment by nurse and physiotherapy staff can help in creating a robust moving and handling plan and maintain the safety of the patient in the healthcare setting.

ANATOMY AND PHYSIOLOGY RECAP

Musculoskeletal system

The musculoskeletal system is composed of muscles, bones, joints, and connective tissues like tendons and ligaments surrounding these structures. These structures function jointly to support the body's weight and to enable movement of the body.

Muscles

Muscles are made up of connective tissue. There are three main types of muscles in our body – voluntary (skeletal) muscles, involuntary (visceral) muscles and heart (cardiac) muscles (Springhouse, 2002). Skeletal muscles are made up of muscle fibres which enable voluntary and reflex movements by muscular contraction to move body parts or move the body as a whole.

Bones

The adult human skeleton has a total of 206 bones and is divided into the axial skeleton and the appendicular skeleton. The axial skeleton consists of the skull, ribcage, sternum and spinal column and forms the axis of the skeleton which anchors the other bones. The appendicular skeleton is comprised of the bones of the limbs and girdles. Where bones meet, joints are formed and connective tissues (i.e., ligaments and tendons) complete the structure of the joints (Marshall et al., 2017). The skeletal functions include support, movement, protection, storage and formation of blood cells.

Joints

Joints are also sometimes called articulations and they are formed where two or more bones meet. Joints can mainly be classified into three types – fibrous joints, cartilaginous joints and synovial joints (Peate, 2017). Fibrous joints are held only by a ligament (dense tissue composed of collagen-rich fibres). Examples of fibrous joints are radioulnar and tibiofibular joints. Cartilaginous joints are made up of cartilage for, e.g., intervertebral joints and symphysis pubis. Synovial joints are very flexible joints comprised of synovial cavity, articular capsule, synovial membrane (which produces synovial fluid) and hyaline cartilage. Examples of synovial joints include elbow joints, shoulder joints, knee joints and hip joints. The main function of joints is in facilitating a range of movements.

Tendons and ligaments

Tendons are composed of fibrous connective tissue that attach muscles to the fibrous membrane covering the bone. When skeletal muscles contract, tendons facilitate movement. Ligaments are also made up of dense fibrous connective tissue. Ligaments are flexible and strong and connect bones to other bones. Ligaments promote movement and stability.

For this chapter, the musculoskeletal function in facilitating movement will be discussed further. The various ranges and degrees of movement occur due to lever systems formed by attachment of ligaments and tendons to bones and muscles. Through leverage, contraction and pulling, several bones can change the direction and strength of motion by forces produced by the skeletal muscles (Peate, 2017). This can result in fine and gross movements through articulation of bones and muscles.

This whole process is coordinated by the brain. The frontal lobe of the brain contains the motor system. The motor system begins with the premotor areas of the brain which are involved in planning and coordinating complex movements. The system ends with the primary motor cortex which sends the final output to the spinal cord to enable contraction and movement of specific muscles. Some key terms associated with musculoskeletal movement are explained below.

KEY TERMS

Abduction: moving a limb or other part away from the midline of the body

Adduction: moving a limb or other part toward the midline of the body

Circumduction: moving a limb in a circle (a combination of extension, flexion, abduction, and adduction)

Eversion: turning a body part outward

Extension: increasing the angle between two adjoining bones

External rotation: moving a body part away from the midline

Flexion: decreasing the angle between two adjoining bones

Internal (medial) rotation: moving a body part toward the midline

Inversion: turning a body part inward

Pronation: turning a body part downward

Retraction and protraction: moving a body part backward and forward

Supination: turning a body part upward

Moreau et al. (2002)

CLINICAL SKILLS RELATED TO MOBILITY AND SAFETY

There are numerous skills related to mobility and maintaining safety and the benefits of keeping moving are manifold. In healthcare settings, focus during acute care is mainly on stabilising the patient medically. This could result in patients spending a number of days on the bed and losing their normal mobility and function. It is important to focus on early mobilisation to promote functioning of the rest of the body organs and to achieve the overall benefits. Delayed mobilisation could result in alteration in skin integrity and development of other physical and mental ill health. Keeping mobile and physically active helps to manage and prevent conditions like cardiovascular diseases, cancer, and diabetes (WHO, 2022). It is equally important that all aspects of care are delivered safely in compliance with the Nursing and Midwifery Council *Code* (2018). This will ensure dependable and professional care delivery for patients. Hence it is very important for nurses and healthcare professionals to understand the skills pertaining to optimising mobility and maintaining safety.

While manual handling is emphasised mainly for adult patients, it is vital to recognise the importance of moving and handling in children's nursing settings. There is significant risk when working with babies, children and children requiring additional support. Some examples of at-risk moving and handling activities in children's nursing include carrying in and out of the car, moving from the floor, hoisting dependent children and handling over cot sides and in incubators. Care should be taken regarding moving and handling neonates, babies, toddlers and children depending on their age, weight and size. Behavioural, emotional and psychosocial factors affecting the handling of children should be considered. The basic principles of performing a manual handling technique safely, described later in this chapter, will also apply to manual handling of children. Where extra support is required for children with disability or special needs, a referral should be made to the occupational therapist and relevant disciplines for the necessary adaptations so that moving and handling can be carried out safely and effectively for the child while maintaining staff safety and wellbeing. The Children Act 1989 & 2004 are care protection frameworks which emphasise including children where possible in decisions related to their care management.

The clinical skills covered in this chapter can be suitably applied to different ranges of patients in various healthcare settings. The focus may differ slightly depending on area of clinical practice or community care. The skills discussed in this chapter should not be considered as comprehensive as there may be other safe methods of assessing and assisting a patient's mobility outside the domain of this chapter.

Use evidence-based risk assessment tools to determine need for support and intervention to optimise mobility and safety: Discussion

Any moving and handling activity should be assessed for risks involved as per the *Manual Handling Operation Regulations Act* (1992). Certain activities could increase the level of risk, including aiding people with activities of daily living like bathing and assisting with transfers. There are two types of assessments – generic and individual (Health & Safety Executive, 2021):

- **Generic risk assessments** cover the environmental and workplace aspects, e.g., the appropriateness of the physical environment, type and frequency of the activity, equipment required, number of staff and emergency procedures. Use of risk assessments ensures safety for staff and patients.
- **Individual risk assessments** cover the moving and handling requirements of the person and include the staff required to mobilise the person, equipment needed etc. These assessments should be person-centered and discussed with the individual as well as the family so that the individual and family are assured of their safety and care.
- **Patient risk assessment tools:** Risk assessments are carried out using tools which enable the assessment to be carried out safely and methodically. Moving and handling risk assessments must be completed on initial assessment or admission and must be reviewed based on any changes in the individual's mobility and functional ability. Using a patient risk assessment and safe handling care plan is also beneficial for all patients in hospital and care settings.

COMPLETING A PATIENT-SPECIFIC MOVING AND HANDLING RISK ASSESSMENT: STEP BY STEP

- Explain the importance of maintaining the moving and handling risk assessment to the person. Involve the family in the process if appropriate.
- Assess what the person is able/unable to do without assistance.
- Assess the person's weight bearing ability and factors affecting mobility including disability, skin condition, history of falls, medical/surgical condition etc.
- Check how the person can reposition themselves in bed.

(Continued)

- Assess the person's ability and cooperation in transferring in and out of bed, in and out of chair etc.
- Establish the number of staff required to manage transfers. If hoists are used, two staff may be required to carry out the activity safely. Follow the local procedures in the care setting regarding safe use of equipment.
- Check the size and weight of the person and verify use of appropriate equipment based on the person's weight and size.
- Where a complex moving and handling assessment is involved, refer to the physiotherapist as appropriate for further advice.
- Complete all the sections of the risk assessment form using evidence from discussion with the person, family, case notes, activity assessments etc.
- Update the risk assessment when there is a change in the person's condition, mobility or functional ability. Review the assessment at least once weekly even if there is no change in the person's condition.

To access the All-Wales patient safe handling risk assessment (as an example), visit: www.nationalbackexchange.org/index.php/docman-utility-menu/177-all-wales-nhs-manual-handling-passport-scheme-revised-2020/file (accessed October 18, 2022).

CASE STUDY

Owen

Owen Jones is a 70-year-old man who has been admitted to a general medical ward due to nausea and fever. He has been unsteady on his feet for the past week and requires assistance of one person to mobilise. He weighs 62kg and has a height of 164cm. He has a history of high blood pressure and falls when attempting to walk. He lives on his own in a ground floor flat and has a daughter who helps with shopping.

Complete a moving and handling risk assessment for Owen using the risk assessment form in the document mentioned above.

USE APPROPRIATE SAFETY TECHNIQUES AND DEVICES: DISCUSSION

For all moving and handling activities, it important to bear principles of safety in mind prior to performing any activity. These principles ensure safety for the person involved as well ensuring that staff can perform the activity without causing undue stress to themselves. Some basic principles for managing a technique safely include:

- Staff involved should maintain a broad base (feet a shoulder's width apart) when performing the activity to maintain stability.
- Staff should maintain the natural shape of the spine and avoid bending, stooping or twisting which could cause cumulative stress to the spine.
- Advise the person to maintain a broad base and to look up and lead with the head when performing activities like sit to stand, transfers, walking etc.
- Ensure the area is clear and clutter free and it is safe to perform the activity.

- Communicate and explain the activity to the person and to the rest of the staff involved.
- Adopt an open palm approach when handling patients to prevent injuries like bruising.
- For activities where the person can initiate the movement, allow the person to start the activity when they are ready while supporting the person as per need.
- For dependent persons, adopt a command for commencing the activity (e.g., 'Ready, steady, move') after explaining the command to the patient and the team member.
- Allow plenty of time and provide ample reassurance to the person if they are anxious or fearful.
- Check the risk assessment and safe handling plan prior to moving the person.
- Follow local protocols for moving and handling during emergency situations.

Most importantly, *consent* is very important to be gained prior to performing any activity or procedure involving the person. Consent involves adults who can make the decision after having the benefits and risks of the procedure or treatment explained to them to get an informed choice. For children, adults who have parental responsibility could give consent (Royal College of Nursing, 2022). For adults who are not capable of giving consent due to lack of ability in decision-making, procedure or treatment could be provided without consent, if it is in the best interest of the person. This falls within the legislation of the Mental Capacity Act (UK Government, 2005). An addition to this Act called Deprivation of Liberty Safeguards (DoLS) applies in England and Wales to protect individuals in care whose ability has been limited by ensuring that it is appropriate and in their best interests. Examples of people who would have consent issues include individuals suffering from dementia, mental health issues and brain disorders.

Safety devices include use of bed rails, use of safety belts (for wheelchairs) and safety alarms for persons at risk of falls. These are used commonly in healthcare settings. Bed rails are most commonly used in hospitals and community settings.

Bed rails, also known as side rails, are generally used to prevent patients falling out of bed thus preventing injury to the patient. Estimates of falls from bed in hospital varies from 20% (Healy and Scobie, 2007) to 70% (Oliver, 2002) which suggests the benefit of use of bed rails where appropriate. The advantages of use of bed rails include feeling a sense of security, prevention of accidental fall when turning or being transported in a bed, enabling turning and repositioning in bed (where bed rails are manufactured to assist with the same) and to provide easy access to bed controls. Disadvantages include feelings of restriction, falls when patients climb over the bedrails, accidental bruises and cuts and causing agitation and preventing independence. A detailed risk assessment should be carried out for all persons requiring use of bed rails. A bed rails risk assessment should be completed on initial contact or on admission to the hospital setting.

The points to consider during a risk assessment include (UK Government, 2021):

- Is it likely that the bed user would fall from their bed?
- If so, are bed rails an appropriate solution or could the risk of falling from bed be reduced by means other than bed rails?
- Could the use of a bed rail increase risks to the occupant's physical or clinical condition?
- Has the bed user used bed rails before? Do they have a history of falling from beds, or conversely of climbing over bed rails?
- Do the risks of using bed rails outweigh the possible benefits from using them?
- What are the bed user's views on using bed rails?
- What configuration of bed, mattress and rail system is being used?

Where use of bed rails is deemed not necessary or unsafe, consider keeping the bed in the lowest position, with frequent patient monitoring, providing mobility aids within easy reach, considering and meeting the needs that the patient would want to get out of bed for, for example toileting, pain, hunger, thirst etc. If the patient is at risk of falls as well as at risk of climbing over the bed rails, it is advisable to nurse them on an ultra low bed with mats next to the bed as long as this does not cause any further risk. Remember that assessing patient risk is very much individualised and patient-centred, and you will need to get support from senior staff members where possible. Include patient and family in decisions taken about them. Follow local policies in relation to nursing care, care planning and decisions related to care.

USE OF BED RAILS FOR AN ADULT PATIENT: STEP BY STEP

- Check the bed rails risk assessment to ensure it is safe to use them for the patient.
- Explain the procedure to the patient and gain consent.
- Provide all necessary items required by the patient within easy reach.
- Pull the bed rails into position and check that they are secure. Check that the patient is comfortable.
- Ensure that the mattress is correctly fitted to prevent entrapment between the mattress and bed rails.
- If it is safe to do so, cover the bed rails with foam padding to avoid accidental bruises and injury to the patient.
- Leave the bed in the lowest possible position when leaving the patient. Provide call bell to the patient if the patient is able to use it safely.
- Document the procedure in the patient's notes.
- Check the patient frequently, attend to toileting and personal care needs regularly and maintain privacy and dignity at all times.

IDENTIFY AND MANAGE RISK OF FALLS AND USE OF MOVING AND HANDLING TECHNIQUES RELATED TO FALLS: DISCUSSION

Conditions that often lead to falls, slips and trips

A fall is commonly defined as an unintentional event which has caused the person to rest or lower to the ground (WHO, 2018).

Ensure the assessment, planning, implementation, and treatment evaluation of falls is robust. Having a more sufficient understanding of the pathology of falls is important for pre- and post-fall management. Falls in older adults, particularly front facing, are often seen as the most common form of injury (WHO, 2018).

Post-operation pain from initial operation period and potential muscle atrophy are common side effects. Individuals not engaging with post-operation exercises are at an increased risk of weakening muscle groups. It is acknowledged that loss of muscle mass is a driving cause for community-related falls in older adult populations (Gawler et al., 2016).

Organic brain disorders

Conventionally neurological issues can be a prime cause for falls, mainly resulting from manifested psychiatric symptomology which in turn causes a number of physical changes. Organic brain syndrome is less a specific neurological diagnosis and more a generalised term for more abnormal symptoms which can impact the nervous system in a litany of ways. Special consideration for and insight into an individual's mental health can help recognise and identify the deteriorating state of an individual. Consider conducting a Mental State Examination (MSE) to ascertain an individual's mental state at that moment. Further psychological tests can and should be considered in the patient's care, particularly if identified with an organic brain disorder.

CASE STUDY

Taylor

Taylor is a 22-year-old transgender man who is acting in a peculiar manner. You notice Taylor is wearing thick layers of clothing when it is very hot on the ward. He also seems distracted, is talking to himself and is dishevelled in presentation. His gait appears to be impacted and he is swaying as he walks. You suspect his mental health is declining and you know from experience this can increase the risk of falling. You wish to assess Taylor and then liaise with the mental health team for further support and review.

Questions

1 Would you know how to conduct a mental state examination?
2 Using the scenario, what terminology would you use to describe Taylor's affect, behaviour and cognition?
3 What could be the potential risks of using inappropriate terminology or missing aspects of a mental state examination?

To find out more about a MSE using the I-AM-A-STAR framework, please follow this link: https://cronfa.swan.ac.uk/Record/cronfa38823 (accessed October 18, 2022).

Obesity

With obesity at its highest level in recent years it is important to consider the wider risks of inactivity within the general population; increased pressure on ligaments and joints with a weakened state of muscle mass can lead to an onset of health-related issues that can exacerbate a risk of falls (Baker, 2022). Obesity is considered a complex social and health issue and over the past four decades we have seen a significant increase in obesity levels in the United Kingdom. In 1980, obesity in England was recorded at 6% for males and 9% for females; compare this to 2019, where 27% of males and 29% females are currently considered obese (Hancock, 2021). This presents further challenges as the extent of the injury and recovery time can be worsened/lengthened due to these circumstances. Falls have been seen to be increased in obese people over the age of 60, but there is a lack of evidence to develop a correlation with fall-related injuries or fractures (Neri et al., 2019).

Malnutrition

Individuals with multiple or co-morbidities are at risk of malnutrition. This can significantly increase risk and likelihood of falls if not managed appropriately. It is important to know why certain aspects impacting nutrition can lead to an increase of falls.

- Chronic conditions can affect the individual's ability to eat and drink, which can predispose people to malnutrition and subsequently a weakened state.
- Changes to daily routines like structured mealtimes caused through health implications can lead to malnourished states and result in a reduced nutritional intake.
- Previous falls or other physical impediments can result in reduced levels of diet and fluid intake, creating more inherent challenges to an individual's life (cooking and its preparation, use of utensils, swallowing and chewing) largely resulting in a likely poorer diet and nutritional intake of key proteins, carbohydrates, vitamins and salts.
- Appetite and taste can change as we age; this often results in older adults not finding mealtimes pleasurable or losing interest in food.
- As we age, the requirements for our bodies change, and the nutrition our body requires can be at risk of being neglected. Dehydration is a large factor in this: it can lead to a lower blood pressure, resulting in dizziness and weakness increasing the risks of falls and trips.

Often falls are associated with the older adult population and sometimes considered a consequence of getting older. We see a greater prevalence of falls within older adults above 65 and it is a common misconception to solely associate aging as the primary cause. It is in fact more a consequence of the general health of the individual. Older adults in excellent health can be at no more of a risk of falls than individuals in their younger years. It is recognised that cognitive changes due to aging are associated with increased falls and we see a prevalence of falls in those over 85, with an increase of white males being at further risk, but this is largely associated with an individual's failing health or diagnosis (Terrosso et al., 2010). Other conditions such as transient ischemic attacks, diabetes, associated mental health issues, alcohol and drug intake (including prescribed medications) are leading causes of increased falls for our patients.

To ensure adequate support is provided to your patients during these events, we must explore common forms of injury and the subsequent issues that can arise from these. It is important that a safe and effective process is followed to ensure high quality care is provided in an appropriate time and manner to manage the incident. Under NICE guidelines, health professionals are recommended to assess for physical and spinal injuries prior to moving (NICE, 2019). We shall now explore how to do this, and once this has been achieved, what else to review and manage during incidents like this.

Consequences of falls

An emphasis on prevention of falls is vital. Falls can be extremely traumatic as well as dangerous for patients. This next section looks at a number of the consequences of a fall on a person.

Spinal cord injuries

Falls such as trips, slips and stumbling are seen to be the leading cause of Spinal Cord Injuries (SCIs) (Chen et al., 2016). A SCI can be fatal to a patient. Poor management of patient safety in this instance can lead to serious consequences ranging from life threating to severe health consequences such as bladder or bowel control, neurological issues and musculoskeletally induced pain. Unexpected movement after a fall can lead to a worsening state of the patient, therefore it is vital that a thorough assessment is undertaken to ascertain the level of risk present prior to movement. This can include a motor assessment, sensory assessment and a fundamental overview assessment (ABCDE).

Head injuries

Falls are the leading cause of Traumatic Brain Injury (TBI), particularly in older adults. TBI may not be the first or initial aspect of care and assessment that would rush through your mind when you are managing an incident. It is, however, important to consider how vital effectively assessing and managing a potential TBI can be in these situations. Frontal temporal injuries are more common and are often found due to the more common forward fall. Intercranial pressure often creates immense stress on the break, causing parts of that brain tissue to die.

As with all good practice, assessment is the initial key to effective management. Consider a neuro assessment approach and think beyond the head. Consider how your patient is following instructions, moving or coordinating their actions. A Glasgow Coma scale is effective in assessing this as it combines both a neurological and motor assessment to ascertain the patient's neuro state.

Glasgow Coma Scale

The Glasgow Coma Scale is a neurological scale which aims to ascertain the consciousness of the patient. This reviews three primary aspects of what is deemed as consciousness: eye movement/opening, verbal response and body response. These factors are then scored out of 15, 15 being normal consciousness and 3 meaning the individual is in a coma (Teasdale, 1974). It is important to remember that while conducting a Glasgow Coma Scale assessment, a person with certain cognitive impairments such as a dementia or learning disability may have an affected score. Falls resulting in suspected brain injury are a common requirement for undertaking a Glasgow Coma Scale assessment, but there are also other reasons why one may be conducted.

These can include:

- Epilepsy
- Trauma such as an intracranial hemorrhage or raised intracranial pressure
- Endocrine or metabolic issues, such as hypoglycemia
- Excessive alcohol poisoning or illicit substance use

It is important to understand the types of conditions and symptoms you may see whilst conducting this assessment. It provides you with a fundamental understanding as to the potential barriers of care and communication that are currently present for the patient. It also allows you to broaden your ability to respond quicker to the needs of the individual.

Soft tissue damage

We can often see several soft tissue injuries during falls. These typically tend to be low on a practitioner's priority list with primary focus being on fracture or spinal injuries. Soft tissue injuries like contusions, strains and sprains, along with bursitis, are common soft-tissue injuries. Awareness of these soft tissue injuries should be considered as they can often invoke pain, discomfort and if not appropriately treated, take a long time to heal. With acute injuries often caused during falls always consider RICE:

1   **Rest.** Ensure you advocate rest initially after the injury has occurred. During the initial stages ensure you are advising your patient to not weight bear on the injury to avoid further complications such as a recurring fall or further strain on the area. It is important that this is not misinterpreted for complete inactivity. Recommend light stretching as this can be beneficial during these stages to promote blood flow to the areas and help the patient acclimatise to the injury's pain.

2   **Ice.** Utilization of ice or cold packs for 20 minutes at a time can be useful to reduce inflammation in the initial stages of the injury. It is important to consider that inflammation is a requirement of the healing process, and this should only be encouraged during the initial event and some hours after if appropriate. If pain persists, further cold packs can be used to assist in pain management.

3   **Compression.** Mainly to prevent blood loss and swelling, consider using bandages on the area to assist in the reduction of both of these and provide the area with additional support.

4   **Elevation.** Used to reduce excessive swelling, raising the injury site can aid in the reduction of pain and unnecessary swelling.

Sprains are a stretch or tear of a ligament which is a strong band of connective tissue which connects the end of one bone to another. The primary function is to support the body's joints. The patella ligament for example plays a role in stabilising and connecting your knee to the femur and the tibia, enabling movement. Common areas of the body that are vulnerable to sprains are typically wrists, ankles and knees. These are common during falls and mainly due to a sharp or unexpected twist of limbs and appendages often seen in falls. This is where extreme tension is placed on the ligament. Harsh impact is also another common cause: outstretched hands can often result in sprains due to the impact caused.

Classification of sprains

A sprain is injury or trauma to the muscles or tendons, which are fibrous cords of tissue which connect muscle to bone. Sprains often occur in the back, arms or legs when individuals fall. Symptoms of sprain often consist of muscle weakness, inflammation and pain.

- **Sprain grade one:** Slight stretching and some damage to the fibers of the ligament.
- **Sprain grade two:** A partial tear of the ligament where laxis can be evident when the joint moves.
- **Sprain grade three:** Typically, we see a complete tear of the ligament causing significant instability and pain for the patient.

Pain can vary in intensity. Bruising, inflammation and swelling are often common occurrences when individuals fall. For patients, significant pain can have several negative factors both physical and psychological, including fear of falling again due to the pain. The fear these falls can invoke can influence individuals to avoid physical tasks, sometimes to their detriment.

Fractures

Most falls statistically do not result in injury. Once a fall occurs, a patient's likelihood of falling increases and so does their risk of injury, particularly if they exhibit clusters of risk factors (NICE, 2018). A person falling can be a result of many different factors: age, impaired gait, cognitive impairment, medication usage. One or more of these (clustering) can result in higher likelihood of falls (NICE, 2018). Common forms of fracture include intertrochanteric hip fractures, neck of femur fractures and distal radius fractures. It is vital that a full head to toe assessment is conducted when looking for both fractures and soft tissue damage. Initial open fractures (the protrusions of bones) are commonly observed, however it is important not to rule out closed fractures. Closed fractures, if not identified, can be damaging to patient recovery, depending on the style of fracture. There are different types and patterns of fractures to be aware of when it comes to individuals falling. Below are some of the common bone fracture categories:

- **Open fracture:** The bone has broken through the skin, or trauma has opened the fracture site. Usually considered a medical emergency.
- **Non-displaced fracture:** The bone fractures, but is still in alignment.
- **Displaced fracture:** An out of alignment fracture where the bone is broken in two or more places.
- **Closed fracture:** The skin around the fracture site is not broken.

Pattern names are given to fracture types. Here are some types of fracture patterns to review:

- **Avulsion fracture:** This is where part of the bone has fragmented from its main mass.
- **Transverse fracture:** Where the fractured bone and the bone's axis are at a right angle from each other.
- **Spiral fracture:** This is where the bone is partially twisted at the breakpoint.
- **Stress line fracture:** Commonly a crack or hairline crack in the bone.
- **Buckled/impacted fracture:** Ends of the fracture are driven into each other.
- **Oblique fracture:** The fracture has resulted in a curved or sloped pattern.
- **Compression fracture (wedge):** Often associated with spinal/vertebrae damage.
- **Comminuted:** A fracture resulting in the bone fragmenting in several places.
- **Linear fracture:** A break that runs parallel to the bone's axis.

Minimal aid for the fallen patient

Communication is key throughout all areas of interventions we are going to review. Patients in these circumstances may be confused, frightened and in pain. This can lead to anger and potential violence, so it is important before starting this process that the patient is in a relatively calmed state and is able to understand and undertake instruction.

Consider:

- Can the patient move unaided?
- Can the patient follow instruction and understand direction?
- Does the patient have the strength and ability to stand from the floor unaided?
- If yes to all and the patient is ready, give verbal instruction and encouragement to move themselves from the floor. Assist in the environment, like moving a chair closer to the individual to sit on but reduce physical contact where possible. Ensure the events are documented and the incident is logged. It would be good practice to evidence how the individual got up.

ACTIVITY: PAUSE AND REFLECT

Why would it be important to document the findings of these considerations in the patient notes? There are a number of different factors as to why documenting these findings are important:

(Continued)

- This assists in your assessment framework and would be considered a primary survey procedure. This enables health professionals to undertake initial assessments to effectively build a baseline of the current presenting health of the patient. This will allow further assessments, planning, interventions and evaluations of care to be carried out more effectively.
- It improves communication across the wider multidisciplinary team.
- It enables health professionals to prioritise care.
- It demonstrates and evidences the level of care provision provided to the individual.
- It can allow teams to carry on delivering a standardised level of care for the patient.

HELP A PATIENT TO STAND WITH MINIMAL ASSISTANCE: STEP BY STEP

- If the patient has been assessed and is safe to rise from the floor, ask them to roll to their side (preferably with their dominant arm free). Instruct the patient to place their free arm palm flat on the ground and their other arm supporting their head.
- Instruct the patient to slowly push themselves up supporting their weight with both arms. Having a wide arm placement (one in line with their shoulder and the other in line with their stomach) creates greater stability and evens out weight distribution, making the task easier.
- Instruct the patient to shift their weight over to bring all four limbs on the ground; this provides greater stability and allows for the next task to be completed with more ease.
- Using your environment, bring a chair up to the front of the patient. Instruct them to place their hands on the arms of the chair; at this point instruct the patient to re-adjust bringing their knees closer, aligning their center of gravity through their knees, hips and head.
- At this stage, bringing a chair behind the patient, instruct them to stand themselves up by pushing on the arms of the chair in front of them. Once standing bring the chair behind them closer and when ready inform the patient they can sit back slowly.
- Look to assess the patient, ensure they are comfortable and conduct the necessary post-falls protocols and assessments depending on need. Patients may have a lot of adrenaline and cortisol rushing through their body after the event. This could possibly induce another fall. Ensure the patient is not unattended directly after a fall.

Emergency care following a falls injury

During an emergency, how we move and handle a patient is the fundamental aspect of the care we provide. It not only affords the patient the dignity and respect they deserve, but it also ensures you and your patient are safe throughout. Moving a patient incorrectly or not adhering to proper procedure could result in patient harm or waste vital minutes that could be required for providing life saving procedures like cardiac or pulmonary resuscitation. Knowing when to move your patient and how is extremely important during these time sensitive incidents. Below is a flow chart depicting four of the most common accidents that a patient may collapse from and their ideal subsequent procedures.

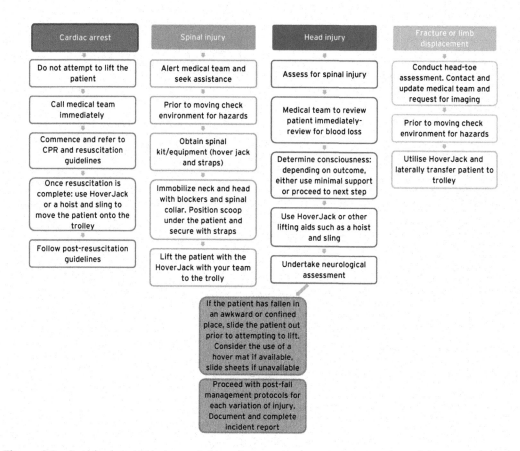

Figure 9.1   Accidents and their procedures

ACTIVITY: PAUSE AND REFLECT

From your clinical experience, have you come across patients who have fallen in the past? What was the process followed by the staff during that time? Specifically, what assessments were carried out?

CASE STUDY

Jay

Jay Rees is a 22-year-old patient who has been admitted to an acute mental health assessment ward due to suicidal behaviours and the presentation of visual and auditory hallucinations. Jay has presented with heightened levels of aggression towards staff over the past week. They weigh 68kg and have recently fallen down a flight of stairs and were found unconscious. It was reported Jay

(Continued)

purposefully fell in an attempt to injure themself. You have just started your shift and discover Jay laying supine on the floor, and they appear to have fallen. You instinctively notice a 4cm laceration on Jay's forehead and note their right leg appears longer than the left.

What assessments would you think to carry out first and what special considerations might you want to think about prior to conducting the assessment?

- Prior to moving forward , an airway, breathing and circulation assessment should be conducted to ascertain the breathing and airway of the patient.
- A head-to-toe assessment establishes further potential injuries: spinal injury assessment/leg fracture.
- Conduct a neurological assessment using the Glasgow Coma Scale.
- Based on the information provided, list your main concerns.

Head trauma

Although individuals may initially present with a soft tissue injury on the forehead of 4cm, it could allude to more severe and potential intercranial pressure, which can lead to brain injury or damage. Special consideration of further neck and spinal injury should be considered (see above discussion).

Left non-displaced fracture

Due to the shortening of the left lower limb, this can be further assessed by application of axial pressure and assessing for pain, additionally assessing for pain during log roll due to the rotation movement of the technique. Consider further assessing by feeling for the distal pulse. Additionally, if Jay is able, consider asking them to slowly perform a slow, straight leg raise from a supine position. Pain will likely hinder this ability further, indicating a fracture.

Pain management post-incident

The patient may be experiencing pain or less traumatic injuries such as bruising or strains. Provide care and support for these in the form of a self diagnostic pain assessment and treatment along with **R**est **I**ce **C**ompression **E**levation (RICE). The patient may or will likely feel embarrassed after the fall. It would be prudent and good practice to ensure time is spent with the patient to note their feelings and reflect with them about the event at a later point.

Patient becoming violent and aggressive

Falls can be frightening experiences for patients. Patients in a frightened state may become aggressive or violent, based on the circumstances. Patients with altered perception or cognitive impairment may also be at a greater risk of becoming violent. This can be a very difficult situation for care staff, particularly when trying to provide support.

Patients with a tendency to become nervous, aggressive, reach out or grab should have care plans or risk management plans in place. It is vital for the care teams to be familiar with these plans and document and record areas of effective management or areas which increase or do little to support the patient.

If a patient has fallen and becomes aggressive whilst staff are intervening, it is important to give that patient space. Staff should not engage in any restrictive practice interventions until the patient has been assessed for spinal or head injury. Allowing the patient space will give both staff and patient time to open a dialogue. Managing environmental risks such as removing any objects that could easily be used as a weapon, other patients or general trip hazards would be a far more productive step to safely manage the area. Talk calmly to the patient and allow time and space for gaps. Contact or over explanative discussion can distress, confuse, or simply frustrate the person further. Allowing the patient space and time will often allow that individual opportunity to process the event and their situation. This can often lead to an opening of dialogue and a request for assistance. Staff should ensure they look to manage their own emotions and behaviours, as situations like these can often leave staff feeling frustrated. Consider changing staff members, to allow for fresh interactions. When approaching, talking to or touching the patient, take care to be gentle, polite and to go at a pace the person is comfortable with, preferably at a 45 degree angle of approach at eye level. If touch is required, ensuring staff maintain flat open palm gestures will reduce the risk of staff inadvertently grabbing the patient (creating a restraint scenario) and will also non-verbally communicate to the person a relaxed and calm manner.

ACTIVITY: HAVE A GO

Can you list two symptoms that could be associated to each of these conditions?

Epilepsy

1:

2:

Raised intracranial pressure

1:

2:

Hypoglycemia

1:

2:

Alcohol poisoning

1:

2:

Advanced Trauma Life Support guidelines should always be followed when in situations of acute severe trauma. Ideally, a full past history around the traumatic incident should be obtained for clinical review. Examination of the spine requires special consideration. Palpation of the nuchal ridge to the first thoracic vertebral will be performed by an appropriate practitioner. When determining acute abnormality, tenderness may be a key indicator; haematoma and involuntary muscle spasms may also be evident. It is important to ensure a continuity of assessment of the cervical structure, this would be achieved by placing opposing thumbs on the spinous process of C2 and systematically placing progressive pressure in a circular manner down the midline. This can be repeated 2–3cm from the midline. Relevant clinical investigations would be requested, for example x-rays by an appropriate practitioner.

USE OF HOVERJACK TO MOBILISE A PERSON FROM THE FLOOR TO TROLLEY USING A LATERAL TRANSFER: STEP BY STEP

A HoverJack is an inflatable device that allows staff to lift a patient without the aid of a lift team. It is a flexible and proactive approach to supporting a fallen patient in both community and clinical settings. Lifting teams can require multiple staff usually starting at four, making the procedure resource-heavy. A HoverJack will typically require two members of staff, not only saving the number of staff required, but also ensuring the patient can be lifted in a steady manner, making the process smoother and more comfortable for the patient due to its consistent singular inflation as opposed to multiple staff attempting to lift simultaneously.

EQUIPMENT

- HoverJack
- HoverMatt
- Hover air supply pump

PROCEDURE

- A minimum of two healthcare practitioners is required to perform this activity for an average-size dependent person.
- Check the moving and handling plan related to the patient to ensure that correct equipment is used to move the person. Ensure that the plan is up to date.
- In the absence of a written plan, obtain information from the person, family, healthcare professional (e.g., physiotherapist) and case notes to establish a correct moving and handling plan and use of appropriate equipment.
- Explain the activity to the person and obtain verbal consent if possible.
- Ensure that the trolley height is correct and suitable for the healthcare practitioners involved in the technique.
- Check the general condition and cleanliness of the equipment and inspect the HoverMatt for any rips, loose stitches and general integrity. Check the HoverJack for safety label and safe working load and ensure that the person's weight is within the safe limits for using the HoverJack. Check that equipment is the correct size for the person. Check the sling for Lifting Operating & Lifting Equipment Regulation (LOLER) inspection label.
- Check any of the other equipment for any sign of wear and tear, damage, safe working load and check that the sling in use is compatible with the hoist. Check the pump and connection leads to ensure that it is working sufficiently. Confirm the LOLER inspection date.
- Roll the person to one side. To do so, one healthcare practitioner should stand on either side of the patient and then kneel. Ask the person to turn their face towards the direction of transfer, cross their arms in front of their body and to bend their farther knee.
- If the person is unable to bend their knee themselves, the healthcare practitioner should facilitate this by placing one hand under the knee and the other hand under the heel or around the ankle and enable the person to bend their knee and hip. The healthcare practitioner facing the person should place their hand closest to the head of the bed on the person's shoulder

and the other hand on the person's hip or thigh. The healthcare practitioner on the other side would also place one hand on the shoulder and the other hand on the hip or thigh laterally.

- Use a command for when you are ready to move, e.g., 'Ready, steady, roll', to turn the person from their back to their side. During the movement the healthcare practitioner on the opposite side of the patient would give a gentle push to the person while shifting the weight from the back foot to the front foot. The healthcare practitioner facing the person would roll the person towards the other healthcare practitioner. If it is not possible to turn the person in this manner, use of equipment – e.g. slide sheets – should be considered to roll the person.

- To fit the deflated HoverJack, first fold the HoverJack in half with labels and straps on the outside. Place the folded HoverJack on the floor as close to the person's back as possible, making sure no straps or plastics are protruding outwards. The person can now roll onto their back. The position of the HoverJack should be checked to ensure that it is correctly under the person.

- The person should be central on the HoverJack and there should be no part of the patient's body over the edges of the HoverJack itself. Alternatively, if the patient has fallen in a confined space, the healthcare practitioners should look to use slide sheets or a HoverMatt to slide the person out to an area where they can be moved. The HoverJack will now be in the correct position to conduct the next steps.

- Whilst you are placing the HoverJack, you can also fit the pat slide and slide sheets between the patient and the HoverJack using the same log roll maneuver. If you are using a HoverMatt, a pat slide or slide sheets will not be required.

- For using HoverJack to lift the person from the floor to trolley, ensure the patient is in a supine position on the jack, fit the straps and secure these across the chest and legs as indicated. Ensure the straps are secured but not restrictive on breathing and airway. The HoverJack straps will become tighter as the Jack inflates, so ensure this is being monitored by both healthcare practitioners.

- One healthcare practitioner should be near the person's head to monitor the lift and reassure the patient; additionally they can monitor airway and breathing. The other healthcare practitioner should be positioned near the foot end to inflate the HoverJack.

- The healthcare practitioner near the head should inform the patient of the maneuver and provide reassurance as required. If the patient is able, have them state when they are ready to commence the maneuver. The other healthcare practitioner should check the red cap valves are closed prior to inflation.

- Do not cap the inflation valve; begin inflation by attaching the air hose to the bottom valve (valve 1). You will inflate all valves starting from the bottom and subsequently moving up. Most HoverJacks have four chambers/valves. Repeat the process for each subsequent chamber until the process is complete.

- During each valve's inflation employ a look, listen and feel technique. **Look:** at the patient rising, once the patient has stopped, it is an indicator that the chamber is full. Additionally check the straps and ensure they are not becoming too tight. **Listen**: as the chamber becomes full, the air filling process will increase in pitch, indicating the chamber is filled with air. **Feel:** the section in question once filled will feel rock hard to touch, giving a lot of resistance. Repeat this process for each chamber prior to moving to the next.

- Once all chambers have been completed, one healthcare practitioner then presses the standby button on the air supply and brings the trolley alongside the hover jack. The healthcare practitioner near the head will never leave the patient at this point. You can move the HoverJack using its handles if bringing a trolley to the patient is impractical. Adjust the trolley height to the HoverJack's height.

(Continued)

- Detach the safety straps of the HoverJack and ensure the air supply hose is attached and on standby. (If you are using a HoverMatt – attach the air hose to the HoverMatt valve.)
- With a healthcare practitioner remaining at the person's head/shoulder, they will inform the patient that the next step will be to move them onto the trolley. Another two staff members will join the team, one going to the same side as the healthcare practitioner near the person's head near the hip, with the other healthcare practitioner going around the trolley side, taking the HoverMatt straps with another member of staff.
- Ensure the trolley brakes are on and that the trolley is as close to the HoverJack as possible. Your team will now slide the patient over to the trolley. It is important one person take the lead in issuing instructions. A 'Ready, steady, slide' command should be given, with the healthcare practitioners on the side of the patient giving a gentle push to the person while shifting their weight from the back foot to the front foot (their hands would be placed on either the person's shoulder or hip in an open palm gesture). The healthcare practitioners facing the person would pull the straps of the HoverMat towards them while shifting the weight from the front foot to the back foot. Balance is key in this maneuver. As the healthcare practitioners pull, they should take a step back, minding their environment and maintaining balance.
- Check that the person is comfortable on the trolley.
- Deflating the HoverMatt, healthcare practitioners can log roll the patient and remove the matt using the same method it was applied. This is done to minimise tissue damage and promote comfort with mobility.

ACTIVITY: PAUSE AND REFLECT

Try and list as many considerations as you can that you need to think about upon finding a person who has fallen.

Considerations

- Is the person unconscious?
- What is their level of consciousness?
- Do they have a head injury and have they taken anticoagulants? (Warfarin, Enoxaparin, Dabigatran, Rivaroxaban, Apixaban.)
- Is there any indication of a major haemorrhage?
- Is the person indicating any chest pain?
- Any other pain identified?
- Is there any limb deformity such as shortening or rotation issues?
- Any observed excessive swelling or bruising evident?
- Does the person present with dizziness or sickness?

USING APPROPRIATE MOVING AND HANDLING EQUIPMENT TO SUPPORT PEOPLE WITH IMPAIRED MOBILITY: DISCUSSION

A person's mobility can be affected, limited or reduced due to several reasons. Impaired mobility can impact on a person's safety and can have a detrimental effect on emotional and mental wellbeing. While a lot of discussion related to impaired mobility is focused on older people, people of other ages can also have mobility issues (Iezzoni et al., 2001). Most mobility issues are associated with physical illnesses while some may be due to mental health issues. There are acute and chronic causes of impairment in mobility (Table 9.1). Following periods of acute illness functional deconditioning can occur in patients in hospital settings. This can happen quite quickly in older persons and may take longer to improve (O'Hanlon and Twomey, 2009).

A range of equipment is available to support people with reduced/impaired mobility. Equipment need varies based on the level of dependence of the person. The following are some categories of patients you may see in any care setting along with equipment that may be used to aid their mobility. Patients are categorised based on their needed level of assistance.

- **Minimum assistance:** Patients in this category may only require verbal prompts for enabling them to mobilise. Others may need the use of walking aids like a walking stick and frames to mobilise whilst having supervision of a healthcare practitioner, support staff or nurse. Some examples of this category are patients whose mobility is mildly affected due to arthritis, minor toe or ankle surgeries or patients who have mild cognitive impairment.
- **Moderate assistance:** Patients in this category require further help to mobilise. This would involve the assistance of two staff with use of additional equipment to assist with the movement. Equipment used could include slide sheets, stand aids and active hoists (see Figure 9.2). Some examples in this category include patients who have suffered a stroke affecting one side of the body, undergone one side amputation or one sided knee surgery.
- **Maximum assistance:** Patients in this category are usually non weight bearing and require maximum help to move. Moving and handling patients in this category would involve use of slide sheets and passive hoists (see Figure 9.3). Some examples in this category include critically ill patients on artificial ventilation, end of life patients and patients with end stage dementia.

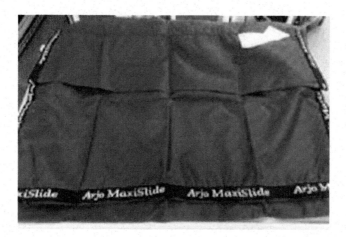

Figure 9.2 Arjo MaxiSlide

ACTIVITY: PAUSE AND REFLECT

From your clinical experience, have you come across patients who fit the categories discussed above? What equipment was used to mobilise those patients?

Table 9.1 Causes of decline in mobility

Neurological	Cardiovascular	Respiratory	Musculoskeletal	Renal	Endocrine	Psychiatric	Medications	Other
Stroke	Angina/angina equivalent	Respiratory tract infection	Osteoarthritis	Chronic kidney disease	Hypothyroidism	Depression	Benzodiazepines (sedation, confusion)	Reduced confidence
Cerebellar dysfunction	Heart failure	Asthma	Rheumatoid arthritis	Renal osteodystrophy	Metabolic syndrome	Anxiety	Opioids (sedation, confusion)	Dehydration
Peripheral neuropathy	Intermittent claudication	Chronic obstructive pulmonary disease	Gout	Urinary infection	Osteoporosis	Substance abuse	Antipsychotics (sedation, extrapyramidal signs)	Visual impairment
Dementia	Thromboembolism	Pulmonary fibrosis	Joint effusion	Incontinence	Addison's disease		Antihypertensives (hypotension, bradycardia)	Carcinoma
Parkinson's disease	Venous or arterial ulceration	Bronchiectasis	Disc prolapse				Diuretics (hypotension)	Cellulitis
Parkinson's plus syndromes	Postural hypotension		Spinal stenosis				Analgesics (sedation, confusion)	Paronychia
Normal pressure hydrocephalus			Myopathy				Statins (causing muscle aches or rhabdomyolysis)	Other ulceration
Myasthenia gravis			Muscular dystrophies				Antihistamines (drowsiness)	
Multiple sclerosis			Peroneal muscle atrophy				Alpha blockers for prostatism (hypotension)	
Motor neurone disease			Polymyalgia rheumatica					
Guillain–Barré syndrome								
Paraneoplastic								

Source: O'Hanlon and Twomey (2009)

Equipment which may be required to help with moving and handling patients include the following (Health and Safety Executive, 2021):

- Suitable walking aids, handrails etc. for people needing minor assistance
- Wheelchairs
- Transfer boards used to assist in moving from and to different furniture (e.g., seat to wheelchair)
- Turntables used to assist in turning people around
- Handling belts to assist residents who can support their own weight, e.g., to help them stand up. These should not be used for lifting
- Slide sheets
- A selection of hoists – e.g., hoists to raise fallen individuals from the floor, standing hoists, mobile hoists etc.
- Lifting cushions used to assist people to get up from the floor or bath
- Bath hoists or bath lifts and/or adjustable height baths
- A sufficient number of slings of different types and sizes
- Electric profiling beds – for dependent/immobile residents
- Bed levers, support rails/poles
- Bariatric equipment (i.e., for use with very heavy people)
- Emergency evacuation equipment

Some skills related to moving and handling of a person are discussed in the previous section. This section will discuss and demonstrate use of appropriate equipment, i.e., slide sheets and passive hoist for moving a person with impaired mobility requiring maximum assistance with mobility needs.

Slide sheets are manual handing equipment required to assist a person to reposition. Slide sheets are made up of non-frictional material promoting ease of movement and preventing strain on the caregiver. Slide sheets are used in pairs and are available as flat slide sheets and roller slide sheets. Some slide sheets are washable, and some are disposable. The choice over the use of washable and disposable slide sheet varies based on departmental policies. As per health and safety regulations slide sheets should be checked prior to each use and periodically according to the Provision and Use of Work Equipment Regulations, 1998.

USE OF FLAT SLIDE SHEETS TO SUPPORT AN IMMOBILE PERSON TO MOVE UP THE BED: STEP BY STEP

PREPARATION

- A minimum of two healthcare practitioners would be required to perform this activity for an average size dependent person. However, refer to the moving and handling risk assessment to ascertain the number of practitioners required for this activity.
- Check the moving and handling plan related to the person to ensure that correct equipment is used to move the person. Ensure that the plan is up to date.
- In the absence of a written plan, obtain information from the person, family, healthcare professional (e.g., physiotherapist) and case notes to establish correct moving and handling plan and appropriate use of equipment.
- Explain the activity to the person and obtain verbal consent.

(Continued)

- Ensure that the bed height is correct and suitable for both healthcare practitioners involved in the technique.
- Check the slide sheet for the integrity of the fabric, stitching, labels, evidence of wear and tear and cleanliness.

PROCEDURE

- The healthcare practitioners should stand on either side of the bed and place the slide sheets on top of the person after obtaining the person's consent. If this is not possible, fold the slide sheet on top of a clean table or bed.
- Fold the slide sheets approximately hand width apart.
- One healthcare practitioner should hold the folded slide sheet in their hand, taking care that their fingers are covered with the sheet, and insert the folded slide sheets under the natural curve of the person's neck or under the person's pillow with the open end on the top facing the head of the bed. The second healthcare practitioner should pull the slide sheet from the other end ensuring that the slide sheets are even on each side of the person. Move the slide sheets gently under the person's shoulders.
- The healthcare practitioners should stand facing the head end of the bed with the fingers of the hand nearer to the person facing up and thumbs tucked in. With the thumbs remaining in tucked position, the healthcare practitioners should hold the rolled bottom side of the slide sheets. The healthcare practitioners' other hands should hold the top flaps of the slide sheets. The health- care practitioners should keep their elbows on the bed so that the slide sheets can be pulled downwards or unraveled towards the bottom end of the bed. The healthcare practitioners' feet should be in walking stance position.
- To fit the slide sheet under the person, the bottom side of the folded slide sheet should be pulled under the person by both healthcare practitioners on either side of the bed.
- It is important that the healthcare practitioners communicate with each other as they unravel the slide sheets. An appropriate command, e.g. 'Ready, steady, pull', should be used when start- ing the activity so that both the healthcare practitioners perform the activity in synchrony. Continue unravelling the slide sheets until the slide sheets are fully under the person. If any difficulty is experienced when fitting the slide sheet under the heavier part of the person's body, push down on the mattress at that level as the slide sheet is pulled under the person.
- To move the person up the bed, the healthcare practitioners should stand at the head end of the bed facing the bottom end of the bed. Hold the top part of the top slide sheet using the hand closest to the person and a maintain a walking stance position.
- Use an appropriate command, e.g. 'Ready, steady, move', to move the person up the bed slowly by the healthcare practitioners transferring their weight from front foot to back foot or step- ping back. Ensure that the activity is done slowly so that the person's head does not reach the headboard.
- Alternatively, the healthcare practitioners should maintain an oblique position (facing the bottom of the bed diagonally) and use both hands to hold the top slide sheet at the shoulder and hip level and move the person up the bed using weight transfer or stepping back as described previously.
- Once the person is in a correct position on the bed, remove the slide sheets. The bottom slide sheet is removed first to minimise direct friction from the slide sheet on the person's body. To remove the slide sheets, one healthcare practitioner should fold the corner of the bottom slide sheet downwards and pass it under the natural curve of the person's ankle. The healthcare prac- titioner on the other side of the bed should take hold of the corner and utilise their body weight to pull the slide sheet while walking up from the foot end to the head end of the bed slowly. This activity should be repeated for the second slide sheet from the opposite side.

POST-PROCEDURE

- Ensure that the patient is comfortable and in the correct position on the bed.
- Leave the bed at a safe height for the person.
- Use bed rails if recommended in the moving and handling plan. A bed rails risk assessment along with the moving and handling plan is required for persons requiring use of bed rails.

To watch this procedure in action, see Go Further at the end of this chapter.

ACTIVITY: PAUSE AND REFLECT

As demonstrated in the procedure above slide sheets are effective equipment for moving and handling immobile persons in bed. Is use of slide sheets beneficial for staff members?

Slide sheets reduce the risk of musculoskeletal issues and improve job satisfaction in nursing practice. More information can be found in the following article:

Alperovitch-Najenson, D., Weiner, C., Ribak, J., and Kalichman, L. (2020) 'Sliding sheet use in nursing practice: An intervention study', *Workplace Health & Safety,* 68 (4): 171–81. doi. org/10.1177/2165079919880566

Passive hoists and slings

Passive hoists are equipment utilised to transfer a person in and out of bed or chair (see Figure 9.3). Various types of hoists are available depending on individual patient need. Some types include mobile

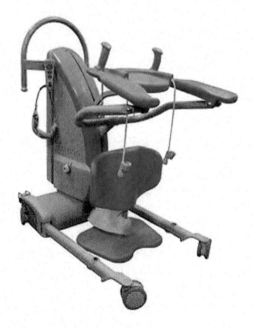

Figure 9.3   Mechanical standing hoist

hoists, gantry hoists, ceiling hoists etc. All hoists are used with special slings which are suitable for use with each type of hoist. Some slings available are loop slings, clips slings, in-situ slings, bath slings, toileting slings and amputee slings. All hoists and slings must be checked six-monthly as per the Lifting Operation and Lifting Equipment Regulation, 1998.

USE OF PASSIVE HOIST TO MOBILISE A PERSON FROM BED TO CHAIR: STEP BY STEP

PREPARATION

- Two healthcare practitioners would be required to perform this activity for an average size dependent person.
- Check the moving and handling plan related to the person to ensure that correct equipment is used to move the person. Ensure that the plan is up to date.
- In the absence of a written plan, obtain information from the person, family, healthcare professional (e.g., physiotherapist) and case notes to establish correct moving and handling plan and use of appropriate equipment.
- Explain the activity to the person and obtain verbal consent.
- Ensure that the bed height is correct and suitable for both healthcare practitioners involved in the technique.
- Check the general condition and cleanliness of the sling and inspect the sling for any rips, loose stitches, and integrity. Check the sling for safety label and safe working load and ensure that the person's weight is within the safe limits for using the sling. Check that the sling is the correct size for the person. Measurement of the sling varies depending on the model and make of the sling. Please follow appropriate measurement guidance as per manufacturer instructions. Check the sling for LOLER inspection label. If using a disposable sling, check the label for the person's name and ensure that the sling has not gotten wet at any point. It is not safe to use a sling which has gotten wet previously due to risks of breakage of sling during use.
- Check the hoist for any sign of wear and tear, damage, safe working load and check that the sling in use is compatible with the hoist. Check the hoist batteries to ensure that it is sufficiently charged. Confirm the LOLER inspection date.

PROCEDURE

- Roll the person to one side on the bed. To do so, one healthcare practitioner should stand on either side of the bed. Ask the person to turn their face towards the direction of transfer, cross their arms in front of their body and to bend their farther knee. If the person is unable to bend their knee themselves, the healthcare practitioner should facilitate this by placing one hand under the knee and the other hand under the heel or around the ankle and enable the person to bend their knee and hip. The healthcare practitioner facing the person should place their hand closest to the head of the bed on the person's shoulder and the other hand on the person's hip or thigh. The healthcare practitioner on the other side would also place one hand on the shoulder and the other hand on the hip or thigh laterally. Both the healthcare practitioners should adopt a walking stance.
- Use a command, e.g., 'Ready, steady, roll', to turn the person from their back to their side. During the movement the healthcare practitioner on the opposite side of the bed would give a gentle push to the person while shifting the weight from the back foot to the front foot. The healthcare practitioner facing the person would roll the person towards the healthcare practitioner while

shifting the weight from the front foot to the back foot. If it is not possible to turn the person in this manner, use of equipment (e.g., slide sheets) should be considered to roll the person.

- To fit the sling, first fold the sling in half with labels and straps on the outside (see Figure 9.4). Place the folded sling on the bed a few centimetres from the person's back with shoulder straps at the level of the person's shoulders (see Figure 9.4). Fold the top leg piece under the person's neck beneath the pillow. Roll the rest of half of the sling over itself until it reaches the person's back. The person can now roll onto their back. The handler on the other side would now pull the leg piece of the sling from under the pillow walking down to the foot end of the bed.

- The position of the sling should be checked to ensure that it is correctly under the person. The leg pieces are then inserted under the person's legs by bending the person's knees as described in the previous step. Alternatively, the healthcare practitioners should cover the clips/loops of the leg piece with one hand and insert it under the natural curve of the person's knee pushing down on the mattress and adjust it in position under the thigh once the clip/loop is passed under the person's knee. The sling would now be in the correct position to attach to the hoist.

- For using a passive mobile hoist to transfer the person from bed to chair, sit the patient up slightly using bed controls if possible. The healthcare practitioners should stand on either side of the bed. One healthcare practitioner should bring the hoist towards the person's bed so that the legs of the hoist are at right angles under the person's bed.

- The healthcare practitioner on the opposite side should steady the spreader bar of the hoist. Adjust the level of the spreader bar using the hoist controls so that the hoist is at a level that allows the

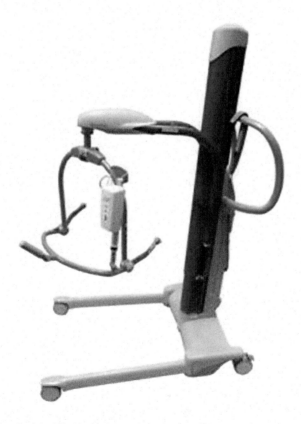

Figure 9.4 Mechanical hoist (seated position maneuvers)

(Continued)

clips or loops of the sling to be attached conveniently. The healthcare practitioners should check the attachments on the opposite side to confirm that it is attached firmly. Before commencing hoisting, place a small roller slide sheet under the person's heel to minimise friction during hoisting.

- Bring the hoist up which will cause tension on the hoist loops/clips and perform a final check to ensure it is safe to continue the activity. Continue the activity by lowering the bed so that the person gets suspended in the sling.

- One healthcare practitioner then moves the hoist away from the bed while the other healthcare practitioner supports the person ensuring that the person's heels are off the bed.

- Spread the legs of the hoist and bring the hoist above the seat of the chair. The healthcare practitioners can stand on either side of the hoist while one healthcare practitioner will bring the hoist down using the controls so that the person is completely sat back in the chair.

To watch this procedure in action, see Go Further at the end of this chapter.

POST-PROCEDURE

- Check that the person is comfortable in the chair.

- Except in-situ slings, all slings should be removed once the person is sat in the chair. This is done to minimise tissue damage and promote comfort. To remove the sling, place the person's one leg on a low footstool to create a gap between the thigh and the chair. Fold the leg piece of the sling away from the patient's skin and move it along the side towards the back of the chair. The leg piece should be folded behind the back of the sling on the person's lower back. Repeat the procedure for the other side.

- Ask the person to lean forward slightly so that the sling can be moved away gently from the person's back. If the person's functions are very limited, consider using a small roller slide sheet to remove the sling from under the person.

ACTIVITY: WHAT IS THE EVIDENCE?

Are there any issues with the use of hoists, which has now become an integral part of delivering health and social care services?

For further information on hoisting, read the article 'Getting to grips with hoisting people', available at https://www.hse.gov.uk/pubns/hsis3.pdf (accessed October 18, 2022).

CHAPTER SUMMARY

This chapter has highlighted some of the key points, skills and procedures related to mobility and safety around mobilising people in care settings. Best practice and up-to-date resources available have been considered and outlined in relation to this area. Anatomy and physiology revision and recap will enable you to acquire depth of knowledge and understanding of the topic. As mobility is a vast subject, further skills related to this need to be developed over the duration of the nursing course and career.

This chapter has discussed mobility and safety procedures and assessments used in care settings. As mentioned in the beginning of the chapter, the discussions and skills detailed in this chapter are non-exhaustive, and a deeper understanding of the practices adopted in the areas you work will further advance your practice and knowledge base. Attending and updating moving and handling courses yearly would enable staff to keep up to date with changes in practice.

ACE YOUR ASSESSMENT

Q1 Which one of the following is not the function of the skeleton?

a Support
b Movement
c Production of glucose
d Production of red blood cells

Q2 Fill in the missing word: Slide sheets are moving and handling equipment required to_____ a person

a lift
b reposition
c weigh
d stand

Q3 Passive hoists are required to assist which of the following categories of patients?

a Moderately dependent
b Minimally dependent
c Independent
d Fully dependent

Answers

1 C
2 B
3 D

GO FURTHER

To gain a better understanding of moving and handling including the relevant legislations related to manual handling, visit and read 'Moving and Handling in Health and Social Care' https://www.hse.gov.uk/healthservices/moving-handling.htm (accessed October 18, 2022).

For safe use of bed rails and to improve your understanding of risk assessment related to the same, look at 'Guidance: Bed rails management and safe use' at https://www.gov.uk/guidance/bed-rails-management-and-safe-use (accessed October 18, 2022).

Watch a passive hoist demonstration video here: https://www.youtube.com/watch?v=M12VEI7ycgE (accessed October 18, 2022).

Watch a slide insertion and repositioning here: https://www.youtube.com/watch?v=cEZBn7Qw74U (accessed October 18, 2022).

Watch a HoverJack demonstration here: https://www.youtube.com/watch?v=1uxIX7XQO8Y (accessed October 18, 2022).

REFERENCES

Arjo (2005) *Arjo Huntleigh Guidebook for Architects and Planners*. Malmö: Arjo. https://www.arjo.com/int/services-solutions/healthcare-solutions/architects-and-planners/ (accessed October 18, 2022).

Arjo (2022) 'Positive Eight'. https://www.arjo.com/int/insights/positive-eight/ (accessed October 18, 2022).

Baker, C. (2022) 'Obesity Statistics (Research briefing)', commonslibrary.parliament.uk, March 16. https://commonslibrary.parliament.uk/research-briefings/sn03336/#:~:text=28%25%20of%20adults%20in%20England,bariatric%20surgery%20and%20international%20comparisons (accessed January 30, 2023).

Chen, Y., Tang, Y., Allen, V. and DeVivo, M.J. (2016) 'Fall-induced spinal cord injury: External causes and implications for prevention', *The Journal of Spinal Cord Medicine*, 39 (1): 24–31. doi.org/10.1179/2045772315Y.0000000007

Gawler, S., Skelton, D.A., Dinan-Young, S., Masud, T., Morris, R.W., Griffin, M., Kendrick, D., Iliffe, S. and ProAct65+ Team (2016) 'Reducing falls among older people in general practice: The ProAct65+ exercise intervention trial', *Archives of Gerontology & Geriatrics*, 67: 46–54.

Hancock, C. (2021) 'Patterns and trends in excess weight among adults in England', UK Health Security Agency Blog, March 4. https://ukhsa.blog.gov.uk/2021/03/04/patterns-and-trends-in-excess-weight-among-adults-in-england/ (accessed October 18, 2022).

Healey, F. and Scobie, S. (2007) *Slips, Trips and Falls in Hospital* (3rd report). NHS National Patient Safety Agency. http://mtpinnacle.com/pdfs/slips-trips-fall-2007.pdf (accessed October 18, 2022).

Health and Safety Executive (2021) 'Moving and handling in health and social care'. https://www.hse.gov.uk/healthservices/moving-handling.htm (accessed October 18, 2022).

Iezzoni, L.I., McCarthy, E.P., Davis, R.B. and Siebens, H. (2001) 'Mobility difficulties are not only a problem of old age', *Journal of General Internal Medicine*, 16 (4): 235–43. doi.org/10.1046/j.1525-1497.2001.016004235.x

Marshall, P., Gallacher, B., Jolly, S. and Rinomhota, S. (2017) *Anatomy and Physiology in Healthcare*. Banbury: Scion.

Moreau, D., Stockslager, J.L., Cheli, R. and Haworth, K. (eds) (2002) *Lippincott Professional Guides: Anatomy and Physiology* (2nd edition). Philadelphia, PA: Wolters Kluwer.

National Institute for Health and Care Excellence (NICE) (2018) *Nice Impact: Falls and Fragility Fractures*. https://www.nice.org.uk/media/default/about/what-we-do/into-practice/measuring-uptake/nice-impact-falls-and-fragility-fractures.pdf (accessed October 18, 2022).

National Institute for Health and Care Excellence (2019) *2019 Surveillance of Falls in Older Patients: Assessing Risks and Prevention* (CG161). https://www.nice.org.uk/guidance/cg161/evidence/appendix-a-summary-of-evidence-from-surveillance-pdf-6784064894 (accessed October 18, 2022).

Neri, S.G.R., Oliveira, J.S., Dario, A.B., Lima, R.M. and Tiedemann, A. (2020) 'Does obesity increase the risk and severity of falls in people aged 60 years and older? A systematic review and meta-analysis of observational studies', *The Journals of Gerontology: Series A*, 75 (5): 952–60. doi.org/10.1093/gerona/glz272

Nursing and Midwifery Council (NMC) (2018) *The Code: Professional Standards of Practice and Behaviour for Nurses, Midwives and Nursing Associates*. London: NMC. https://www.nmc.org.uk/globalassets/sitedocuments/nmc-publications/nmc-code.pdf (accessed October 18, 2022).

O'Hanlon, S. and Twomey, C. (2009) 'Mobility impairment in older adults', *InnovAiT*, 2 (9): 546–50. doi.org/10.1093/innovait/inp102

Oliver, D. (2002) 'Bed falls and bedrails – What should we do?', *Age and Ageing*, 31 (1): 415–18.

Peate, I. (2017) 'The skeletal system', in I. Peate and M. Nair (eds), *Fundamentals of Anatomy and Physiology for Nursing and Healthcare Students* (3rd edition). Oxford: Wiley. pp. 165–96.

Royal College of Nursing (RNC) (2022) 'Consent', rcn.org.uk. https://www.rcn.org.uk/clinical-topics/Consent-in-England-and-Wales (accessed January 30, 2023).

Springhouse (2002) *Lippincott Professional Guides: Anatomy & Physiology*. Philadelphia, PA: Wolters Kluwer.

Social Care Institute for Excellence (SCIE) (n.d.) *Deprivation of Liberty Safeguards (DoLS)*. https://www.scie.org.uk/mca/dols# (accessed December 2022).

Teasdale, G. and Jennett, B. (1974) 'Assessment of coma and impaired consciousness: A practical scale', *Lancet*, 304: 81–4.

Terroso, M., Rosa, N., Torres Marques, A. and Simoes, R. (2014) 'Physical consequences of falls in the elderly: A literature review from 1995 to 2010', *European Review of Aging and Physical Activity*, 11: 51–9. https://doi.org/10.1007/s11556-013-0134-8

UK Government (1991) *The Children Act 1989 (Commencement and Transitional Provisions) Order 1991*. https://www.legislation.gov.uk/uksi/1991/828/made (accessed October 18, 2022).

UK Government (2004) *Children Act 2004*. https://www.legislation.gov.uk/ukpga/2004/31/contents (accessed October 18, 2022).

UK Government (2005) *Mental Capacity Act 2005*. https://www.legislation.gov.uk/ukpga/2005/9/contents (accessed October 18, 2022).

UK Government (2014) *The Health and Social Care Act 2008 (Regulated Activities) Regulations 2014*. https://www.legislation.gov.uk/ukdsi/2014/9780111117613/regulation/12 (accessed October 18, 2022).

UK Government (2021) 'Guidance: Bed rails management and safe use', gov.uk, January 12. https://www.gov.uk/guidance/bed-rails-management-and-safe-use (accessed October 18, 2022).

World Health Organization (WHO) (2018) 'Falls: Ageing and health', who.int, April 26. https://www.who.int/news-room/fact-sheets/detail/falls (accessed October 18, 2022).

World Health Organization (2022) 'Physical activity', who.int, October 5. https://www.who.int/news-room/fact-sheets/detail/physical-activity (accessed October 18, 2022).

RESPIRATORY CARE

10

GABBY WILCOX

ANNEXE B NURSING PROCEDURES

8.1   Observe and assess the need for intervention and respond to restlessness, agitation and breathlessness using appropriate interventions
8.2   Manage the administration of oxygen using a range of routes and best practice approaches
8.3   Take and interpret peak flow and oximetry measurements
8.4   Use appropriate nasal and oral suctioning techniques
8.5   Manage inhalation, humidifier and nebuliser devices
8.6   Manage airway and respiratory processes and equipment
2.9   Collect and observe sputum specimens

——— LEARNING OBJECTIVES ———

After reading this chapter, you should be able to:

- Identify the main functions of the respiratory system
- Discuss a variety of common respiratory interventions
- Understand the clinical skills required for this area of patient care

STUDENT VOICE

Understanding what affects a person's breathing and how we can help them with it is vital. The respiratory system is complicated but once you understand it, all the interventions make sense.

Craig, 3rd year, Adult Health

INTRODUCTION

We take breathing for granted, but any disruption can be frightening and unpleasant for patients in our care. The respiratory system has a vital role to play in providing oxygen to the whole body and affects all the other systems. Many health conditions directly affect the respiratory system but others, even if they seem unrelated, will still have some effect on the patient's breathing. Patients both in hospital and at home, across all age ranges, will need some type of respiratory intervention at times. A good foundation in the parts and functions of the respiratory system will allow you to assess and manage patients with breathing problems. The chapter covers evidence-based practice and best practice in relation to the respiratory needs of patients.

ANATOMY AND PHYSIOLOGY RECAP

The respiratory system enables movement of air into the body so that oxygen can be transported by the bloodstream and delivered to the tissues to allow aerobic energy production.

Air enters the lungs via the nose and mouth and travels through the pharynx, larynx and trachea. The trachea then divides at the carina and forms the right and left main bronchus of each lung. The left lung has two lobes, and the right lung has three. The bronchi subdivide into smaller airways known as bronchioles which eventually end in an alveolus – a tiny air sac lined with a single cell epithelial wall and surrounded by numerous capillaries (tiny blood vessels). The human body contains millions of alveoli which give a large surface area for gas exchange to take place from the lungs into the bloodstream and back. The lungs are lined with a double layer of smooth membrane – the parietal pleura lines the thoracic cavity and the lung itself is lined with the visceral pleura. Pleural fluid between the membranes reduces friction by allowing them to slide over each other and creates a surface tension which holds the two pleurae together and helps prevent the lungs from collapsing.

Overview and function of respiratory system

The respiratory system is responsible for delivering oxygen to the cells of the tissues, and for removing carbon dioxide from the body. Oxygen is vital for cells to function, and in using it they produce carbon dioxide (a waste product) which needs to be removed. To transport the gases to and from the tissues the respiratory system works closely with the cardiovascular system. This allows homeostasis to be maintained for optimum health.

For the respiratory system to work effectively, four distinct functions are necessary:

- Pulmonary ventilation
- External respiration
- Gas transport
- Internal respiration

Ventilation

Pulmonary ventilation refers to the act of breathing; the physical movement of air in and out of the lungs. It is a mechanical process consisting of inspiration (breathing in) and expiration (breathing out).

Inspiration is active and results from contraction of the diaphragm which moves downwards at the same time as contraction of the intercostal muscles lifts the sternum and ribs upwards and outwards. This causes the lungs to expand and increase in volume, which decreases the pressure in the lungs compared to the air outside. This pressure gradient draws air into the lungs which the body can use for respiration (Cathala and Costa, 2019).

Expiration is mainly passive and happens when the diaphragm relaxes along with the intercostal muscles, which reduces the lung volume and pushes air out of the lungs. Normal breathing is therefore negative pressure ventilation as the air is drawn into the lungs by the negative pressure gradient.

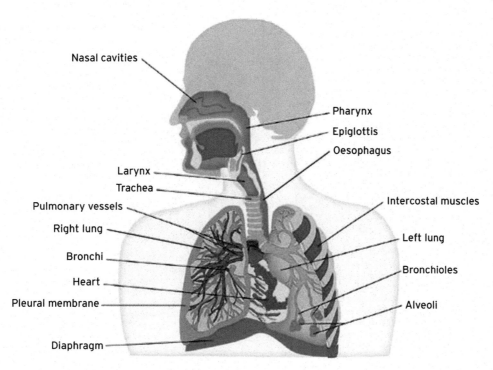

Figure 10.1   The respiratory system

Room air contains 21% oxygen, as well as nitrogen (79%), carbon dioxide (0.03%) and other rare gases (0.03%) (Preston and Kelly, 2017).

Several other factors also influence airflow:

- Lung compliance, which means the ease with which the lungs expand and stretch.
- Airway resistance, which is governed by the diameter of the airways which can be changed by the smooth muscle lining them. Bronchoconstriction (narrowing of the airways) can increase resistance and therefore reduce airflow and bronchodilation (widening of the airways) will do the opposite.
- Alveolar surfactant, a vital fluid that lines each alveolus to prevent them from collapsing during expiration.

Breathing is controlled by the respiratory centres in the brainstem which is stimulated by changes in the pH (the acid-base balance) of the blood to either increase or decrease the respiratory rate and depth.

Respiration: External

Respiration refers to the process of gas exchange inside the body. This is divided into external respiration which occurs between the lungs and the bloodstream, and internal respiration which happens between the bloodstream and the cells within tissues and organs. External respiration means the diffusion of oxygen from the alveoli into the tiny capillaries surrounding each alveolus to then be taken to the left side of the heart and pumped around the body. Carbon dioxide, which is a waste product of respiration, diffuses from the capillaries into the alveoli to be exhaled. This diffusion is driven by the concentration gradient

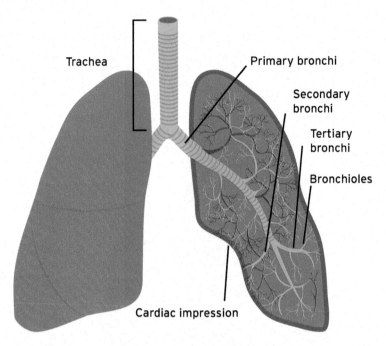

Figure 10.2   The lungs

of oxygen across the membrane that divides the alveoli from the capillary. Blood in the pulmonary artery (travelling from the right side of the heart to the lungs) is low in oxygen and high in carbon dioxide because it has been returned from the tissues where oxygen has been used up and carbon dioxide has

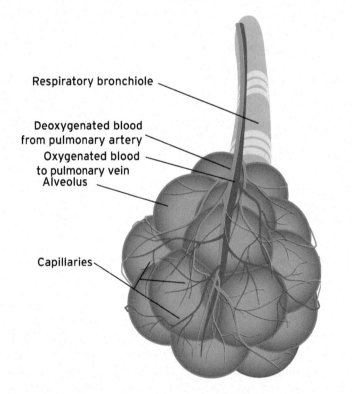

Figure 10.3   Anatomy of alveoli

been produced. The partial pressure of oxygen is higher in the alveoli, so oxygen passively moves from the alveoli into the capillaries, whereas the partial pressure of carbon dioxide is higher in the capillaries and therefore diffuses passively into the alveoli in the opposite direction.

Gas transport

This refers to the process of carrying oxygen from the lungs to the tissues, and carbon dioxide back from the tissues to the lungs. Oxygen is transported by binding to molecules of haemoglobin which are travelling in the bloodstream, and then separates when it reaches the tissue to diffuse into the cells. Each haemoglobin can carry four molecules of oxygen at which point it is fully saturated (Cook et al., 2020).

Respiration: Internal

Internal respiration means the gas exchange that takes place in the cells. Cells need oxygen to produce adenosine triphosphate which is the energy source needed to power all the cell's functions. This process is called aerobic respiration and produces carbon dioxide as a waste product. Due to this, the concentration of oxygen is lower in the tissues than the blood, and the concentration of carbon dioxide is higher in the tissues than the blood. As blood travels through the capillaries, oxygen and carbon dioxide follow the concentration gradient and diffuse between the blood and the tissues. As the gases diffuse down the concentration gradient from high pressure to low pressure, oxygen diffuses from the blood into the tissues and carbon dioxide in the opposite direction from the tissues into the blood.

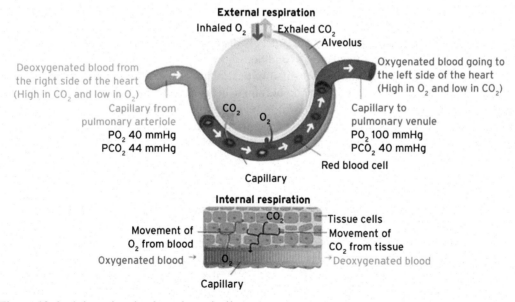

External respiration

Inhaled O_2 Exhaled CO_2

Alveolus

Deoxygenated blood from the right side of the heart (High in CO_2 and low in O_2)

Capillary from pulmonary arteriole
PO_2 40 mmHg
PCO_2 44 mmHg

CO_2 O_2

Oxygenated blood going to the left side of the heart (High in O_2 and low in CO_2)

Capillary to pulmonary venule
PO_2 100 mmHg
PCO_2 40 mmHg

Red blood cell

Capillary

Internal respiration

CO_2

Tissue cells

Movement of O_2 from blood

Movement of CO_2 from tissue

Oxygenated blood O_2

Deoxygenated blood

Capillary

Figure 10.4   Internal and external respiration

KEY TERMS

Apnoea: absence of breathing

Compliance: the expandability of the airways, how stiff the airways are

(Continued)

Diffusion: the movement of a substance from an area of high concentration to an area of low concentration

Dyspnoea: difficulty in breathing

Homeostasis: the maintenance of the optimum internal environment for the body, meaning the body is constantly adjusting to maintain the optimum temperature, pH and other factors

Hypercapnia: a build-up of carbon dioxide in the blood

Hypoxaemia: low oxygen levels in the arterial blood

Hypoxia: low oxygen supply to a tissue of the body

Resistance: the resistance to airflow in the respiratory tract is affected by the diameter of the airways and the flow of air

Respiration: the process of gas exchange between the air and the body's cells. External respiration is when gas enters the bloodstream from the lungs and internal respiration is when gas enters the cells from the bloodstream

Ventilation: the movement of air from the atmosphere into the lungs

---

CLINICAL SKILLS RELATED TO RESPIRATORY CARE

As outlined in the introduction, the topic of the respiratory system and breathing is vast. Oxygen is vital to survival and helps the cells of the body produce energy via aerobic respiration. Anaerobic respiration without using oxygen is less efficient. Any disruption to the body's supply of oxygen will rapidly lead to deterioration of the patient's condition.

The clinical skills covered below are essential in developing and expanding your knowledge and practice in this area, and they are skills you should aim to develop throughout the full duration of your programme of study. Fundamental skills learnt in year one will be expanded upon in years two and three and even beyond into your early years of registration. The focus may differ slightly dependent on your clinical placement areas or areas you ultimately choose to work in.

Assessing breathlessness: Discussion

Breathlessness is also known as dyspnoea or shortness of breath and can be a feature of many different physical and mental health conditions. Breathlessness is normal in healthy people after vigorous physical exertion; however, it should resolve once the activity is stopped. Breathlessness in unwell patients, or when it is sudden or prolonged, is debilitating and distressing and is usually the result of a complex interaction between physiological, psychological and social factors. Interestingly, patients with similar levels of lung function report widely varied perception of their breathlessness which reinforces the subjective nature of the symptom.

Note this is not a comprehensive list and many other factors or a combination of factors may influence a patient's respiratory function.

When assessing a patient who is breathless, it is important to consider all contributing factors.

A comprehensive assessment should include:

- The patient's subjective perception of their breathlessness and any change from their normal baseline. This may include use of a self-reporting scale such as the Medical Research Council Dyspnoea Scale (Fletcher et al., 1959).

Table 10.1 Causes of breathlessness

Type	Conditions
Respiratory	Asthma Chronic Obstructive Pulmonary Disease (COPD) Pneumonia Croup Bronchiectasis Bronchiolitis Pulmonary embolus Respiratory infection
Cardiac	Heart failure Arrhythmia
Psychological	Anxiety Panic attacks
Other	Obesity Smoking Scoliosis Anaemia

- Objective measurements such as respiratory rate, oxygen saturations, spirometry and peak expiratory flow measurements.
- Observation of the patient for accessory muscle use, visibly increased work of breathing and the presence of cyanosis.
- Be mindful that cyanosis presents differently in different patients. Skin tone of the patient can have an impact on what you will see and how it will be assessed. In patients with darker skin tones this may be less obvious – observe the colour of the nails and mucous membranes and document any abnormalities.
- Listening to any audible chest sounds and chest auscultation (covered in detail in Chapter 1).
- In children you should observe any recessions (drawing in) of the sternum or between the ribs.
- Document any contributing factors such as environmental exposure to irritants and living conditions.

ACTIVITY: PAUSE AND REFLECT

Many factors can affect a patient's breathing. Consider Denzil, a 78-year-old retired builder who was exposed to asbestos during his working life. He lives in social housing and has reported mould on the walls of his house to the local authority. He smoked 20 cigarettes a day for 35 years and has recently cut down to 5 a day. He lives in an area with high levels of air pollution near a busy motorway. He keeps racing pigeons and cares for them daily.

Think about which of these factors might impact his breathing and how their effects could be minimised.

Table 10.2   The Medical Research Council Dyspnoea Scale (Fletcher et al., 1959; used with the permission of the Medical Research Council)

Grade	Degree of breathlessness related to activities
1	Not troubled by breathlessness except on strenuous exercise
2	Short of breath when hurrying or walking up a slight hill
3	Walks slower than contemporaries on level ground because of breathlessness or has to stop for breath when walking at own pace
4	Stops for breath after walking about 100 metres or after a few minutes on level ground
5	Too breathless to leave the house, or breathless when dressing or undressing

It is important to remember that restlessness or agitation may be the first sign of hypoxia or dyspnoea especially in non-verbal patients, and tremor and myoclonic jerks (involuntary muscle twitches) can be a sign of a build-up of carbon dioxide which may occur with inadequate breathing.

Sternal and/or intercostal recessions in children occur because their chest wall is more flexible and can be drawn inwards when the child is working very hard to breathe. This is a sign of significantly increased work of breathing in a child. Children are usually alert and interact with their environment when feeling well so be very cautious when assessing a lethargic quiet child with breathing difficulties. Head bobbing and grunting in infants are also signs of increased work of breathing.

A multidisciplinary, holistic approach is recommended to manage breathlessness. Any medical condition which is affecting the patient's breathing should be identified and optimised where possible with both medications and non-pharmacological strategies. The medications used will depend on the underlying condition, but most patients will also benefit from cognitive and behavioural strategies to manage their symptoms.

ACTIVITY: PAUSE AND REFLECT

Assessment of breathlessness is usually subjective for the patient and varies widely according to their perception. Why do you think it is important for patients to self-assess their breathing? Do you think this makes it a more or less accurate assessment? How might a patient's culture and beliefs impact their self-assessment of breathlessness?

OXYGEN THERAPY: DISCUSSION

Oxygen is essential for the body to function at a cellular level. Some conditions such as asthma and COPD directly affect oxygenation, whereas in other acute conditions, oxygen consumption may be increased due to changes in the patient's metabolic rate and in response to acute physical stress.

Oxygen is considered a drug and therefore must be prescribed correctly and administered by a competent health professional. Supplemental oxygen is required by any patient who is experiencing hypoxaemia (low levels of oxygen in the blood) and should be administered to achieve a target range of oxygen saturation, which should be identified on the oxygen prescription (see clinical skills video 'Managing the administration of oxygen' below).

In an emergency, high flow oxygen can be given without a prescription but must be titrated to target saturations once the patient has been assessed and stabilised.

Oxygen saturations refer to the percentage of haemoglobin molecules in the blood that are fully saturated with oxygen and normal levels are 95–100%. The most accurate method to measure oxygen saturations is with Arterial Blood Gas (ABG) analysis (O'Driscoll et al., 2017), however, this is an invasive test that is often painful and needs to be done by a competent practitioner so in practice most patients will have their peripheral oxygen saturations measured using pulse oximetry (see Chapter 2, The Importance of Assessment). Patients in acute areas should have their observations measured regularly using a track and trigger system (such as NEWS2) and have the amount of oxygen they are receiving recorded along with any device used to administer it.

Hypoxaemia is harmful to patients, however over-oxygenation can be detrimental, too, so most patients will have a target saturation range of 94–98% prescribed, unless they are at risk of hypercapnic respiratory failure in which case target saturations may be 88–92% or another individualised range.

ACTIVITY: WHAT IS THE EVIDENCE?

A large systematic review and meta-analysis in 2018 showed that untargeted oxygen therapy increased patient mortality in a large range of conditions, without improving other outcomes, even when adjusted for age, sex and socio-economic status (Chu et al., 2018).

Hypercapnic respiratory failure (also called Type 2 respiratory failure or CO_2 retention) means hypoxaemia with an elevated level of carbon dioxide in the blood. This can only be detected on an ABG and is more common in patients with chronic lung conditions. If the patient is in hypercapnic respiratory failure, giving too much oxygen may lead to depression of their respiratory drive and cause them to stop breathing. High concentrations of oxygen can be toxic after long-term therapy so it is important to administer the minimum oxygen possible while still maintaining the target saturations.

CASE STUDY

Lloyd

Lloyd is a 55-year-old long distance lorry driver who has COPD and uses inhalers. In the last six months Lloyd has had several hospital admissions with shortness of breath and has been referred to the community respiratory team. Icheku is with their practice supervisor and visits Lloyd at home. Lloyd explains his breathing is feeling 'tight' again and that he has run out of inhalers. The house smells of cigarette smoke. Lloyd's son is present and says that Lloyd doesn't understand why his breathing has gotten worse over the last few months.

Questions

1   How should Icheku assess Lloyd?
2   How can Icheku explain what COPD is to Lloyd's son?
3   What treatment is Lloyd likely to need?
4   What other topics might Icheku discuss with Lloyd at this visit?

(Continued)

Answers

1   An ABCDE assessment should be done initially (Cathala and Moorley, 2020). The assessment of airway and breathing should consider the presence of wheeze, coughing, sputum production and Lloyd's perceived degree of breathlessness. Subjective assessments including his oxygen saturations and respiratory rate are an important part of this assessment, and some community respiratory nurses carry portable spirometers to assess lung function. A detailed history of Lloyd's signs and symptoms will be needed and their impact on activities of daily living.

2   Icheku can explain that COPD is a progressive chronic condition that is characterised by limitations of airflow that cannot be fully reversed. COPD is the name given to a group of lung conditions that cause similar symptoms, which includes emphysema (damage to the alveoli causing them to be enlarged and less efficient for gas exchange), chronic bronchitis (long-term inflammation of the airways with increased mucous production) and chronic asthma. It is common in older adults and is often caused by smoking. The main symptoms are cough, sputum production and gradually worsening shortness of breath. As the disease progresses the patient may be prone to episodes of temporary worsening of symptoms known as an exacerbation, which may be caused by a bacterial or viral infection (an infective exacerbation of COPD) or by an environmental trigger such as smoking or pollutants (a non-infective exacerbation of COPD).

3   Pharmacological management will usually include inhaled short-acting bronchodilators via inhaler or nebuliser with oral corticosteroids which will be weaned carefully once the condition improves. They will only be prescribed antibiotics if there is a likelihood of bacterial respiratory infection. Exacerbations of COPD may need to be managed with oxygen if needed, titrated to achieve oxygen saturations between 88 and 92%. If Lloyd requires oxygen, he will need to be admitted to hospital in the first instance and can be assessed later for the need for long-term oxygen therapy (LTOT) at home, however this will only be an option if no one in the home smokes cigarettes, due to the flammability of oxygen.

4   If Lloyd is well enough to be monitored and treated at home, Icheku will need to address several aspects of health and living arrangements. Lloyd seems to need more education and information about the disease along with advice on recognising and managing an exacerbation. Other factors can be considered such as exercise, nutrition, vaccination advice and the nurse could consider referral for various psychological and behavioural interventions. Lloyd should be advised to stop smoking and avoid cigarette smoke in the environment – a referral for smoking cessation can be done via the GP, and his son should also be encouraged to stop if he smokes. Lloyd should also be advised on the importance of any prescribed medication and any barriers to their use should be explored.

Oxygen devices and equipment

Oxygen can be given using a variety of devices and equipment, which can be substituted and titrated to achieve target oxygen saturations. This means that nurses must be familiar with a range of equipment and confident in calculating the amount of oxygen provided by each type. Room air provides 21% oxygen and there are a variety of devices available to give higher percentages of inspired oxygen. The amount of oxygen given is expressed as the fraction of inspired oxygen (FiO_2) and written as a percentage.

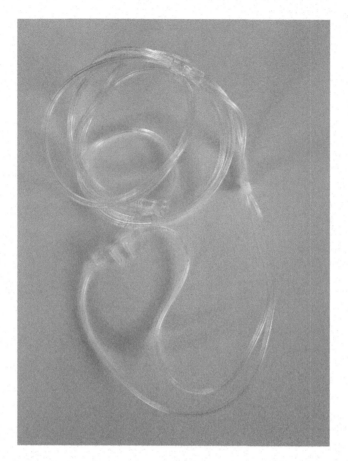

Figure 10.5   Nasal cannula

Nasal cannula

This consists of plastic oxygen tubing formed into two prongs which are inserted into the nostrils. The device wraps around the top of the ears and is adjusted under the chin. It is lightweight and more comfortable than a facemask, and allows the patient to eat, drink and talk unimpeded. However, it is only suitable for patients requiring low FiO_2 as flow rates over 6L/min are not recommended, and preferably should be under 4L/min.

Simple face mask

A simple semi-rigid plastic mask is usually used for moderate flow rates (5–10L/min) which delivers approximately 40% to 60% FiO_2 depending on the patient's respiratory rate and pattern. This means that the exact FiO_2 the patient receives may not be accurate and therefore these are only suitable for short-term use (such as in post-operative recovery units).

At flow rates of less than 5L/min it is possible for exhaled carbon dioxide to build up in the mask and therefore another device should be used for patients at risk of hypercapnic respiratory failure or those requiring lower flow rates.

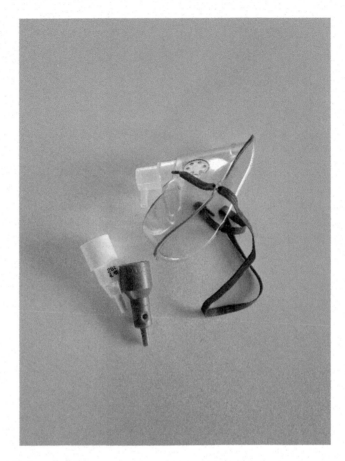

Figure 10.6   Simple face mask

Venturi face mask (fixed performance system)

This is similar in appearance to a simple face mask; however, it has a Venturi adaptor attached between the mask and the tubing which ensures the delivery of an accurate FiO_2 regardless of the patient's respiratory rate and depth. This makes it the preferred option for patients requiring longer term oxygen therapy and allows much more precise titration. It is also more suitable for patients at risk of hypercapnic respiratory failure as it is easier to titrate the FiO_2.

The adaptors are colour-coded and labelled with both the FiO_2 it provides and the flow rate required to achieve this.

Reservoir mask (non-rebreathe mask)

A reservoir mask is used when oxygen concentrations over 60% are required. It consists of a semi rigid plastic mask with the addition of a reservoir bag with a one-way valve which ensures the patient is breathing only from the reservoir containing high concentration oxygen. There are also one-way valves on the outer mask, meaning exhaled gas containing carbon dioxide does not build up in the mask.

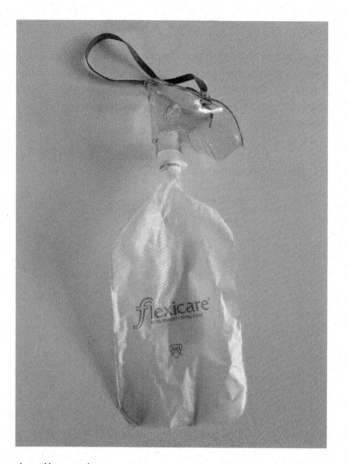

Figure 10.7 Non-rebreathe mask

The reservoir must be inflated with oxygen before the mask is put on the patient. At flow rates of 10–15L/min, a reservoir mask will deliver 60% to 90% FiO_2. When such high oxygen concentration is required the patient is acutely unwell and rapid assessment is required in case of further deterioration. Many healthcare organisations allow the administration of 15L of oxygen using a reservoir mask in an emergency by a registered nurse via a Patient Group Direction (PGD). PGDs are written instructions which allow the administration of certain medications in planned circumstances by registered professionals.

ACTIVITY: CRITICAL THINKING

When you are registered, you may be assessing acutely hypoxic patients with chronic lung conditions such as COPD. These patients are at risk of Type 2 (hypercapnic) respiratory failure, which means that too much oxygen can depress their respiratory drive and stop them breathing. However, in an emergency the nurse can only administer high flow oxygen with the reservoir mask. How would you approach this situation?

Oxygen for children or patients with complex needs

Many children find oxygen masks and devices threatening and uncomfortable. To encourage cooperation and reduce their anxiety it may be more acceptable to ask their parent or carer to hold the mask or tubing near the patient's face allowing 'blow-by' oxygen administration. This is obviously less consistent and accurate than other methods of oxygen delivery but may be useful in cases where a low concentration of oxygen is needed.

Table 10.3   Flow rates and oxygen delivery of devices

Device	Flow rate (in L/min)	Percent of FiO_2 delivered
Nasal cannula	1	25%
• 25%-45% O_2 delivery	2	29%
• Can be drying at high flow rates	3	33%
• Patient can eat, drink and talk	4	37%
	5	41%
	6	45%
Simple facemask	6	35%
• 35%-60% O_2 delivery	7	41%
• Not very accurate delivery	8	47%
• Can be humidified	9	53%
	10	60%
Reservoir mask (non-rebreathe mask)	10	80%
	15	100%
• For high O_2 concentrations		
Venturi mask	2	24%
• Accurate delivery of FiO_2	4	28%
	8	35%
	8	40%
	12	60%

WATCH THE VIDEO

MANAGING THE ADMINISTRATION OF OXYGEN

Watch along as you read through this step by step procedure by scanning the QR code with your smartphone camera or via https://study.sagepub.com/rowberry.

OXYGEN THERAPY: STEP BY STEP

EQUIPMENT

- Oxygen supply (wall supply or in a cylinder)
- Oxygen flow meter
- Appropriate oxygen device and tubing
- PPE

COMMENCING OXYGEN THERAPY

- Explain the procedure to the patient and gain consent. Provide a chaperone if required. Ensure you have the knowledge and competence to perform the skill and are familiar with local policy.
- Assess the patient's condition and ensure observations have been taken recently and documented. Assess the level of oxygen required and select an appropriate device.
- Check there is a written prescription for oxygen therapy with a documented target saturation range for titration.
- Gather the equipment needed including selected device, and make sure that pulse oximetry equipment is available.
- Attach the device via the oxygen tubing to the oxygen supply and commence at the appropriate flow rate. If using an oxygen cylinder, ensure there is sufficient oxygen available.
- Apply the device to the patient's face as per the manufacturer guidelines and adjust to fit comfortably.
- Check the patient is comfortable and give reassurance if needed.
- Document the commencement of oxygen therapy and the inspired oxygen concentration (FiO_2) in the patient's notes.
- Monitor the patient's response to oxygen therapy and titrate FiO_2 to achieve the target saturation levels. Allow several minutes after each change to observe the response. Document all adjustments to the FiO_2 and the patient's saturation levels.

MANAGING A PATIENT RECEIVING OXYGEN THERAPY

- Continue to monitor your patient, performing observations regularly according to local policy. Record the FiO_2, flow rate and device used along with the saturations.
- Consider the need for humidification if the patient is likely to need oxygen for more than 24 hours.
- Help the patient to reposition regularly to promote comfort and maximise ventilation.
- Monitor potential pressure areas where the device is in contact with the patient's skin such as behind the ears and record their condition.
- Administer other respiratory therapies according to the patient's care plan, such as nebulisers and other relevant medications.
- Promote adequate fluid intake and observe the oral and nasal cavity for dryness. Provide water-based lubricant if the oxygen is drying out the mucosa and consider humidification.
- Observe and document any secretions, obtain samples if required and consider referring to physiotherapy if the patient has difficulty clearing secretions.
- Observe for signs of deterioration including changes in respiratory rate, reduced saturations, increased work of breathing or respiratory effort, drowsiness, tremor or confusion and escalate concerns according to local policy.
- Titrate FiO_2 (changing device if necessary) to maintain saturations within target range. Allow several minutes after each change to observe the response. Document all adjustments to the FiO_2 and the patient's saturation levels.

(Continued)

DISCONTINUING OXYGEN THERAPY

- Once the saturations have remained stable in the target range on the lowest FiO_2 available, consider removing the device.
- Monitor saturations for several minutes after discontinuing oxygen therapy and recheck regularly.
- Document the removal of oxygen and the patient's saturations.

HUMIDIFICATION

Humidification should be considered for all patients who receive supplemental oxygen for any length of time. As air enters the respiratory tract it is warmed and humidified in the nasal passages. The respiratory tract is lined with cilia – these are epithelial cells that are covered in tiny hairs which remove mucous and secretions. If these become dry, they can't work as efficiently, and the secretions become thicker and are not removed as easily which can predispose to infection. For patients with a tracheostomy or an endotracheal tube humidification is essential, as the tube will bypasses the upper airway passages where humidification takes place. To avoid this and to increase patient tolerance of oxygen therapy, a variety of humidification devices are available.

Heat and Moisture Exchange (HME) filters can be used in the circuit and contain a pleated fabric that conducts heat, often with a bacterial filter. The material retains expired heat and moisture and allows it to return to patient in the next inspiration. Bubble humidifiers bubble oxygen through water at room temperature and humidification chambers force oxygen through a warm reservoir of water.

ACTIVITY: WHAT'S THE EVIDENCE?

The British Thoracic Society guidelines (O'Driscoll et al., 2017) suggest that bubble bottle humidification should not be used as no benefit has been demonstrated in two trials (Campbell et al., 1988; Andres et al., 1997), and in a third trial the bottles were a source of bacterial contamination (Cameron et al., 1986).

PEAK EXPIRATORY FLOW MEASUREMENT: DISCUSSION

A patient's Peak Expiratory Flow Rate (PEFR) is a pulmonary function test that measures the maximum flow (in litres per minute) of a forced expiration from fully inflated lungs. It is most often used in patients with asthma to measure the extent of airflow obstruction during an asthma attack. Normal measurements are usually around 400–700L/min but vary according to the patient's size, sex and age. Many patients will know their usual measurement, and the difference from this during an acute obstructive exacerbation is very useful to determine the severity of the attack, but if this information is not available the expected best can be calculated. Peak flow measurement is easy to perform and interpret providing the patient is properly prepared and serial recordings can quantify the severity of airway obstruction and record the patient's response to treatment.

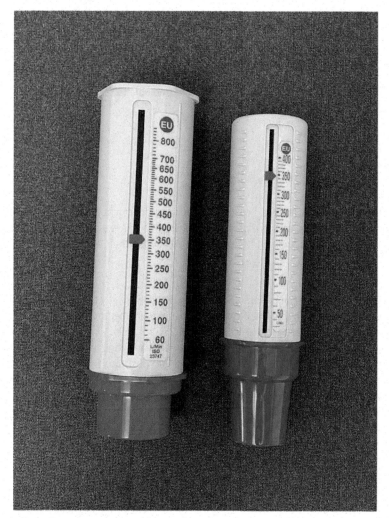

Figure 10.8 Peak flow meter

Source: Wikimedia Commons/Whispyhistory (CC BY-SA 4.0)

WATCH THE VIDEO

TAKING PEAK FLOW RECORDINGS

Watch along as you read through this step by step procedure by scanning the QR code with your smartphone camera or via https://study.sagepub.com/rowberry.

PEAK EXPIRATORY FLOW MEASUREMENT: STEP BY STEP

Make sure the patient is standing or sitting up straight and able to take a deep breath.

EQUIPMENT NEEDED

- Peak flow meter
- Mouthpiece
- Peak flow chart to record the measurement

Note that if the patient is so short of breath that they can't perform a peak flow measurement you should abandon it and ensure they are assessed promptly as this is a sign of a severe exacerbation. Distressing the patient by insisting on the task will only worsen their symptoms.

PROCEDURE

- Explain the procedure to the patient and gain consent. Demonstrate the procedure if the patient is unfamiliar. Provide a chaperone if required. Ensure you have the knowledge and competence to perform the skill and are familiar with local policy.
- Ask the patient for their best peak flow measurements and their most recent results.
- Assist the patient to position themselves in an upright position.
- Ensure the peak flow meter is held horizontally and the needle is at zero, unimpeded by the patient's fingers.
- Ask the patient to take a full deep breath, then immediately place their mouth around the mouthpiece.
- Ask the patient to blow into the meter with their maximum force.
- Note the reading, then return the needle to zero.
- Allow the patient to rest briefly, then repeat until you have three readings.
- Record the best of the three readings on the peak flow chart and report any concerns.
- Clean and store or dispose of the peak flow meter according to the manufacturer instructions and local infection prevention and control policy.

CASE STUDY

Jameela

Jameela is 13 years old and has come to the Children's Emergency Department after feeling short of breath while playing netball at school. The patient is accompanied by their mother. On arrival Jameela is distressed and pale and you can hear a wheeze on exhalation. Jameela has a history of two similar episodes that were less severe and did not require hospital attendance, and oxygen saturations are 92% on air. The doctor is present and thinks this is probably an acute asthma attack.

Questions

1　How will you assess Jameela?
2　How will you explain what is happening to Jameela and Jameela's mother?
3　How will you expect the doctor to manage the care?

Answers

1 Jameela will need to be assessed rapidly using the ABCDE approach giving particular attention to the airway and breathing. In addition, an increasing heart rate corresponds to increased
   severity of an asthma attack, so this must be recorded accurately. A peak flow reading is very
   useful but as Jameela does not have an existing diagnosis of asthma they may not know their
   usual measurement and you will need to compare it to the expected peak flow reading for their
   age and size. It is likely the doctor will need to take an arterial blood gas sample. This can be
   taken from the radial artery and is a painful procedure, but in some clinical areas a capillary
   sample can be taken from the finger or ear lobe, which is better tolerated, especially in children
   and younger adults.

2 You can explain that asthma is a common chronic condition affecting the breathing which is
   often diagnosed in childhood. It is characterised by inflammation and constriction of the airways
   and common symptoms are shortness of breath and chest tightness with wheeze and coughing
   that often get worse at night. An asthma attack is when these symptoms temporarily get worse.

3 Management of an asthma attack depends on the severity of the exacerbation. The severity of
   an exacerbation is graded as follows:

Table 10.4 Asthma severity

Severity	Explanation
Life threatening	PEFR (peak flow rate) less than 33% best or predicted, *or* oxygen saturation of less than 92%, *or* altered consciousness, *or* exhaustion, *or* cardiac arrhythmia, *or* hypotension, *or* cyanosis, *or* poor respiratory effort, *or* silent chest, *or* confusion
Severe	PEFR 33-50% best or predicted (at least 50% best or predicted in children) *or* respiratory rate of at least 25/min in patients over 12 years, 30/min in children between 5 and 12 years and 40/min in children between 2 and 5 years *or* pulse rate over 110/min in patients over 12 years, 125/min in children between 5 and 12 years and 140/min in children between 2 and 5 years *or* inability to complete sentences in one breath or accessory muscle use *or* inability to feed (infants) with oxygen saturation of at least 92%
Moderate	PEFR more than 50-75% best or predicted best (at least 50% best or predicted best in children) and normal speech, with no features of acute severe or life-threatening asthma
Mild	An asthma exacerbation with no features of moderate, severe or life-threatening asthma

Source: National Institute of Clinical and Health Excellence (NICE) (2021)

NICE guidance is prepared for the National Health Service in England. All NICE guidance is subject
to regular review and may be updated or withdrawn. NICE accepts no responsibility for the use of its
content in this product/publication.

Treatment of an asthma exacerbation usually involves inhaled bronchodilators via inhaler or
nebuliser and oral corticosteroids. If the patient is hypoxic they should be given oxygen and this
should be titrated to achieve oxygen saturations of 94-98%. Frequent observations (according to
the local track and trigger policy, or a minimum of every 30 minutes) and serial blood gases should
be done to monitor the response to treatment. If the patient does not begin to improve with treatment, specialist help from intensive care should be sought.

ACTIVITY: WHAT'S THE EVIDENCE?

Research has found that nebuliser therapy is not as efficient as using an inhaler with a spacer device when administering bronchodilators for children with asthma and showed an 80% decrease in hospital admission (Iramain et al., 2019). This is hypothesised to be because more of the drug is deposited in the lungs when using an inhaler and spacer, but the authors describe resistance to this from healthcare professionals in more severe cases because nebulisers can be driven by oxygen. The researchers state that if the patient is hypoxic, they can be given oxygen via a nasal cannula while using the inhaler and spacer, which is actually more effective.

FRACTIONAL EXHALED NITRIC OXIDE (FENO)

Another test that may be used in respiratory assessment is Fractional Exhaled Nitric Oxide (FeNO). Nitric oxide levels in exhaled air can be high where there is airway inflammation such as in asthma. The patient will be asked to exhale into a mouthpiece attached to a monitor, and this is often used as part of an initial asthma diagnosis. It also has some use in ongoing monitoring of patients with asthma.

AIRWAY DEVICES

Airway obstruction is a medical emergency and dealing with it is covered in Chapter 4. However, airway devices may be used outside of emergency situations, or may be used to allow suctioning to clear secretions. Oropharyngeal and nasopharyngeal airways are known as airway adjuncts and can be very useful tools in certain situations. It is helpful for nurses to have confidence in sizing and inserting airway adjuncts as they may be required in a variety of settings.

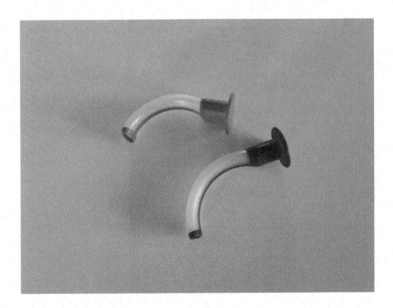

Figure 10.9   Oropharyngeal airway

Oropharyngeal airway

An oropharyngeal airway (often known as an OP airway or a Guedel airway) is a curved rigid plastic tube designed to maintain an open channel between the tongue and the hard palate. It has a flange at the oral end and is flattened to conform with the airway. Oropharyngeal airways come in a variety of sizes ranging from premature infants to large adults. They can be sized by lining the airway up along the cheek to ensure it equals the distance from the patient's front teeth to the angle of the jaw.

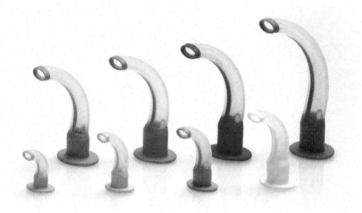

Figure 10.10   Sizing an oropharyngeal airway

Source: Wikimedia Commons/Intersurgical Ltd (CC BY-SA 3.0)

Oropharyngeal airways are designed to be used in unconscious patients only – if it is inserted into a semi-conscious patient it may stimulate coughing or vomiting or cause laryngospasm. As a general rule, if the patient doesn't tolerate an oropharyngeal airway then they don't need one!

OROPHARYNGEAL AIRWAY INSERTION: STEP BY STEP

- If possible, explain the procedure to the patient and gain consent. Provide a chaperone if required. The patient's conscious level may fluctuate, informed consent may not always be possible. Ensure you have the knowledge and competence to perform the skill and are familiar with local policy.

- Ensure the airway is clear of debris, use suction if necessary.

- Insert the airway past the teeth and gums: in adults, insert it upside down initially and then rotate it 180° as you pass halfway in order to reduce the risk of pushing the tongue back and down. In children, especially infants, there is a greater risk of damaging the soft palate so it can be inserted the right way up and slid backwards over the tongue – using a tongue depressor may help.

- If placement is correct, the airway flange should lie flat along the teeth or gums and any airway obstruction should be relieved.

- Reassess your patient's breathing and document the insertion.

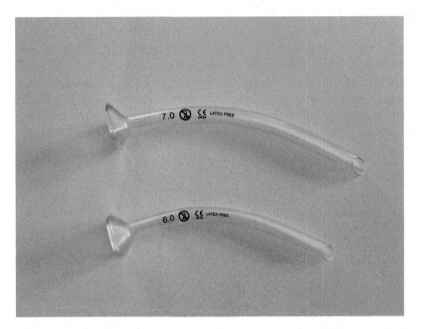

Figure 10.11   Nasopharyngeal airway

Nasopharyngeal airway

Nasopharyngeal airways (or NP airways) can be used in conscious patients and therefore have much wider uses than oropharyngeal airways. They consist of a long flexible plastic tube with a flange at the nose end and a bevel at the tip. They come in a range of sizes according to their diameter and the length increases with the width. The length can be sized by lining the airway up along the cheek to ensure it equals the distance from the patient's nostril to the angle of the jaw.

Caution should be used if the patient has a suspected base of skull fracture, and insertion can often cause bleeding initially, so be aware of any clotting disorders or anticoagulation medication your patient might be taking. Nasopharyngeal airways are invaluable when used to provide a channel for suctioning secretions from the pharynx (detailed below) especially in a frail patient or a patient with a weak cough.

—— NASOPHARYNGEAL AIRWAY INSERTION: STEP BY STEP ——

- Explain the procedure to the patient and gain consent. Provide a chaperone if required. Ensure you have the knowledge and competence to perform the skill and are familiar with local policy.
- Lubricate the airway with a water-based lubricant.
- Insert the airway with the bevel end first, with the bevel opening towards the septum.
- Slide with a rotating motion backwards and down along the floor of the nostril (pushing it up will cause trauma) until the flange is against the nostril.
- If an obstruction is felt, try the other nostril with the same technique.
- Reassess your patient's breathing and document the procedure.

AIRWAY SUCTIONING

Suctioning of the pharynx to remove secretions or other material from the patient's upper airway is an invasive procedure. The pharynx may be accessed via the mouth using a rigid Yankauer suction catheter, or via the nose using a soft suction catheter. Suctioning may be done to remove secretions, sputum, saliva, blood, vomit or any other foreign material and is indicated in any of the following situations: if the patient is unable to cough and clear their airway independently; if secretions are retained in the upper airway; or in an emergency situation.

Indications for pharyngeal suctioning include:

- Visible secretions in the airway
- Patient reports presence of secretions
- Suspected aspiration of gastric or upper airway secretions
- Unrelieved coughing
- Obvious increased work of breathing or agitation
- Auscultation of coarse, gurgling breath sounds

However, there are risks associated with pharyngeal suctioning so it should only be done as and when necessary – rather than as a routine, regular procedure. Risks include causing hypoxia if the suctioning is prolonged; damage to the oral/nasal mucosa from the catheter tip; and distress or discomfort to the patient. It is also possible to cause laryngeal spasm or (especially with the nasopharyngeal route) vagal nerve stimulation which can lead to bradyarrhythmia and even death.

Therefore, the nurse must consider several key points before suctioning a patient:

- Is there a true need for suctioning? Production of large amounts of sputum does not necessarily mean that the patient can't clear their secretions independently.
- How great is the risk of harm compared with the potential benefit of suctioning? Alternative strategies to loosen and clear secretions should be considered, as well as any higher risk factors, for example if the patient takes regular anticoagulant medications.
- Does the patient understand and consent to the procedure? Suctioning is unpleasant and invasive, and a patient may decline to have the procedure. It may also be necessary to use suctioning to clear a patient's airway when they are unable to give informed consent. Wherever possible the patient's wishes must be respected.

Many patients may require suction, for a wide variety of reasons. A patient may have an inadequate cough if they are exhausted or have an altered level of consciousness, or a patient with an impaired swallow reflex after a stroke may be more likely to have secretions pool at the back of their pharynx and need assistance clearing them.

Alternative strategies to manage secretions may not completely avoid the need for suctioning but may at least reduce the frequency it is required. Ensuring the patient is well hydrated and performing good oral care to prevent the oral cavity drying out can help prevent upper airway secretions crusting, and humidification of the patient's oxygen, if used, can also contribute. Providing good pain relief and promoting mobilisation and regular repositioning will help the patient expectorate their secretions more effectively. Referring for chest physiotherapy can help with various techniques to aid secretion clearance and several types of medication can help loosen or reduce the amount of secretions produced.

Suction pressures should be as low as possible while still removing secretions to avoid damage to the mucous membranes, and the maximum recommended pressure varies according to the patient's age. For nasopharyngeal suctioning, the soft suction catheters used are supplied in varying sizes which can also be selected according to the patient's age.

Table 10.5 Suction pressure and catheter size by age

Age	Suction pressure range	Nasopharyngeal suction catheter size
Neonate	60-80 mmHg (8-11 kPa)	5-6 Fr
Infant	80-100 mmHg (11-13 kPa)	6-8 Fr
Child	100-120 mmHg (13-16 kPa)	8-10 Fr
Adult	120-150 mmHg (16-20 kPa)	10 Fr

Suction should only be applied while the catheter is being withdrawn, and the whole procedure should take no more than 15 seconds in adults, no more than 10 seconds in children, and no more than 5 seconds in neonates and infants to minimise the risk of hypoxia.

Oral suctioning

Oral suctioning is usually done using a rigid plastic suction catheter with a curved tip, known as a Yankauer. There is a port on the side of the Yankauer which means that suction is only applied when the port is occluded, allowing the nurse more control. Oral suctioning is usually done only as far as the mouth and pharynx are visible and therefore carries low risk of contaminating the lower airways. Standard ANTT is recommended, but exceptions may occur in certain settings, so local policy should be followed.

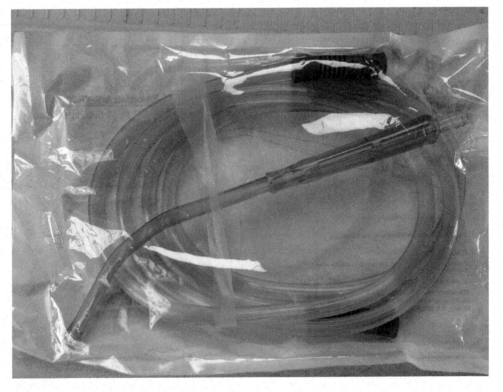

Figure 10.12 Yankauer suction catheter

Source: Wikimedia Commons/Thomasrive (CC BY-SA 3.0)

— WATCH THE VIDEO —

ORAL AND NASAL SUCTION

Watch along as you read through this step by step procedure by scanning the QR code with your smartphone camera or via **https://study.sagepub.com/rowberry**.

— ORAL SUCTIONING: STEP BY STEP —

EQUIPMENT NEEDED

- Wall suction device or portable suction unit with canister and tubing
- Yankauer suction catheter
- Jug or basin and water
- Appropriate PPE including a visor/eye protection (due to risk of splashing)
- Drape or towel to cover the patient's clothing

PROCEDURE

- Explain the procedure to the patient and gain consent. Provide a chaperone if required. Ensure you have the knowledge and competence to perform the skill and are familiar with local policy.
- Position the patient. If they are conscious, place the patient in Fowler's or semi-Fowler's position. If they are unconscious, place them onto their side facing you.
- Drape the towel over the patient's chest to protect their clothes.
- Check and adjust the suction pressure to the recommended range according to the patient's age.
- Wash hands and gather the equipment.
- Don PPE including non-sterile gloves.
- Open the Yankauer catheter and attach the base to the suction tubing.
- Ask the patient to take some deep breaths and cough to encourage secretions to loosen and gather in the back of the mouth.
- Insert Yankauer into the side of the patient's mouth without applying suction until you reach the back of the visible oropharynx.
- Slowly withdraw the Yankauer while applying suction by occluding the port, rotating slightly to avoid mucosal damage.
- Slide the Yankauer into the other side of the mouth and follow the same procedure.
- If the secretions are thick, flush the Yankauer by dipping it into the basin of water and applying suction.

(Continued)

- Discard of the Yankauer in clinical waste; dispose of other items according to local policy.
- Remove PPE and wash hands.
- Document the procedure in the patient's notes, recording the date and time; the reason for suctioning; the amount, colour and consistency of the secretions; and any problems encountered.

Nasal suctioning

Nasopharyngeal suctioning is done with a soft suction catheter passed via the nose into the nasopharynx to clear secretions. If a patient will need regular nasopharyngeal suctioning, consider the use of a nasopharyngeal airway. This is a thin sheath inserted into one nostril using lubrication and allows repeated suctioning with less discomfort and trauma associated with their use (see above). Insertion can be uncomfortable, but they are usually well tolerated once in-situ. As the catheter may access the lower airways and inadvertently cause contamination, ANTT should be used during nasopharyngeal suctioning.

NASAL SUCTIONING: STEP BY STEP

EQUIPMENT NEEDED

- Wall suction device or portable suction unit with canister and tubing
- Soft suction catheter of appropriate size
- Jug or basin and water
- Appropriate PPE including eye protection (due to risk of splashing) and at least one sterile glove
- Drape or towel to cover the patient's clothing

PROCEDURE

- Explain the procedure to the patient and gain consent. Provide a chaperone if required. Ensure you have the knowledge and competence to perform the skill and are familiar with local policy.
- Position the patient. If they are conscious place the patient in Fowler's or semi-Fowler's position. If they are unconscious, place them onto their side facing the nurse.
- Drape the towel over the patient's chest to protect their clothes.
- Check and adjust the suction pressure to the recommended range according to the patient's age.
- Wash hands and gather the equipment.
- Don PPE including non-sterile gloves and place a small amount of water-based lubricant on the sterile field.
- Open the suction catheter and attach the base to the suction tubing.
- Apply a sterile glove to the dominant hand and use it to withdraw the end of the catheter from the packaging.
- Ask the patient to take some deep breaths and cough to encourage secretions to loosen and gather in the back of the mouth.
- Using the dominant hand, lubricate the tip of the catheter and insert it into the patient's nasal passage (without applying suction) aiming towards the corner of the opposite eye and to the

floor of the nose, rotating gently. If resistance is felt, do not force the catheter but withdraw slightly and continue. If unable to advance the catheter, withdraw and attempt to insert into the other nostril.

- Once at the level of the pharynx, slowly withdraw the catheter while applying suction by occluding the port, rotating slightly to avoid mucosal damage.

- If the secretions are thick, flush the catheter by dipping it into the basin of water and applying suction.

- Wrap the catheter around your dominant hand and remove from the suction tubing and discard in clinical waste; dispose of waste according to local policy.

- Remove PPE and wash hands.

- Document the procedure in the patient's notes, recording the date and time; the reason for suctioning; the amount, colour and consistency of the secretions; and any problems encountered.

SPUTUM SAMPLE: DISCUSSION

A specimen from the respiratory tract can be used to identify infection, tuberculosis and lung cancer. The specimen can confirm the presence of bacterial, viral or fungal infection and allows the causative organism to be identified so that treatment can be tailored specifically.

Sputum specimens are indicated when the patient has signs of a respiratory tract infection such as a productive cough, and also if there are signs of sepsis or the patient has a high temperature of unknown origin.

Mucous production in the respiratory tract is normal, with the purpose of trapping debris and inhaled particles including bacteria and humidifying air as it enters the respiratory tract. However, sputum production is not normal and has an underlying cause such as smoking, cystic fibrosis, chronic lung disease or infection.

It is important to document the type, consistency and amount of sputum a patient expectorates when possible, as some characteristic features may help to identify the cause of excess sputum production.

Table 10.6 Types of sputum and possible causes

Type	Characteristics	Pathology associated
Blood	Blood stained or clots present	Pulmonary embolus, malignancy, clotting disorders
Mucoid	Clear, grey or white	Asthma or COPD
Purulent	Thick, yellow or green	Infectious cause – abscess, pneumonia
Serous	Frothy, sometimes pink	Pulmonary oedema

If the patient is conscious and has a good cough, then they can directly expectorate into the specimen container. Therefore, it is essential to explain the difference between sputum and saliva, as if the specimen contains saliva this will not be representative of the organisms in the lungs. If the patient is unable to produce the specimen independently then the nurse can consider using oro- or nasopharyngeal suction to obtain it using a sputum trap which connects into the suction tubing and catches the sputum during suctioning.

ACTIVITY: PAUSE AND REFLECT

Obtaining a sputum sample may be unpleasant for your patient. How would you approach this with an elderly patient who has dementia? How could you explain this procedure simply and put your patient at ease, to obtain an adequate sample for analysis?

Sputum traps can also be used in the suction circuit to obtain a specimen from a ventilated patient via their endotracheal or tracheostomy tube. If the patient's secretions are particularly thick or sticky, consider using nebuliser therapy to loosen the secretions, and ensure that the patient is receiving adequate pain relief to allow full chest expansion and an effective cough.

SPUTUM SAMPLE: STEP BY STEP

EQUIPMENT NEEDED

- Universal container
- PPE including eye protection in case of droplets

PROCEDURE

- Explain the procedure to the patient and gain consent. Provide a chaperone if required. Ensure you have the knowledge and competence to perform the skill and are familiar with local policy.
- Position the patient in Fowler's or semi-Fowler's position.
- Wash hands and don PPE.
- Ask the patient to take several deep breaths and cough, expectorating into the container.
- Seal the container, dispose of waste, remove PPE and wash hands.
- Label the container before leaving the patient.
- Document the procedure in the patient's notes, recording the date and time; the reason for obtaining the specimen; the amount, colour and consistency of the secretions; and any problems encountered.

CHAPTER SUMMARY

This chapter has recapped respiratory anatomy and physiology and has examined the relevant clinical skills required to meet a patient's respiratory needs. A good understanding of the respiratory system and confidence with these skills will allow the nurse to support patients with a range of needs across a variety of clinical areas. Care should be taken to familiarise yourself with any local policy.

ACE YOUR ASSESSMENT

Q1   What is internal respiration?

   a   Gas exchange between the alveoli and the bloodstream

   b   Breathing

   c   Gas exchange between the bloodstream and the cells

   d   The movement of air in and out of the lungs

Q2   What is Type 2 respiratory failure?

   a   Hypoxia

   b   Hypoxia with hypercapnia

   c   An asthma attack

   d   Emphysema

Q3   When should you suction a patient?

   a   Every 4 hours if they can't cough

   b   Only if they are unconscious

   c   When they show clinical signs of secretions

   d   Never

Q4   What oxygen can be administered by a registered nurse in an emergency?

   a   Whatever the patient needs to maintain saturations over 94%

   b   None unless there is a prescription

   c   2L/min via nasal cannula

   d   15L/min via a reservoir mask

Answers

1   A

2   B

3   C

4   D

GO FURTHER

An excellent textbook on respiratory nursing is:

Preston, W. and Kelly, C. (2017) *Respiratory Nursing at a Glance.* Chichester: Wiley Blackwell.

The Khan Academy website has some videos on the respiratory system which will help you understand lung physiology:

https://www.khanacademy.org/test-prep/mcat/organ-systems/the-respiratory-system/v/inhaling-and-exhaling (accessed October 20, 2022).

For more information on how cyanosis and other skin changes appear in skin of different colours, the following reference is very useful:

Makwende, M., Tamony, P. and Turner M. (2020) *Mind the Gap: A Handbook of Clinical Signs in Black and Brown Skin.* https://www.blackandbrownskin.co.uk/mindthegap (accessed October 20, 2022).

REFERENCES

Allibone, E., Soares, T. and Wilson, A. (2018) 'Safe and effective use of supplemental oxygen therapy', *Nursing Standard*, 33 (5): 43–50.

Andres, D., Thurston, N. and Brant, R. (1997) 'Randomised double-blind trial of the effects of humidified compared with nonhumidified low flow oxygen therapy on the symptoms of patients', *Canadian Respiratory Journal*, 4: 76–80.

Cameron, J., Reese, W. and Tayal, V. (1986) 'Bacterial contamination of ambulance oxygen humidifier water reservoirs: A potential source of pulmonary infection', *Annals of Emergency Medicine*, 15: 1300–2.

Campbell, E., Baker, M. and Crites-Silver, P. (1988) 'Subjective effects of humidification of oxygen for delivery by nasal cannula: A prospective study', *Chest*, 93: 289–93.

Cathala, X. and Costa, A. (2019) 'Anatomy and physiology', in Moorley, C. (ed.) *Introduction to Nursing for First Year Students*. London: Sage. pp. 112–41.

Cathala, X. and Moorley, C. (2020) 'Performing an A–G patient assessment: A practical step-by-step guide', *Nursing Times*, 116 (1): 53–5.

Chu, D., Kim, L.-Y., Young, P., Zamiri, N., Almenawer, S., Jaeschke, R. [...] and Alhazzani, W. (2018) 'Mortality and morbidity in acutely ill adults treated with liberal versus conservative oxygen therapy (IOTA): A systematic review and meta analysis', *The Lancet*, 391 (10131): 1693–705.

Conway, J., Fleming, J. and Perring, S. (1992) 'Humidification as an adjunct to chest physiotherapy in aiding tracheo-bronchial clearance in patients with bronchiectasis', *Respiratory Medicine*, 86: 109–14.

Cook, N., Shepher, A. and Boore, J. (2020) *Essentials of Pathophysiology for Nursing Practice*. London: Sage.

Fletcher, C., Elmes, P., Fairbairn, A. and Wood, C. (1959) 'The significance of respiratory symptoms in the diagnosis of chronic bronchitis in a working population', *British Medical Journal*, 2 (5147): 257–66.

Iramain, R., Castro-Rodriguez, J., Jara, A., Cardozo, L., Bogado, N., Morinigo, R. and De Jesus, R. (2019) 'Salbutamol and ipratropium by inhaler is superior to nebuliser in children with severe acute asthma exacerbation: Randomised clinical trial', *Pediatric Pulmonology*, 54: 372–7.

Jevon, P. and Ewens, B. (2012) *Monitoring the Critically Ill Patient* (3rd edition). London: Wiley Blackwell.

Lister, S., Hofland, J. and Grafton, H. (2020) *The Royal Marsden Manual of Clinical Nursing Procedures* (10th edition). Chichester: Wiley Blackwell.

McKinney, A. (2012) 'Acute exacerbation of chronic obstructive pulmonary disease', in K. Page and A. McKinney, *Nursing the Acutely Ill Adult Case Book*. Maidenhead: Open University Press. pp. 41–8.

Medical Research Council (1959) *MRC Breathlessness Scale*. London: Medical Research Council.

National Institute for Health and Care Excellence (NICE) (2021) *Asthma: Diagnosis, Monitoring and Chronic Asthma Management* (NG80). NICE, March 22. https://www.nice.org.uk/guidance/ng80/resources/asthma-diagnosis-monitoring-and-chronic-asthma-management-pdf-1837687975621 (accessed October 20, 2022).

National Institute for Health and Care Excellence (2022) 'Acute exacerbation of asthma', NICE, April. https://cks.nice.org.uk/topics/asthma/management/acute-exacerbation-of-asthma/ (accessed October 20, 2022).

O'Driscoll, B., Howard, L., Earis, J. and Mak, V. (2017) 'BTS guideline for oxygen use in adults in healthcare and emergency settings', *Thorax*, 72: ii1–ii90.

Preston, W. and Kelly, C. (eds) (2017) *Respiratory Nursing at a Glance*. Chichester: Wiley Blackwell.

Resuscitation Council UK (2021) *The ABCDE Approach*. London: Resuscitation Council UK.

Shepherd, E. (2017) 'Specimen collection 4: Procedure for obtaining a sputum specimen', *Nursing Times*, 113 (10): 49–51.

PREVENTING AND MANAGING INFECTION

11

LISA DUFFY AND LEE GAUNTLETT

NMC STANDARDS COVERED IN THIS CHAPTER

ANNEXE B NURSING PROCEDURES

9.1   Observe, assess and respond rapidly to potential infection risks using best practice guidelines
9.2   Use standard precautions protocols
9.3   Use effective aseptic, non-touch techniques
9.4   Use appropriate personal protection equipment
9.5   Implement isolation procedures
9.6   Use evidence-based hand hygiene techniques
9.7   Safely decontaminate equipment and environment
9.8   Safely use and dispose of waste, laundry and sharps

LEARNING OBJECTIVES

After reading this chapter, you should be able to:

- Discuss the transmission of infection
- Identify risks and evidence-based measures used to prevent and control infection in line with NMC standards
- Highlight the key principles of standard and transmission-based infection control precautions
- Observe, assess and respond rapidly to potential infection risks using best practice guidelines

STUDENT VOICE

Infection prevention and control prevents harm to our patients. It is the responsibility of all student nurses to understand and promote good practice.

Mohammed, 1st year, Mental Health

INTRODUCTION

Infectious diseases are caused by microscopic organisms (such as viruses or bacteria) which are passed from one person to another, or from an animal to human (and vice-versa). Whilst some organisms cause us little to no harm, others cause significant morbidity and mortality. The battle between humans and infectious diseases has continually shaped our history; the bubonic plague of the middle ages, the HIV epidemic and the Covid-19 pandemic are just a few examples. Even before the Covid-19 pandemic, in 2019 lower respiratory tract infections were the fourth leading cause of death worldwide, with 2.6 million lives lost (WHO, 2020).

The aim of the chapter is to introduce you to Infection Prevention and Control (IPC), and to Healthcare Associated Infections (HCAI) and the consequences of risk assessment. The various topics and activities are to help you to piece together theoretical learning underpinning IPC practice. They highlight your responsibilities as a student nurse and are to be used alongside infection prevention proficiencies for practice. Effective infection prevention and control requires knowledge about what is meant by infection, prevention and control and the:

- main routes to infection
- extent of the problem
- main causes and types of HCAI
- modes of transmission in healthcare settings
- main principles and methods for HCAI prevention and control.

As nurses and students, it is important that we use evidence-based, best practice approaches for meeting the needs for care and support with the prevention and management of infection, accurately assessing the person's capacity for independence and self-care and initiating appropriate interventions. Evidence-based informed IPC practice is essential for maintaining a safe environment for everyone and reducing the risk of the spread of infection and infectious diseases. Preventing harm to patients, health workers and visitors due to HCAIs is fundamental to achieve safe quality care and reduce antimicrobial resistance. Similarly, preventing and reducing the transmission of infectious diseases that cause global threats, such as coronaviruses, influenza or influenza-like infectious diseases and other emerging pathogens, is essential.

Healthcare associated infections

What is an HCAI? According to WHO (2010), a HCAI is defined as an infection acquired in a hospital by a patient who was admitted for a reason other than that infection and/or an infection occurring in a patient in a hospital or other facility in whom the infection was not (latently) present at admission. This includes infections that are acquired in the hospital, but appear only after discharge, as well as occupational infections among healthcare staff.

Why is discussing HCAIs important? A European study found that for every 20 patients hospitalised, at least one acquired an HCAI which was preventable (Haque et al., 2018). Firstly, it is essential to prevent HCAIs because the spread of these infections results in avoidable death and harm to patients, increases patient suffering and prolongs hospital stays/treatment. Secondly, increasing numbers of infections are caused by pathogens resistant to conventional antimicrobials. Alarmingly, more than 70% of HCAIs caused by bacterial infections are resistant to treatment by drugs; reducing healthcare associated infections will reduce the need to use our precious antimicrobials and will preserve their effectiveness.

The Covid-19 pandemic has demonstrated the need for effective IPC practice in both hospital and community settings. Implementation of key IPC practice (included in this chapter) will continue to be vital in mitigating the risk of transmission of harmful microorganisms to both patients and staff. The costs associated with treating patients suffering from HCAI are significant. Longer hospital stays and the need for a higher level of care add to healthcare budgets, as well as the economic burden borne by patients and families.

GO FURTHER

The IGH podcast is produced by Liverpool University. This episode discusses antimicrobial resistance and infection prevention, with added discussions from Dr Jennie Wilson, Vice President of the Infection Prevention Society:

https://podcasts.apple.com/gb/podcast/antimicrobial-resistance-and-infection-prevention/id1377675093?i=1000451255987

MICROBIOLOGY - INTRODUCTION

KEY TERMS

Bacteria: single-cell organisms, encapsulated in a cell wall

Flora: naturally occurring or indigenous microorganisms

Fungi: spore-producing organisms which feed on organic matter

Prions: misfolded proteins, which are disruptive to normal biological processes

Protozoa: single-cell parasitic organisms which feed on organic matter

Virus: infectious agent which replicates inside the living cells of an organism

To meet the NMC standard 9.1 this section will explain how microbiology forms the basis for IPC practice. In the field of nursing you are studying, a fundamental knowledge of microbiology will help you to consider and explain to your patients the rationale for any infection control practice or care given.

People, like all animals in existence, are not sterile. We all contain countless bacteria and other microbes within our skin, mouth and bowel for example. These normally found microbes are broadly termed normal human flora or commensals. We need to consider the significance of this in sickness and in health as well as within the healthcare practice. We will also consider the events that lead to an infection occurring, including when the normal flora can cause problems.

Microbiology

The normal flora of humans is exceedingly complex. It consists of more than 200 species of bacteria and may be influenced by many things. Factors that can influence it include genetics, age, gender, stress, nutrition, diet, and even if a person has pets or not (Ward, 2016). Microbiology is the study of microscopic organisms, i.e., those not seen by the naked eye. Within healthcare generally these microscopic organisms (microorganisms) are divided into the following main groups:

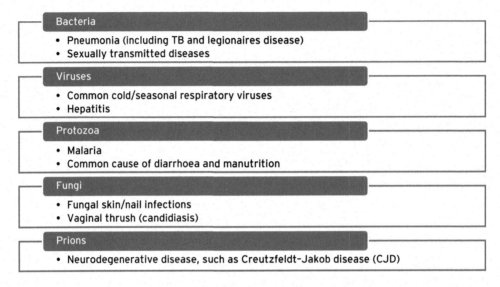

Bacteria
- Pneumonia (including TB and legionaires disease)
- Sexually transmitted diseases

Viruses
- Common cold/seasonal respiratory viruses
- Hepatitis

Protozoa
- Malaria
- Common cause of diarrhoea and manutrition

Fungi
- Fungal skin/nail infections
- Vaginal thrush (candidiasis)

Prions
- Neurodegenerative disease, such as Creutzfeldt-Jakob disease (CJD)

Figure 11.1   Five main groups of microorganisms, with common pathologies

These microorganisms exist everywhere, on us, inside us and within the environment we live in, but not all of them have the potential to cause harm. Organisms that have the potential to cause harm can be present in or on the human body without causing the body to react. The bacteria will still reproduce and multiply but will not stimulate the immune system. When bacteria is present, but not causing symptoms of illness, we call this colonisation. In fact, it has been shown that having a varied colonisation is beneficial to the human body (Weyrich et al., 2015).

Sometimes, normal flora can cause problems, as can microorganisms that are not normally found on us. An infection happens when a microorganism invades any part of the human body and causes the immune system to react. This reaction will then be perceived as symptoms. Symptoms can vary by microorganism type as well as by the location within which the microbe is found. For example, an infection by the common cold will cause a cough and a runny nose – both of which are a part of the respiratory system.

When a microorganism that is a part of the normal flora causes an infection, we call this an endogenous infection. If the microorganism comes from the environment, it is termed exogenous.

As healthcare professionals we can cause infections within our patients, and therefore hygiene is important. For example, improper hand washing can contaminate a healthy wound and compromise its healing, an exogenous infection. Not only can people transfer microbes between them, but so can other surfaces like beds, tables and so on. Of course, microbes can also be spread via air in the form of droplets. HCAIs are an exogenous source and come from staff or equipment (Blaser, 2016).

This is an important concept to acknowledge because interventions which are carried out to help a patient can ultimately become harmful. There are numerous examples of this like an infection of a central line (a catheter used for delivery of medication into the vein above the heart), a urinary tract infection caused by a urinary catheter, and so on. We can take steps to minimise the risk of iatrogenic infections by adopting Aseptic Non-Touch Technique (ANTT).

Conversely the eradication of the normal human flora via the improper use of antibiotics and poor heralding of antimicrobial stewardship can also lead to harm in our patients, as is the case with a clostridium difficile infection, discussed later within this chapter. This is why a good grounding in the knowledge of microbiology is required to navigate pertinent components which will minimise harm to our patients and lead to their benefit.

The diagram below shows the normal distribution of human flora and identifies where it is found. While these microorganisms are harmless in these sites, if they are transferred to another site in the body, they have a potential to cause infection.

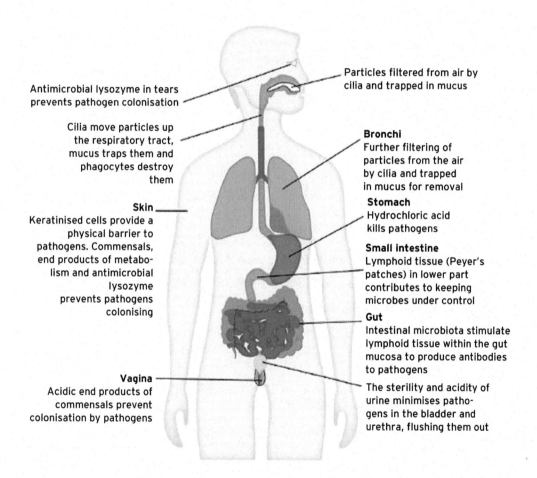

Figure 11.2   Physical and biochemical barriers to infection

Commensals have a range of functions within the human body. They can take residence (space) and take the nutrients in and from their area and hence stop other pathogenic organisms from multiplying and causing infection. Gut commensals are a good example of this.

Bacteria cause the following type of infections and range from local/mild infections to life threatening systemic infections.

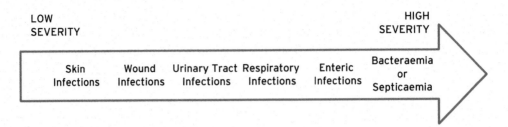

Figure 11.3 Common infection types and severity of disease

Differentiation of bacteria – bacteria shapes

By identifying the species of bacteria, we are able to determine their characteristics, what types of infection they likely to cause, and how to treat these.

The shape (also known as morphology) is one of the more easily distinguishable properties of bacteria which allow scientists to differentiate between them. If we can identify a specific bacterium, or indeed broadly define some of its characteristics, then we are much more able choose appropriate antibiotic drugs to treat bacterial infections. The key terms box below defines the shape names attributed to bacteria.

KEY TERMS

There are four main classifications of bacteria shapes:

Bacilli: rod-shaped bacteria (also Streptobacilli – a chain of rod-shaped bacteria)

Cocci: spherical or round bacteria (also Streptococcus – a chain of spherical bacteria)

Spiral: as the name suggests, spiral-shaped bacteria

Vibrio: comma-shaped, or kidney-bean-shaped bacteria

Differentiation of bacteria – Gram staining

Unlike human cells, a bacterial cell contains a cell wall outside the cell membrane. This is useful for us because it provides another way in which we can identify the bacterium. Some bacteria have thick cell walls due to thick layers of peptidoglycan and thin walls due to thin layers. Hans Christian Gram developed a method in 1884 which can exploit this; it is now named 'Gram staining' in his honour. Typically, the cells are stained with different dyes. The bigger crystal violet (purple) dye is trapped within the thick cell wall, and stains it purple. This dye is not trapped in a bacterium with a thin cell wall. Another dye is then used to stain the cells red or pink. A thick cell walled bacteria is classed as Gram positive and stains purple. A thin cell walled bacteria is Gram negative and stains red (Tripathi and Sapra, 2021).

In clinical practice, most sputum, wound and tissue samples which are processed in the laboratory undergo Gram staining as it is a cheap and quick test to perform which can provide some useful information to the healthcare professionals. While it does not precisely identify a bacteria species, it can allow identification of the cell wall type, and therefore influence the choice of antimicrobial drug used. Prescribing an antibiotic medication which is better at treating a specific group of bacteria (such as Gram-positive bacteria) is preferable to treating with a broader 'empiric' antibiotic medication.

KEY TERMS

Empiric antibiotic therapy: antibiotics administered without culture or identification of infection. Overuse of empiric antibiotic therapy can lead to antibiotic resistance.

Common commensals and their locations

It is useful to know where certain bacteria live. This knowledge can guide us when making clinical decisions. The table below summarises some of the common locations and related bacteria within the human body.

Table 11.1   Common human commensals and their locations

Location	Name
Skin	Staphylococcus, micrococcus, diptheroids, gram negative bacilli
Oral cavity and pharynx	Alpha and beta haemolytic streptococci, staphylococcus, pneumococcus
Gastrointestinal	Enterococcus, pseudomonas, streptococcus, lactobacillus
Genital tract	Lactobacillus, streptococcus

Source: Adapted from Davies (1996)

It may not be immediately apparent why the commensal location is important. As an example, lets consider that a patient who is very unwell from an infection has blood cultures taken. These are samples of blood from the patient which are then grown in a special medium in a lab to try and grow whichever bacteria are present. The blood cultures grow a species called *Staphylococcus aureus*. This bacteria is known to potentially cause infective endocarditis, an infection of the heart valves or inner lining of the heart. It is a common commensal of skin. This may therefore lead to an examination of the patient's skin, and identification of a wound or cut which may have led to the infection.

Clinically significant bacteria

Now we know a little about bacteria shapes and Gram staining, we can use these terms of differentiation to describe common bacteria that cause HCAI infection and are often seen in clinical practice.

Staphylococcus aureus

Often found in as part of the normal skin flora, Staphylococcus aureus may cause many superficial skin infections, such as cellulitis, impetigo and abscesses which are of low severity. In the hospital setting (within a more susceptible patient population) Staphylococcus aureus can cause pneumonia, infective endocarditis, and sepsis.

Its name is suggestive of some of its physical properties. The 'coccus' part of its name means it is spherical or round-shaped, with the 'aureus' part named after a golden Roman coin which relates to the characteristic 'golden crust' often observed on the skin lesions it causes. It is a Gram-positive organism.

Most strains of Staphylococcus aureus are sensitive to common antibiotics (such as Flucloxacillin); however, some strains are much more resistant to antibiotics. Those strains resistant to the antibiotic meticillin are termed meticillin-resistant Staphylococcus aureus (MRSA) and often require different types of antibiotics to treat them. In a susceptible patient (i.e., those who have undergone surgery, have underlying illness or indwelling devices) MRSA can cause significant harm and prove difficult to treat.

Streptococcus

Infrequently found on the skin, Streptococcus bacteria typically causes pathogenic infections. While the Stretococcus pygenes is the dominant species, a sub-type called Group A Streptococcus is commonly found in the throat and oral cavity.
Its name is suggestive of some of its physical properties. 'Streptococcus' is a chain of spherical bacteria, while 'pyogenes' means pus-producing. It is a Gram-positive organism.
Common types:

- Streptococcus pyogenes
- Group A Streptococci
- Streptococcus pneumonia

Neisseria meningitidis

Typically found within mucosal nasopharynx surfaces, this Gram-negative diplococcus commensal has the potential to cause a serious infection known as meningitis which is associated with worldwide morbidity and mortality. Meningitis is a serious infection of the protective membranes around the brain and the spinal cord, known as the meninges.

Symptoms of meningitis include fatigue, pyrexia, headache, neck stiffness, sensitivity to light (photophobia), coma and death. It is associated with a non-blanching rash known as petechiae. Although Neisseria meningitidis can cause meningitis, it can also be caused by other bacteria and viruses.

Clostridioides difficile (C. difficile) formally known as Clostridium difficile

Clostridioides difficile is a Gram-positive bacillus that forms spores. It produces two toxins termed A and B and is a common cause of antibiotic-associated diarrhoea. It is thought that it may be a part of the normal flora (Barbut and Petit, 2001). This is important because a C. difficile infection can develop following taking antibiotics because these antibiotics eradicate commensals which are otherwise in competition with C. difficile. This can result in infection and can cause serious illness and inflammation of the colon via the toxins it produces. This is known as colitis and this can progress to severe swelling and rupture (toxic megacolon). Because the bacteria turn into spores, they are resistant to some cleaning products and alcohol hand gels and can live on surfaces for a long time.

Escherichia coli (E. coli)

Escherichia coli is a Gram-negative bacillus that is a part of the gastrointestinal flora. Different species of E. coli exist and can cause various infections. They are a common cause of urinary tract infections and can also cause pelvic inflammatory disease. Typically, the bacteria ascend the perineum and enter the bladder via the urethra, though within the healthcare setting they can enter the bladder via the insertion of a urinary catheter. Certain strains can also cause gastrointestinal infections and cause symptoms such as diarrhoea. One strain called E. coli 0157 can cause a bloody diarrhoea and a condition called haemolytic uraemic syndrome where the blood vessels within the kidneys are damaged leading to blood clots within the kidneys and ultimately kidney failure. This infection is typically acquired from poorly cooked beef.

Figure 11.4 Significant bacteria

Viruses

Examples of viral infection: Common cold, Influenza, Covid-19, Hepatitis, Chickenpox, HIV.

A virus is a very small microbe, much smaller than a bacterium, and is composed of genetic material within a protective protein coat. It cannot reproduce on its own and relies on cells to copy itself. Because a virus does not have the components of a cell, antibiotics do not kill it. Antiviral medications and vaccinations work to reduce the severity of a viral disease or sometimes prevent infection. Viruses outnumber bacteria manyfold. They can cause various symptoms, such as the flu caused by the influenza virus, and can also lead to cancer as is the case in human papilloma virus leading to cervical cancer, among others.

Viruses are spread via numerous ways:

- Droplet or aerosol inhalation (e.g., rhinovirus, Covid-19)
- Infected water or food digestions (e.g., Hepatitis A)
- Sexual transmission or direct transfer from infected blood (e.g., HIV, Hepatitis B)
- Animal vectors (e.g., Yellow Fever, Rabies)

There are too many viruses in existence to discuss each individually within the scope of this book, however some are discussed below.

Common cold (Rhinovirus)

The rhinovirus is a usual cause of the common cold. The main route of entry into humans is via the respiratory system. It causes symptoms of a runny nose, cough and sneezing. There are many different serotypes of rhinovirus and immunity to one does not mean immunity to another. A rhinovirus particle contains RNA within capsid proteins.

The virus has evolved to attach itself to receptors on its host cell, allowing it to cross the cell membrane and deliver its genetic material to the genetic replication zone in the cytoplasm where it replicates itself.

Hepatitis

Hepatitis means inflammation of the liver and there are various causes of this. Certain viruses can induce inflammation of the liver; they are called Hepatitis viruses. Different Hepatitis viruses exist (Hepatitis A–E).

Hepatitis A is a spherical shaped virus with single stranded RNA. It is typically transmitted via the faecal–oral route from an infected person but can also be transmitted via ingestion of contaminated food and water. Most people with Hepatitis A will recover from the infection via their immune system and subsequently gain immunity to it. Rarely, people with Hepatitis A can develop sudden liver failure, otherwise known as fulminant hepatitis and die from this. A vaccine against Hepatitis A is available.

Hepatitis B is an icosaherdral virus with circular double stranded DNA. It is typically transmitted via contact with infected blood or other fluids that contain it. It can cause acute as well as chronic hepatitis. Hepatitis B can be cleared via the immune system but if it persists for more than six months it is considered a chronic infection. In adults chronic hepatitis develops in approximately 5% of cases but in childhood and infancy in about 95% of cases. Chronic hepatitis can cause damage to the liver and lead to cirrhosis, which can in turn lead to a cancer of the liver known as hepatocellular carcinoma. Because hepatitis is spread via contact with blood, it can be transmitted through inoculation with a contaminated needle within the community and also within the hospital, through needle stick injuries for example. It can be prevented by vaccination.

Hepatitis C is a spherical virus with single stranded RNA. It is typically transmitted via exposure to contaminated blood such as in needle sharing, blood transfusions that have not been screened and unsafe sexual practices. Hepatitis C can cause both acute and chronic hepatitis. Approximately 30% of people will spontaneously clear the infection within six months and medication can cure up to 95% of infections. 70% of people that do not spontaneously clear the virus and don't have treatment go on to develop chronic hepatitis which can lead to cirrhosis and ultimately hepatocellular carcinoma. Currently there is no vaccine against this virus (WHO, 2021).

Hepatitis D is a circular single stranded RNA virus. This virus requires the presence of Hepatitis B for its replication. This means that people are infected either simultaneously or after infection with Hepatitis B. Patients who undergo haemodialysis or those who share needles are at a higher risk of Hepatitis D. Hepatitis D and B coinfection is considered the most severe form of chronic hepatitis. This is because patients quickly develop liver related complications which result in death or develop hepatocellular carcinoma. Treatment for Hepatitis D has limited efficacy. It can however be prevented by Hepatitis B vaccination (WHO, 2021).

Hepatitis E is an icosahedral spherical virus containing single stranded RNA. It is mainly transmitted via the faecal–oral route and via contaminated water. It is predominantly cleared by the immune system, though those who are at risk, such as those who are immunocompromised, can develop serious infection. Hepatitis E infection can lead to fulminant hepatitis. A vaccine exists but is not yet available worldwide.

Protozoa

Examples of protozoal disease: Trichomonas, Amoebic dysentery, Giardiasis, Malaria.

Protozoa are single-celled organisms which are predominantly free-living in water and the surrounding environment. Protozoal infections are not common in the UK, as they tend to be more prevalent in tropical and sub-tropical regions. Most protozoa infect humans opportunistically and cause particularly severe disease in the immunocompromised (such as patients with HIV/AIDS or undergoing cancer treatment). Of all the parasites, malaria causes the most significant burden of disease, affecting around 241 million individuals worldwide in 2020 (WHO, 2022).

Many protozoa are transmitted by ingestion of contaminated food or water. This is most significant in developing nations, affecting the poorest and most vulnerable in global society.

Malaria

─────────────────────── **KEY TERMS** ───────────────────────

Anaemia: a lack of red blood cells to carry oxygen to the body's tissues

Febrile: showing the signs of a fever

Rigors: feeling of cold/shivering, with a rise in body temperature

Malaria is an acute febrile illness which presents as fever, headache, and rigors within 10–15 days of infection by the plasmodium parasite. If left untreated, the symptoms can progress and eventually lead to death. The World Health Organization (2022) estimated that 627,000 people died of malaria in 2020 alone.

Malaria parasites are transmitted by a bite from an infected female mosquito. An infected mosquito (known as a vector) lands on a human host and attempts to feed. The parasite enters the blood stream and resides briefly within the human host's liver, before moving inside red blood cells to multiply. As the infection grows, red blood cells become engorged with the multiplying parasite, leading to cell rupture. The red cell destruction causes symptomatic anaemia, with the by-products of destruction leading to host toxicity. The result of these changes can be catastrophic, causing respiratory distress, altered blood coagulation and organ failure.

Climate is key to the geographic distribution of malaria. Without sufficient rainfall the mosquito cannot survive, and without a hot climate, the parasites cannot survive within the mosquito. Sub-Saharan Africa has ideal conditions for the parasite and mosquito, meaning transmission occurs all-year round without significant seasonal variation, and that the African continent has a dispropor-tionally high share of the global disease burden.

Giardiasis

Giardiasis is the name given to the diarrhoeal disease caused by the Giardia protozoa parasite. Giardia species are highly infective; initially spread by human contact with infected faeces or animals. It can also be transmitted human-to-human and isolated outbreaks are frequently linked to infected water sources and swimming pools!

The Giardia protozoa lives within the gastrointestinal tract of its infected host. It causes profuse diarrhoea which can last 1–3 weeks. The diarrhoea itself can contain 'Giardia cysts', which are the highly infectious form of the species, which can be easily released into the local environment by improper waste or sewerage handling, leading to further infection of humans and animals. Treatment is 'supportive', meaning that fluid and electrolyte losses (from loose stools) must be replaced while the disease runs its course. Without prompt rehydration, Giardiasis can be fatal.

ACTIVITY: PAUSE AND REFLECT

Diarrhoeal illness remains a leading cause of death of children under 5, with approximately 1014 children dying each day worldwide (WHO, 2020).

Fungi

Examples of fungal disease: Candidiasis, Aspergillosis, Athlete's foot, Ringworm.

There are thousands of species of fungi, however few are a significant cause of disease in humans. Most commonly, fungal infections manifest in the skin and nails, causing minimal harm. However, it is estimated that the global burden of fungal disease may affect up to 1 billion people a year (Bongomin et al., 2017). Systemic fungal infection is more commonly seen in patients with significant concurrent illness (such as those in intensive care), or within susceptible groups, such as the immunocompromised.

This means patients in hospital or receiving treatment in the community are a significant 'at-risk' group.

Fungi can divide into two groups, the branched filamentous form (imagine a tree branch), or as a yeast (a spherical form). The branched filamentous type multiplies by asexual reproduction and the formation of sacs which contain and disperse fungal spores into the immediate vicinity. These spores can commonly be inhaled (causing lung infection) or infiltrate open wounds. The yeast type multiplies by division, however depending on temperature and environment, can also form hyphae (branch-like filaments of fungus) to propagate.

KEY TERMS

Mycosis: a disease caused by infection with a fungus

Propagate: breed or spread

Subcutaneous: under the skin

Yeast: spherical, single cell organism

There are three broad types of fungal infection:

1   **Superficial mycosis** – fungus growing on the body surface, such as skin, hair and mouth. Examples of this include oral candidiasis, vaginal candidiasis (thrush) and tinea pedis (athlete's foot). These are usually low severity infections. In the example of oral candidiasis, this is often caused by inhaled steroid medications and concurrent antibiotic use eliminating the normal oral flora, allowing candidiasis to propagate.
2   **Subcutaneous mycosis** – fungus growing in deeper layers of skin and nails. These are often caused by skin penetration (from intravenous lines infected with candida).
3   **Systemic mycosis** – opportunistic fungus infections within deep structures/organs. These are more common in patients who are immunosuppressed or on concurrent antibiotic treatment. Common examples are systemic candidiasis or histoplasmosis, fungus spores found in bird and bat droppings.

Candida

Candida is a type of yeast, and the most common cause of fungal infections worldwide (Bongomin et al., 2017). Many species cause little harm and some form part of the normal skin flora. The overall rate of candidaemia infection in England was 3.5 per 100,000 in 2020 (Public Health England, 2021), illustrating the low incidence of infection which was more common in the over-75 age group.

Candida appears as large white colonies on the skin. White spots found within oral mucosa are often termed as 'oral candidiasis' or 'oral thrush' and can be found in other locations such as the genitals or armpits. Oral candidiasis can be distressing for patients; the colonies can cover the tongue and oral mucosal layer, changing the taste of food and drink and causing discomfort. These superficial infections can easily be treated with topical mouth washes or over-the-counter creams.

Ringworm

Ringworm is not a worm, it's a fungus! The name describes the characteristic ring-shaped lesions often seen on the skin. The infection is most commonly seen in young children and adolescents; however, all age groups can be affected. Individual risk factors include excess sweating/poor hygiene, diabetes, and immunodeficiency.

Often caused by the fungal species *T. rubrum*, ringworm is spread by the shedding of fungal spores onto skin. Transmission is facilitated by a warm, moist environment and is further aided by household crowding or sharing of clothes and bath towels.

The lesions can be treated directly with a topical anti-fungal cream (bought from a pharmacy) and the risk of further transmission reduced by avoiding close contact with susceptible individuals and improvements in personal hygiene and laundry.

ACTIVITY: HAVE A GO

For a microorganism to establish itself within a human host, it first must gain entry to the body. List as many physiological and external entry sites and mechanisms to the human body as you can. To start things off, three have been listed for you.

1. Skin	7.	13.
2. Conjunctiva	8.	14.
3. Animal bite	9.	15.
4.	10.	16.
5.	11.	17.
6.	12.	18.

Answers

Mouth, nose, contaminated food/water, sharing needles (illicit drug use), inhalation, nail bed, wound, surgical procedure, indwelling devices (such as catheter or IV cannula), sexual transmission, anus, urethra, vagina, placenta (mother-to-foetus transmission), contaminated blood (e.g., blood transfusion or splash of blood to eyes), needle stick injury.

UNDERSTANDING INFECTION

Virulence

KEY TERMS

Virulence: the ability to cause infection depends on virulence. Factors that influence this ability include:

- Size of dose of inoculation (entry into body)
- Ability to invade host tissues
- Ability to damage host tissues
- Ability to grow/multiply/escape and disseminate

Before infection happens, the susceptible host must be exposed to the *virulence* of a pathogen following the steps outlined in Figure 11.5.

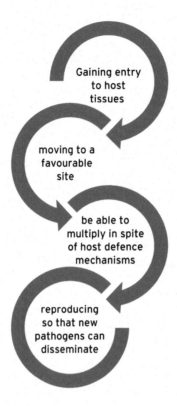

Figure 11.5 Path of virulence

Being aware of the signs and symptoms of infection

The common signs and symptoms of infection are outlined in Figure 11.6.

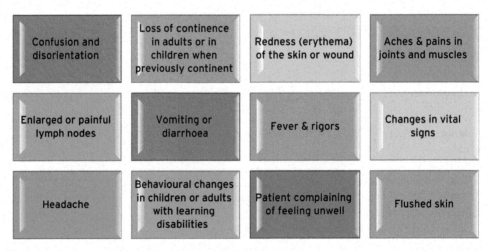

Figure 11.6 Common signs and symptoms of infection

The chain of infection

The chain of infection illustrated in Figure 11.7 comprises six links of a chain that represent the events required to initiate an infection. If any one link of the chain is removed, then infection will not occur. This can assist nurses to ensure risk assessing all aspects of care and using IPC practice that reduces risk (breaks the chain by removing links).

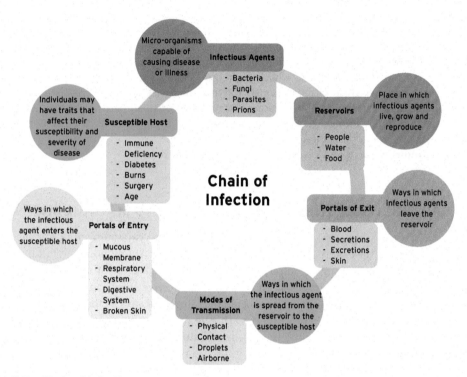

Figure 11.7   Chain of infection

Source: WikiMedia Commons/Genieieiop (CC BY-SA 4.0)

Visit https://www.niinfectioncontrolmanual.net/basic-principles for more information on the basic principles of infection prevention and control.

ACTIVITY: PAUSE AND REFLECT

Obrey is a 69-year-old African Caribbean male with sickle cell disease who has a vancomycin-resist-ant enterococcus-infected pressure ulcer wound.

Consider each link of the chain of infection individually and reflect on how you would address each one.

Routes of transmission

This next section will discuss what IPC practice and skills are needed in more detail to break the chain of infection.

Microorganisms can spread from one individual to another and cause infection (or colonisation). Transmission is through:

- **Person-to-person transmission**: (Direct contact) can occur when microbes present in blood or other bodily fluids of a patient are transmitted to a healthcare worker (or vice versa) through contact with a mucous membrane or breaks (cuts, abrasions) in the skin.
- **Indirect (contact) transmission:** Infections can be transmitted indirectly through devices such as thermometers, stethoscopes, other inadequately decontaminated equipment, medical devices or toys, which healthcare workers pass from one patient to another. This is probably the most common mode of transmission in healthcare settings.
- **Droplet transmission:** Respiratory droplets carrying pathogens are generated when an infected person coughs, sneezes, or talks, as well as during procedures such as suctioning or intubation.
- **Airborne transmission**: Occurs through the dissemination of either airborne droplet nuclei (particles arising from desiccation of suspended droplets) or small particles in the respirable-size range containing infectious agents that remain infective over time and distance (e.g. spores of Aspergillus spp. and Mycobacterium tuberculosis).
- **Percutaneous exposure:** Occurs through contaminated sharps.

CLINICAL SKILLS REQUIRED TO PREVENT AND MANAGE INFECTION

The clinical skills covered below are essential in developing and expanding your knowledge and practice in this area. These are skills you should aim to develop throughout the full duration of your programme of study. They are applicable to all nurses regardless of their field of practice. Although this chapter provides information on safe and effective infection control practice, it is important to remember that local policies and guidance should always be followed and all nursing staff have a duty to be aware of, and comply with, the organisation's requirements when working in a placement area. Finally, during unprecedented times it is essential that local government guidance is adhered to.

Note on terminology: throughout this section the word 'patient' is used in general, but this can refer to a client, service user or care home resident.

Standard Infection Control Precautions (SICPs)

SICPs are the fundamental infection prevention and control measures necessary to reduce the risk of transmission of infectious agents from both recognised and unrecognised sources of infection. SICPs are to be used by all staff, in all care settings, at all times, for all patients, whether infection is known to be present or not, to ensure the safety of those being cared for, staff and visitors in the care environment.

Sources of (potential) infection include blood and other body fluids, secretions or excretions (excluding sweat), non-intact skin or mucous membranes and any equipment or items in the care environment that could have become contaminated.

Application of SICPs during care delivery is determined by an assessment of risk to and from individuals and includes the task, level of interaction and/or the anticipated level of exposure to blood and/or other body fluids.

It is important, however, that staff ensure that standard infection prevention control precautions are used for all patients regardless of their status. These precautions include hand hygiene, use of gloves, aprons and occasionally masks and eye protection, following a risk assessment to identify the risks of exposure to blood, body fluids and microorganisms.

The ten do's to prevent infection

1 Patient assessment for infection risk
2 Hand hygiene
3 Respiratory and cough hygiene
4 Personal protective equipment
5 Safe management of care equipment
6 Safe management of care environment
7 Safe management of linen
8 Safe management of blood and body fluid spillages
9 Safe disposal of sharps
10 Occupational safety: Prevention and exposure management

We will now look at each of these in further detail.

1 Patient assessment for infection risk

The need for correct patient placement and the associated assessment for infection is a requirement of The Health and Social Care Act (2008) (Department of Health, 2015a). In response to this, the Code of Practice on the Prevention and Control of Infections (Department of Health, 2015a) provides guidance on how providers should interpret and meet the requirement on cleanliness and infection control to comply with the law.

Patients must be promptly assessed for infection risk on arrival at the care area (if possible, prior to accepting a patient from another care area) and should be continuously reviewed throughout their stay. This assessment should influence placement decisions in accordance with clinical/care need(s). This assessment for infection risk must be undertaken. This ensures both the appropriate placement of the patient and that appropriate precautions are taken. This applies to all admissions, transfers and discharges to all health and social care facilities including:

- Admissions to hospital and inter hospital transfers
- Transfers from or to another care home
- Attending for treatment or support in another health or adult social care setting

Patients who may present a cross-infection risk include those:

- with diarrhoea, vomiting, an unexplained rash, fever, or respiratory symptoms
- who have had a previously positive test for a Multi-drug Resistant Organism (MDRO) (e.g. MRSA)
- who have been hospitalised outside the designated area (such as part of the country or nationally) within the last 12 months.

DEFINITIONS OF RISK

CONFIRMED RISK

A 'confirmed risk' patient is one who has been confirmed by a laboratory test or clinical diagnosis, e.g. Covid-19, Meticillin-resistant Staphylococcus aureus (MRSA), Multi-resistant Gram-negative bacteria (MRGNB), Pulmonary Tuberculosis (TB), scabies, seasonal influenza and enteric infections (diarrhoea and/or vomiting) including Clostridioides difficile (formerly known as Clostridium difficile).

For Covid-19, please refer to national infection prevention and control guidance.

(Continued)

SUSPECTED RISK

A 'suspected risk' patient includes an individual who is awaiting a laboratory test and/or result or clinical diagnosis to identify reported symptoms of infections/organisms or those who have been in recent contact/close proximity to an infected person.

NO KNOWN RISK

A 'no known risk' resident does not meet either of the criteria above.

There are evidence-based national and local algorithms and pathways within guidance for specific infections and/or symptoms that help to determine categories of risk. For example see p.8 of Public Health England's *Guidelines for PHE Health Protection Teams on the Management of Outbreaks of Influenza-like Illness (ILI) in Care Homes* (2020). https://assets.publishing.service.gov.uk/government/uploads/system/uploads/attachment_data/file/932991/Guidelines_for_the_management_of_out-breaks_of_influenza-like_illness_in_care_homes_05_11_2020.pdf (accessed October 21, 2020).

FOR SPECIALIST AREAS

NEONATAL/SPECIAL CARE BABY UNIT

More information can be found in the National Infection Prevention and Control Manual: *Infection Prevention and Control Within Neonatal Settings (NNU)* (2020). https://www.nipcm.hps.scot.nhs.uk/addendum-for-infection-prevention-and-control-within-neonatal-settings-nnu/ (accessed October 21, 2020).

COMMUNITY SETTINGS

More information can be found in the NHS's *Patient Placement and Assessment for Infection Risk* (2021). https://www.infectionpreventioncontrol.co.uk/content/uploads/2021/05/DC-07-Patient-placement-April-2021-Version-2.00.pdf (accessed October 21, 2020).

If a neonate is considered to be a cross infection risk, then the clinical judgement of those involved in the management of the baby should assess the placement by prioritising the incubator/cot in a suitable area pending investigation, i.e. place in a single room or cohort area/room with a wash hand basin. In addition, incubators/cots should not be placed near any water source where spraying or splashing may occur.

2 Hand hygiene

WATCH THE VIDEO

HANDWASHING

Watch along as you read through this step by step procedure by scanning the QR code with your smartphone camera or via https://study.sagepub.com/rowberry.

Hand hygiene is an essential element of infection control activities because the hands are the most common means in which microorganisms, particularly bacteria, can be spread and subsequently cause infection, especially for those patients who are most susceptible.

Most healthcare associated infections are preventable through good hand hygiene – effective hand decontamination/cleaning hands at the right times and in the right way (WHO, 2011).

Continuous risk assessment must be used to inform hand hygiene practice and always undertaken by all staff to eliminate the risks of cross-infection. Therefore, you must assume that every person you encounter could be carrying potentially harmful microorganisms that could be transmitted and cause harm to others. Hand hygiene is one of the elements of Standard Infection Control Precautions. As such, carrying out effective hand hygiene at the correct point in care is important in improving patient safety and contributing to breaking the chain of infection at every opportunity.

To ensure optimum safety and effective hand hygiene the following points should be considered:

1   Use of a recommended product
2   Application of the correct hand hygiene technique
3   At precise moments in time (using the five moments of hand hygiene; see below)

Hand hygiene is equally important in all healthcare settings. It may be more difficult to achieve in the community setting, but is still essential!

Micro-organisms on the hands fall into two categories.

1   **Transient skin flora**

These are carried temporarily and consist of microorganisms acquired on the hands through contact with other sites on the same individual, from other people, or from the environment. They are easily acquired by touch, and readily transferred to the next person or surface touched, so may be responsible for the transmission of infection. Removal of transient microorganisms is therefore essential in preventing cross-infection, and their removal is easily achieved by washing with soap and water, the use of alcohol rub or hand sanitizing wipes.

2   **Resident skin flora**

These are microorganisms which live permanently in deep crevices and hair follicles, known as skin flora. Most are bacteria of low pathogenicity. They are not readily transferred to other people, and most are not easily removed by washing with soap. They do not need to be removed from the hands during routine clinical care. During invasive procedures, for example minor surgery, there is a risk that resident microorganisms may enter the patient's tissues and cause an infection.

Five moments of hand hygiene

GO FURTHER

Watch the following YouTube video:

RITM DOH (2019) '5 moments of hand hygiene in an inpatient setting', RITM DOH (YouTube video), May 6. https://www.youtube.com/watch?v=XsfKM-YINOE (accessed October 21, 2022).

Read the following poster:

World Health Organization (2009) 'Your 5 Moments for Hand Hygiene'. https://cdn.who.int/media/docs/default-source/integrated-health-services-(ihs)/infection-prevention-and-control/your-5-moments-for-hand-hygiene-poster.pdf?sfvrsn=83e2fb0e_16 (accessed October 21, 2022).

The World Health Organization (WHO) produced the model *5 Moments for Hand Hygiene*. To fully understand the 'five moments' and to ensure that the principle can be applied in all care environments, it is important to be aware of the concept of the 'service user zone'. Staff need to clean their hands at the 'point of care', as well as when they enter and leave the service user's 'zone'. Healthcare workers must decontaminate their hands before and after all contact with service users and whenever hands are visibly soiled.

ACTIVITY: PAUSE AND REFLECT

Returning to the need to risk assess, consider:

- What activity has just been undertaken?
- What activity is about to be undertaken?

Principal hand hygiene can be achieved by hand washing with soap, by the use of alcohol-based hand rub or by the use of hand sanitising wipes. Alcohol-based hand rub is an acceptable alternative to hand washing between caring for different service users or between different caring activities for the same service user as long as the hands are not grossly soiled. They must be free of dirt and organic material.

Risk assessment is needed when determining what hand hygiene product to use. The recommendations in the WHO Guidelines (2021a) on hand hygiene in healthcare are:

- Before routine clinical work begins, remove all wrist and hand jewellery and cover cuts and abrasions with waterproof dressings; ensure that you keep fingernails short; false nails should not be worn.
- While in clinical practice, wash hands with soap and water whenever they are visibly dirty or visibly soiled with blood or other bodily fluids and after using the toilet.

Washing hands with liquid soap and water is paramount when exposure to potential spore-forming pathogens is suspected/proven. During outbreaks of Clostridioides difficile or any other gastrointestinal infection such as Norovirus, hand washing with soap and water is preferred.

It is acceptable that you can use an alcohol-based handrub as the preferred means for routine hand antisepsis when hands are not visibly soiled; if an alcohol-based handrub is not available, wash hands with soap and water.

As we have determined, handwashing is vital. There are three levels of hand hygiene which can be used in clinical settings. These are illustrated in the following table.

Table 11.2   Three levels of hand hygiene

Hand hygiene type	Purpose/method
Social	Meant to clean the hands of physical dirt and debris, as well as some transient bacteria/organisms. It is sufficient for most daily activities. In clinical areas liquid soap should be used (typically in wall mounted dispensers).

Hand hygiene type	Purpose/method
Antiseptic	A more stringent procedure compared to social washing, designed to eliminate microorganisms from the hands. Indicated for 'high-risk' areas or patient groups, and before undertaking any invasive procedures. For example: • Immunocompromised patients • Intensive care/critical care areas • Insertion of urinary catheter, intra-venous cannula • During outbreaks of infection • When treating patients with multi-resistant bacteria Use an antimicrobial detergent **OR** soap & water followed by alcohol rub on dried hands. Please refer to local departmental policy for procedure.
Surgical	The most stringent type of handwashing. Surgical hand decontamination is necessary when a greater level of hand and forearm disinfection is required (prior to invasive surgical procedures). Antiseptic liquids such as iodine or chlorhexidine 4% scrub should be used. A sterile towel must be used for drying. Please refer to local departmental policy for procedure.

Conducting a risk assessment based on the care activity will determine the level of hand hygiene and product you should use.

Transient bacteria are not part of the 'normal flora'. They are bacteria (may also be viruses, etc.) that staff pick up transiently (temporarily) during the course of their work, e.g. when making beds, bed bathing, giving commodes, moving and handling patients or contaminated equipment, collecting patient dishes. In most clinical practice areas, a social hand wash process is adequate – this means using an excellent technique with plain liquid soap and water. This will remove transient bacteria picked up from the environment.

They are carried on the skin surface and, therefore, are easy to pass on from patient to patient. With a good hand hygiene technique, they are easy to remove.

Examples of transient bacteria include E.coli, MRSA, Clostridioidesdifficile spores, Norovirus, and many others.

Resident bacteria are 'normal skin flora'. They are part of each person's natural defence mechanisms.

They are found on the surface, just below the uppermost layer of skin. They are not as easily removed as transient bacteria. These resident bacteria can pose a threat where staff are looking after vulnerable patients or susceptible sites (e.g. invasive devices or wounds).

Examples of resident bacteria include staphylococcus epidermidis (we all carry this bacterium) and staphylococcus aureus (about one-third of the population carry this bacterium).

A hygienic/aseptic hand wash/antiseptic will remove transient bacteria and reduce the level of resident bacteria. This is done by using the same excellent technique, but using:

• an antibacterial liquid soap, e.g. a Chlorhexidine based product
• or normal soap and water followed by alcohol rub, applied to dry hands
• or only alcohol rub (providing hands are physically clean to begin with).

Surgical scrub is a 2–5-minute precise technique performed prior to all surgical/invasive procedures. It is not taught as part of this chapter. Senior staff in specialist clinical areas teach this technique.

Equality and diversity considerations

Individuals with a cognitive impairment or a lack of mobility may need additional support to undertake hand washing and decontamination and other practices to reduce the risk of infection.

Nurses need to be aware of the cultural preferences of colleagues and patients in relation to hand hygiene. Religious beliefs and rituals can be a source of concern in relation to hand hygiene and the use of alcohol hand products for hand decontamination. Most participants in a study indicated that alcohol hand hygiene product use by Muslims is appropriate, regardless of the associated prohibition of alcohol ingestion (Khuan et al., 2018).

ACTIVITY: PAUSE AND REFLECT

From your experience or your learning, what other factors prevent effective handwashing/hygiene?

Community perspective

Hand hygiene practice in the patient's own home should follow the same principles highlighted in the previous section. However, with risk assessment in mind, there is a risk that hand wash facilities in the patient's own home will not be to the same standard as a hospital setting. To minimise risks, in such areas where hand washing facilities are substandard, ensure you carry liquid soap and disposable handtowels. Alternatively, 70% alcohol-based hand gel/rubs and/or wipes or hand sanitising wipes should be used until skin is completely dry.

3 Respiratory and cough hygiene

The phrase 'coughs and sneezes spread diseases' was first used in the 1918–1920 influenza pandemic in the USA. It was designed to encourage good public hygiene and to prevent the further spread of infection within the population. The message remains pertinent within a modern healthcare setting and within the wider area of public health.

When a person with a respiratory infection coughs or sneezes, potentially millions of infectious particles are released into the air. They can be spread person-to-person, by being immediately inhaled by other people close by, or they can be spread indirectly by contaminating surrounding surfaces. Research suggests some viruses can live on surfaces for long periods of time, with influenza persisting on an inanimate surface for four weeks (Valtierra, 2008).

A cough does not necessarily come as a consequence of a respiratory infection – they can be caused by a number of non-infections/non-transmissible causes:

1   Respiratory irritants, such as smoke, dust and chemicals
2   Aspiration of food/fluids into the lungs
3   From prescription medications (Ramipril, a medication used for blood pressure control, often causes a cough)
4   Medical conditions such as pulmonary oedema or respiratory cancers

Numerous respiratory pathogens (for example, Pertussis, Rhinovirus or Covid-19) are spread by coughing, sneezing or being in close proximity to infected individuals and breathing their exhaled air. To prevent this, the following steps are recommended for any individuals with a suspected respiratory infection, to prevent transmission:

1   Cover mouth and nose when coughing/sneezing. If possible, use a disposable tissue.
2   Dispose of tissues in a suitable receptacle (preferably a non-touch waste bin in a healthcare setting).
3   Use appropriate hand hygiene (as outlined in the section on hand hygiene above).
4   Provide conveniently placed alcohol hand gel and handwash facilities (in a healthcare setting).
5   If access to water and hand washing facilities are unavailable, use alcohol-based gel or hand wipes.
6   Keep contaminated hands away from the eyes, nose and mouth.

Use of masks

A medical/surgical mask (fluid resistant/repellent) is theoretically sufficient to prevent droplet infection, whereas a respirator (filter) is needed to prevent airborne infection and needs to be close fitting. In terms of face mask use, the physical barrier may also prevent contact transmission such as hand to face, mouth, or nose. Many more staff are now used to the regular use of masks in clinical practice areas. However, they can become a barrier to effective communication.

ACTIVITY: PAUSE AND REFLECT

Consider the ways communication can be enhanced when staff and patients are required to wear masks.

4 Personal protective equipment

WATCH THE VIDEO

DONNING AND REMOVING PPE

Watch along as you read through this step by step procedure by scanning the QR code with your smartphone camera or via https://study.sagepub.com/rowberry.

PERSONAL PROTECTIVE EQUIPMENT: STEP BY STEP

The most commonly used Personal Protective Equipment (PPE) are gloves, disposable aprons, and face protection. Selection and use of PPE is based on a risk assessment process. The task or situation will determine the choice of PPE in relation to risk of transmission of microorganisms to the patient or carer; risk of contamination of healthcare practitioners' clothing and skin by patients' blood or body fluids; and suitability of the equipment for proposed use.

•   Don appropriate gloves.

(Gloves must be worn for invasive procedures, contact with sterile sites and non-intact skin or mucous membranes, all activities that have been assessed as carrying a risk of exposure to blood or body fluids, and when handling sharps or contaminated devices.)

- Don (put on) immediately before an episode of patient contact or treatment.
- Remove as soon as the episode is completed.
- Gloves to be changed between each caring episode.
- Dispose in accordance with local policy for waste management.
- Hands must be decontaminated immediately after gloves have been removed.

(Sensitivity to natural rubber latex in patients, carers and healthcare workers must be documented, and alternatives to natural rubber latex gloves must be available.)

Sterile versus non-sterile gloves

There are two main categories of gloves used in UK health: non-sterile examination and sterile procedure gloves. They are covered by two different European directives to ensure that they meet the necessary quality standards. Some gloves used in healthcare may be labelled to more than one directive and it is important to consider the differences between the two standards to ensure you have the right glove available for your requirements.

The RCN (Tools of the Trade Guidance for healthcare staff on glove use and the prevention of contact dermatitis) supports the evidence-based approach taken by the HSE. Key issues to consider when deciding on the choice of gloves include the following, and form the basis of a risk assessment for glove use:

- Task to be performed
- Anticipated contact and compatibility with chemicals and cytotoxic drugs
- Latex or other sensitivity
- Glove size required
- Your organisation's policies for creating a latex-free environment

Gloves should never be used as an alternative to hand hygiene which is a central part of standard infection control precautions (Loveday et al., 2014). Gloves act as a physical barrier to prevent contamination of hands by blood and body fluids, chemicals, and microorganisms. The integrity of any glove cannot be taken for granted, and staff should be aware that complete protection or contamination prevention of their hands cannot be guaranteed.

Prolonged use of gloves can increase the risk of work-related dermatitis because of exposure to the material or the chemicals used to manufacture gloves.

Other PPE

- Aprons (vary in design, used for a number of clinical procedures)
- Gowns (used often in operating theatres and ICU)
- Eye protection (should be used based on risk assessment of the task)
- Head protection (should be used based on risk assessment of the task)
- Footwear (should meet health and safety requirements and be suitable for the task)

PPE TIPS

- Keep your hands away from your face whilst wearing PPE.
- If gloves become torn or heavily contaminated, stop the procedure as soon as it is safe to do so, move away from the patient, remove your gloves, and decontaminate your hands before applying clean gloves.
- Limit the surfaces touched in the patient environment.
- Perform hand hygiene after removing each item of PPE.
- All PPE should be discarded as infectious waste.
- Remove gloves, aprons/gowns and eye protection before leaving the patient room.
- Fluid-repellent masks/respirators should be removed immediately outside the patient room.

5 Safe management of care equipment

Cleaning

This process involves 'fluid' – usually detergent and water (or fluid-based disposable wipes) – and 'friction' – the mechanical or physical removal of organic matter including dirt, debris, blood, and bodily fluids. Micro-organisms are removed rather than killed.

To monitor that cleaning is effective, the cleaned surface or equipment should be checked to see if it is visibly clean, i.e. that it is free from dust, dirt, debris, blood, and bodily fluids.

Care equipment can be easily contaminated with blood, other body fluids, secretions, excretions, and infectious agents. Consequently, it is easy to transfer infectious agents from communal care equipment during care delivery.

Physically remove contaminants including dust, soil, large numbers of microorganisms and the organic matter that protects them. Appropriate cleaning products must be provided including appropriate equipment to physically clean where necessary.

Suitable protective clothing must be provided and worn.

Mops and buckets must be thoroughly cleaned after use and stored dry.

The 'S' shape cleaning method ('S' shape method refers to the movement the hand makes when cleaning a surface, starting at the back of the surface making a continuous 'S' shape towards the edge of the surface) can be adopted for many practices. This can be utilised to minimise recontamination of an area and transfer of microorganisms. Equally, it is important to clean from top to bottom and clean to dirty.

Dusting technique should not disperse the dust (i.e. use damp cloths/dusting devices). High horizontal surfaces should be cleaned first.

Floors should be cleaned last, with adequate signage placed while floors are cleaned and drying to prevent slips, trips and falls on wet floors. Once floors are completely dry, signs must be removed as they present a trip hazard.

Using detergent and water may be enough in foyers, offices, corridors and other 'low risk' environments.

Barriers to effective cleaning must be removed:

- Damaged equipment must be condemned or repaired
- Avoid unnecessary clutter
- Manufacturers should provide equipment that is easy to decontaminate

However, the use of disinfection may also be needed in many healthcare environments. Cleaning is a pre-requisite to effective disinfection. Mechanical cleaning technology is used in some instances to ensure an effective cleaning process is completed prior to disinfection. Mechanical processes are preferable, and all parameters of the process can be controlled.

Disinfection

Disinfection is the process of eliminating or reducing harmful microorganisms from inanimate objects and surfaces. A disinfectant must be made up at the right concentration and have contact with a surface for a specified time. The surface needs to remain wet for that time. Staff should know the contact times for the disinfectants in use locally. Products that ease the application such as wipes with realistic contact times for use in a busy healthcare environment should be considered. Manufacturer instructions should always be followed.

- Reduces the number of microorganisms to a safe or relatively safe level.
- Bacterial spores are not usually destroyed (unless specific sporicidal products are used).

Use of chemical disinfection is far less robust than thermal disinfection and is usually used for complex surgical instrumentation such as instruments that are delicate, expensive, and which have long, intricate, narrow lumens. Training is required to ensure competency using the product and process.

Checklist for use of disinfectant

- Check disinfection is appropriate for care equipment/surface being disinfected.
- Pre-clean items and use clean containers.
- Totally immerse items or total area coverage.
- Use recommended dilution and exposure time.
- Do not store used disinfectants, discard as advised by manufacturer instructions.
- Rinse thoroughly with water.
- Remember protective clothing/COSHH regulations.

Use of wipes for the decontamination of equipment

- Increasingly being used to decontaminate low risk patient equipment or environmental surfaces.
- Dirt removal should be considered the main purpose of a detergent wipe; antimicrobial activity (because of the inclusion of a disinfectant) may be of use in some circumstances.
- Always follow specific manufacturer decontamination instructions.
- The appropriate selection of disinfectant wipes is important, as infection prevention efforts may be compromised if the wipe is not fit for its intended purpose.

Tips for clinical placement

- Be aware of who cleans what, when and how.
- Familiarise yourself with a decontamination policy and/or any manufacturer's guidelines issued to ensure that appropriate decontamination of equipment takes place.
- Report inadequate standards and defects in equipment and decoration that might impact on cleaning to relevant personnel. Establish the method to be used.

Questions to be asked

- What is the purpose of the device?
- Are there manufacturer reprocessing instructions?

- Can the item be reprocessed?
- Are the resources and facilities required for cleaning, disinfection, or sterilization available locally?
- How soon will the device be needed?

Assessment to be carried out

- Is it an invasive device?
- In contact with mucous membranes, skin, body fluids or potentially infectious material?
- Can it be cleaned properly and does the SSD have the available resources for cleaning and sterilization of the item? Look at what is available.
- Can the item be sent to a central department for processing, such as an SSD, or does it have to be processed at the point of use?
- Are there sufficient devices for the number of patients requiring its use?

Table 11.3 below will assist in assessing the level of decontamination required.

Sterilisation

The process of killing all microorganisms through physical or chemical means. Sterilisation is used only for critical items, i.e. objects or instruments that enter or penetrate sterile tissues, cavities, or the bloodstream.

Decontamination

Cleaning, disinfection and sterilisation are all decontamination processes. In the context of the environment or non-critical equipment (i.e. equipment or devices that are in contact with intact skin only), the term usually refers to cleaning and disinfection, either using separate cleaning and disinfecting agents in a two-step process, or a '2 in 1' product that cleans and disinfects in one step.

The following table provides the category of risk, indication of use, level of decontamination process and method.

Table 11.3 Decontamination of medical devices

Category of risk	Indication	Level of decontamination required	Examples of medical devices	Method/process
High Risk (critical)	Penetrate skin/mucous membranes (Items that are involved with a break in the skin or mucous membrane or entering a sterile body cavity)	Sterilization	Surgical instruments, implants/ prostheses, rigid endoscopes, syringes, needles	Autoclave Sterile single-use
Medium Risk/ Intermediate (semi-critical)	Contact with mucous membrane/ non intact skin	Disinfection (high level)	Respiratory equipment, non-invasive flexible endoscopes, bedpans, urine bottles	Autoclave Chemical disinfection
Low Risk (non-critical)	Used on intact skin	Clean (visibly clean)	Blood pressure cuffs, stethoscopes	Wash with detergent and water

Source: Adapted from World Health Organization (2016)

— **GO FURTHER** —

Read the following document:

World Health Organization (WHO) (2016) *Decontamination and Reprocessing of Medical Devices for Health-care Facilities*. Geneva: WHO. https://apps.who.int/iris/bitstream/handle/10665/250232/9789241549851-eng.pdf (accessed October 21, 2022).

Medical devices labelled 'for single use'

Devices labelled 'for single use' are designed by manufacturers with the intention of not being reused. For example, single-use injection syringes should never be re-used because the risk of infection is very high. Sterile, single-use injection devices include sterile hypodermic syringes, sterile hypodermic needles, auto-disable syringes for vaccination purpose, syringes with a reuse prevention feature for general purpose, and syringes with needlestick prevention/safety features (e.g. safety syringes) for general purposes.

ACTIVITY: PAUSE AND REFLECT

How will you know if an item is for single use?

Single-patient use means the medical device may be used for more than one episode of use on one patient only; the device may undergo some form of reprocessing between each use.

Medical devices labelled as 'For single patient' use can include nebuliser tubing / masks and some infusion equipment.

6 Safe management of care environment

The National Standards of Healthcare Cleanliness (NHS England, 2021) apply to all healthcare settings – acute hospitals, mental health, community, primary care, dental care, ambulance trusts, GP surgeries and clinics, and care homes, regardless of the way cleaning services are provided.

These standards provide clear advice and guidance to ensure health professionals have a generic understanding of what is needed to ensure a clean healthcare setting. In addition, the evidence-based framework gives an opportunity to assess risks and to determine the efficacy of cleaning services and processes.

Providing and maintaining effective cleaning in healthcare is complex and challenging; it should not be underestimated. The role of the nurse involves responsibilities to ensure cleaning-related risks are identified, minimised, and managed through a process of monitoring and reporting with the guidelines maintained within an organisation.

The starting point to meeting this responsibility is for a nurse to gain an understanding of both the terms cleaning, disinfection, decontamination, and sterilisation and the different stages involved in each process.

7 Safe management of linen

Within healthcare the term 'linen' can include all reusable textile items requiring cleaning/disinfection via laundry processing including:

1   Bed linen: blankets, counterpanes, cot sheets and blankets, duvets, duvet covers, pillowcases and sheets (woven, knitted, half sheets, draw and slide sheets); blankets; curtains; hoist slings
2   Patient clothing: gowns, nightdresses and shirts, pyjama tops and bottoms
3   Staff clothing: scrub suits/theatre attire, tabards, uniforms
4   Towels

Local policy requires the use of standard precautions to be used when handling linen and segregation of used linen is based on risk assessment.

Clean linen

- Should be stored in a designated clean area, preferably an enclosed cupboard.
- If clean linen is not stored in a cupboard, then the trolley used for storage must be designated for this purpose only and covered with an impervious covering that is able to withstand decontamination.

Used linen

This is linen not identified as infectious. It should be placed in a white impermeable bag for dispatch to the laundry. A risk assessment should be taken to ensure the containment of soiled and fouled linen is not compromised. Ensure a laundry receptacle/trolley is available as close as possible to the point of care for immediate linen removal.
   Do not:

- rinse, shake or sort linen on removal from beds/trolleys
- place used linen on the floor or any other surfaces, e.g. a locker/table top
- re-handle used linen once bagged
- overfill laundry bags.

All staff at local level should be trained in the correct coding and bagging procedures to ensure that sharps, clinical waste, and non-clinical waste do not return to the laundry.

Infectious linen

This is linen risk assessed as being used by a patient who is known or suspected to be infectious and/or linen that is contaminated with blood and/or other body fluids, e.g. faeces, vomit, blood or urine:

- Place directly into a water-soluble/alginate bag and secure; then place into a plastic bag (e.g. clear bag) and secure before placing in a laundry receptacle. This applies also to any item(s) heavily soiled and unlikely to be fit for reuse.
- Used and infectious linen bags/receptacles must be tagged (e.g. ward/care area and date).
- Store all used/infectious linen in a designated, safe, lockable area whilst awaiting uplift. Uplift schedules must be acceptable to the care area and there should be no build-up of linen receptacles.

—————————————— GO FURTHER ——————————————

For more information on the decontamination of linen for health and social care, read the following article:

Department of Health (2016) *Health Technical Memorandum 01-04: Decontamination of linen for health and social care: Management and provision.* https://www.england.nhs.uk/wp-content/uploads/2021/05/Mgmt_and_provision.pdf (accessed October 21, 2022).

8 Safe management of blood and body fluid spillages

Spillages of blood and other body fluids may transmit blood borne viruses such Hepatitis B and C. Appropriate personal protective equipment (e.g., non-sterile disposable gloves/aprons) must be worn when dealing with blood and body fluid spillages.

Spillages must be decontaminated and cleaned up immediately by staff trained to undertake this safely. If the spillage is extensive or splashing is likely to occur while cleaning up, additional PPE should be worn (e.g. eye and face protection).

Organic matter should be removed using disposable absorbent towels before disposal into the appropriate healthcare (clinical) waste category. The area should be disinfected using appropriate granules or solution (e.g. chlorine releasing agents) prepared in accordance with the manufacturer instructions and left for the required contact time. Then the area should be cleaned using water and general-purpose detergent and dried or allowed to air dry.

All waste materials such as contaminated paper towels and used PPE should be disposed of as healthcare (clinical) waste after use. Hand hygiene should be performed.

Responsibilities for the decontamination of blood and body fluid spillages should be clear within each area/care setting.

If superabsorbent polymer gel granules for containment of bodily waste are used, these should be used in line with national guidance.

In Scotland refer to the *National Infection Prevention and Control Manual.* https://www.nss.nhs.scot/antimicrobial-resistance-and-healthcare-associated-infection/national-policies-guidance-and-evidence/national-infection-prevention-and-control-manual/#:~:text=The%20National%20Infection%20Prevention%20and%20Control%20Manual%20%28NIPCM%29,and%20supporting%20tools%20for%20infection%20prevention%20and%20control (accessed October 21, 2022).

In England refer to *Risk of Death and Severe Harm from Ingesting Superabsorbent Polymer Gel Granules.* https://www.cas.mhra.gov.uk/ViewandAcknowledgment/ViewAlert.aspx?AlertID=102937 (accessed October 21, 2022).

9 Safe disposal of sharps

—————————————— GO FURTHER ——————————————

The following YouTube videos provide further guidance on the safe disposal of sharps. Remember to always check with local policy when disposing of sharps:

NHS Fife (2019) 'Guide to setting up a sharps disposal box and what to do in the event of a sharps injury', NHS Fife (YouTube video), March 20. https://www.youtube.com/watch?v=h6iGpcMymkY (accessed October 21, 2022).

The First Aid Show (2015) 'Needle stick and sharps injuries', The First Aid Show (YouTube video), October 6. https://www.youtube.com/watch?v=q2ticCkMsAO (accessed October 21, 2022).

10 Occupational safety: Prevention and exposure management (including sharps)

The safe use and disposal of sharps

Health-care providers should be aware of the significant problem of needle-stick injuries. The use of the following practices is recommended to avoid these injuries:

- Keep handling of sharps to a minimum.
- Do not recap, bend, or break needles after use.
- Discard each needle directly into a sharps container at the point of use immediately after use.
- Do not overfill a sharps bin (do not fill above level indicated on the container).
- Do not leave a sharps bin where children can reach it.
- Needles collected from patients should be placed in a sharps container inside a safe box to minimise the risk to community pharmacists.
- Always report injuries from needles in line with local policy.

Transmission Based Precautions (TBPs)

Use best practice guidelines in order to observe, assess and respond rapidly to potential infection risks. It is important to recognise that there are times when SICPs may be insufficient to prevent cross transmission of specific infectious agents or situations. Consequently, additional precautions need to be taken and TBPs need to be used by all staff when caring for patients with a known or suspected infection or colonisation or within a defined area.

IPC advice, practice, care and support should be both age appropriate and culturally appropriate.

Infection Prevention: Summary

In order to minimise the incidence of HCAI:

- Know the main guidelines in each of the clinical environments where you are working.
- Accept responsibility for minimizing opportunities for infection transmission.
- Apply standard and transmission-based precautions.
- Let staff know if supplies are inadequate or depleted.
- Educate patients and their families/visitors about clean hands and infection transmission (WHO, 2021a).

CASE STUDY

Advice for visitors

A group of visitors from China are visiting a patient you are working with on a hospital ward. The group had arrived in the UK three weeks ago when one member became unwell and was admitted to hospital. Only one member of the visitor group speaks English.

Questions

1   What advice will you give the visitors?
2   How will you do this?

Equality and diversity considerations:

Pay extra attention to patients, staff and visitors with additional needs such as physical, sensory or learning disabilities, as well as people who do not speak or read English. Language barriers should not be a reason for not providing advice.

Information regarding the cause or likely cause of infection should be cascaded to other members of the team verbally and where appropriate in inpatient documentation on a need-to-know basis. Signs on doors and any labels in notes should be used sensitively ensuring that patient confidentiality is maintained and no discrimination results from any action.

Local risk assessment and practical management should be considered, ensuring this is a pragmatic and proportionate response, including the consideration of whether there is a requirement for visitors to wear PPE.

Visitors entering a segregated/cohort area must be instructed on hand hygiene. They must not visit any other care area.

Decisions to suspend or restrict visitors will depend on local circumstances and risk assessment.

TBPs involve providing a single room for the patient to be physically cared for in a room of their own. This may involve the patient not being allowed to leave during the duration of the precautions. While a single room may be welcomed by some patients in the short term, the denial of social interaction with anyone other than the staff during a longer hospital stay is often devastating for many patients. Additional support could involve the additional time required to provide psychological support. The person/patient or nominated other should be involved in the risk assessment and decision-making process in relation to isolation, and a plan to address psychological isolation agreed. Consideration should be given to capacity and understanding of the need to isolate and this needs to be reassessed regularly. People may become disorientated and anxious and need reassurance and to be provided with information.

ASEPTIC NON-TOUCH TECHNIQUE

WATCH THE VIDEO

ASEPTIC NON-TOUCH TECHNIQUE

Watch along as you read through this step by step procedure by scanning the QR code with your smartphone camera or via **https://study.sagepub.com/rowberry**.

ANTT refers to aseptic non-touch technique. ANTT is an international set of principles aiming to:

- Standardise practice using an evidence-based approach.
- Support healthcare workers, including nurses, to practice safely and effectively.
- Increase patient safety by reducing the risk of introducing infection into a susceptible body site during procedures such as intravenous therapy, wound care, and urinary catheterisation.

What is ANTT?

ANTT uses a defined framework and is a relatively new approach to undertaking aseptic techniques. This standardised approach, developed in University College Hospital (UCH) London, has been shown to significantly improve the aseptic technique of healthcare workers and reduce the numbers of HCAIs.

ANTT is a core nursing and medical skill that defines the infection prevention and control methods and precautions necessary during invasive clinical procedures to prevent the transfer of microorganisms to 'key' or sterile body sites from healthcare professionals, procedure equipment or the immediate environment to a patient.

The ANTT framework is based upon the goal of asepsis rather than sterility and the approach is gauged on the technical difficulty of each procedure rather than the diagnosis or age of the patient.

CHAPTER SUMMARY

As we have seen in the past, the spread of dangerous infections can be very quick and difficult to control and can have devastating consequences for those we care for, particularly in vulnerable groups. This chapter has provided an overview of Infection Prevention and Control (IPC) measures and some of the considerations needed in clinical practice. This is a vast area and additional personal reading is recommended. IPC specialist nurses can be contacted in all clinical areas of nursing for advice and guidance whenever needed; it is highly advisable to contact them for their subject matter expertise in this area. Ensuring you have knowledge of local policy is vital in this, and all other areas of clinical skills.

Handwashing is the single most effective measure we can take to ensure we reduce the risk to patients, staff and visitors. Maintaining high standards of hand hygiene, and encouraging others to do so, is vital.

ACE YOUR ASSESSMENT

Q1   What does HCAI stand for?

    a   Healthworker cross association of infection

    b   Health care associated infection

    c   Health cross contamination associated infections

(Continued)

Q2   Identify the four main bacteria shapes.

    a   Bacilli, Cocci, Spiral, Vibrio

    b   Bassillus, Central, Spiral, Viral

    c   Bacilli, Central, Spiral, Vibrio

Q3   Identify common signs and symptoms of infection.

    a   Aches, low temp, pain

    b   Aches, fever, flushed skin

    c   Confusion, pain, high BP

Q4   What does PPE stand for?

    a   Protective personal entries

    b   Protection, personal, equipment

    c   Personal protective equipment

Answers

1   B

2   A

3   B

4   C

REFERENCES

Barbut, F. and Petit, J.-C. (2001) 'Epidemiology of Clostridium difficile-associated infections', *Clinical Microbiology & Infection*, 7 (8): 405–10.

Blaser, M. (2016) 'Antibiotic use and its consequences for the normal microbiome', *Science*, 352 (6285): 544–5.

Bongomin, F., Gago, S., Oladele, R. and Denning, D. (2017) 'Global and multi-national prevalence of fungal diseases-estimate precision', *Journal of Fungi*, 3 (4): Article #57.

Davies, C. (1996) *Medical Microbiology* (4th edition). Galveston, TX: University of Texas Medical Branch.

Department of Health (2015a) *Health and Social Care Act 2008 – Code of Practice on the Prevention and Control of Infections and Related Guidance*. London: Department of Health. https://www.gov.uk/government/publications/the-health-and-social-care-act-2008-code-of-practice-on-the-prevention-and-control-of-infections-and-related-guidance (accessed October 21, 2022).

Department of Health. (2015b). *Response to the Consultation on The Health and Social Care Act 2008 Code of Practice for Prevention and Control of Infections and Related Guidance*. London: Department of Health.

Haque, M., Sartelli, M., McKimm., J. and Abu Bakar, M. (2018) 'Health care-associated infections – an overview', *Infection and Drug Resistance*, 11: 2321–33.

Khuan, N., Shaban, R. and Van De Mortel, T. (2018) 'The influence of religious and cultural beliefs on hand hygiene behaviour in the United Arab Emirates', *Infection, Disease & Health*, 23 (4): 225–36.

Loveday, H., Wilson, J., Pratt, R., Golsorkhi, M., Tingle, A., Bak, A., [...] and UK Department of Health (2014). epic3: National evidence-based guidelines for preventing healthcare-associated infections in NHS hospitals in England. *Journal of Hospital Infections*, 86 (Supplement 1): S1–70.

NHS England (2021) *National Standards of Healthcare Cleanliness 2021*. england.nhs.uk, May 4. https://www.england.nhs.uk/publication/national-standards-of-healthcare-cleanliness-2021/ (accessed October 21, 2022).

Public Health England (2021) *Laboratory Surveillance of Candidaemia in England: 2020* (Health Protection Report Volume 15 Number 15). gov.uk, September 14. https://assets.publishing.service.gov.uk/government/uploads/system/uploads/attachment_data/file/1017262/hpr1521_cnddm20_final4.pdf (accessed October 21, 2022).

Royal College of Nursing (RCN) (n.d.) *Tools of the Trade*. https://www.rcn.org.uk/Professional-Development/publications/tools-of-the-trade-uk-pub-010-218 (accessed December 2022).

Tripathi, N. and Sapra, A. (2021) *Gram Staining*. Treasure Island, FL: StatPearls Publishing. https://www.ncbi.nlm.nih.gov/books/NBK562156/ (accessed October 21, 2022).

Valtierra, H. (2008) 'Stability of viral pathogens in the laboratory environment'. *Applied Biosafety*, 13 (1): 21–6.

Ward, D. (2016) *Microbiology and Infection Prevention and Control for Nursing Students (Transforming Nursing Practice Series)*. London: Learning Matters.

Weyrich, L., Dixit, S., Farrer, A. and Cooper, A. (2015) 'The skin microbiome: Associations between altered microbial communities and disease', *Australian Journal of Dermatology*, 56 (4): 268–74.

World Health Organisation (WHO) (2010) 'The burden of health care-associated infection worldwide', who.int, April 29. https://www.who.int/news-room/feature-stories/detail/the-burden-of-health-care-associated-infection-worldwide (accessed October 21, 2022).

World Health Organisation (2011) *Report on the Burden of Endemic Health Care-Associated Infection Worldwide*. Geneva: World Health Organization. https://apps.who.int/iris/bitstream/handle/10665/80135/9789241501507_eng.pdf (accessed October 21, 2022).

World Health Organization (2016) *Decontamination and Reprocessing of Medical Devices for Health-care Facilities*. Geneva: World Health Organization. https://www.who.int/publications/i/item/9789241549851 (accessed October 21, 2022).

World Health Organization (2020) '*The Top 10 Causes of Death*,' who.int, December 9. https://www.who.int/news-room/fact-sheets/detail/the-top-10-causes-of-death#:~:text=Lower%20respiratory%20infections%20remained%20the%20world%E2%80%99s%20most%20deadly,than%20in%202000.%20Neonatal%20conditions%20are%20ranked%205th (accessed October 21, 2022).

World Health Organization (2021a) *Hand Hygiene: Why, How & When?* Geneva: World Health Organization. https://www.afro.who.int/sites/default/files/pdf/Health%20topics/Hand_Hygiene_Why_How_and_When_Brochure.pdf (accessed October 21, 2022).

World Health Organization (2021b) 'Immunization coverage', who.int, July 14. https://www.who.int/news-room/fact-sheets/detail/immunization-coverage (accessed October 21, 2022).

World Health Organization (2022) 'Malaria', who.int, July 26. https://www.who.int/news-room/fact-sheets/detail/malaria (accessed October 21, 2022).

END OF LIFE CARE

12

HYWEL THOMAS, DEB MCNEE, ALISON YOUNG, WENDY MASHLAN, JULIE HAYES AND NICOLA DAWKINS

NMC STANDARDS COVERED IN THIS CHAPTER

PLATFORM 3 ASSESSING NEEDS AND PLANNING CARE

3.4 Understand and apply a person-centred approach to nursing care, demonstrating shared assessment, planning, decision making and goal setting when working with people, their families, communities and populations of all ages.

3.6 Effectively assess a person's capacity to make decisions about their own care and to give or withhold consent.

3.7 Understand and apply the principles and processes for making reasonable adjustments.

3.8 Understand and apply the relevant laws about mental capacity for the country in which you are practising when making decisions in relation to people who do not have capacity.

3.14 Identify and assess the needs of people and families for care at the end of life, including requirements for palliative care and decision-making related to their treatment and care preferences.

PLATFORM 4 PROVIDING AND EVALUATING CARE

4.9 Demonstrate the knowledge and skills required to prioritise what is important to people and their families when providing evidence-based person-centred nursing care at end of life including the care of people who are dying, families, the deceased and the bereaved.

PLATFORM 5 LEADING & MANAGING NURSING CARE AND WORKING IN TEAMS

5.4 Demonstrate an understanding of the roles, responsibilities, and scope of practice of all members of the nursing and interdisciplinary team and how to make best use of the contributions of others involved in providing care.

PLATFORM 7 COORDINATING CARE

7.4 Identify the implications of current health policy and future policy changes for nursing and other professions and understand the impact of policy changes on the delivery and coordination of care.

ANNEXE B NURSING PROCEDURES

3 Use evidence-based, best practice approaches for meeting needs for care and support at the end of life, accurately assessing the person's capacity for independence and selfcare and initiating appropriate interventions.

10.1 Observe, and assess the need for intervention for people, families and carers, identify, assess and respond appropriately to uncontrolled symptoms and signs of distress including pain, nausea, thirst, constipation, restlessness, agitation, anxiety and depression.

(Continued)

10.2 Manage and monitor effectiveness of symptom relief medication, infusion pumps and other devices.

10.3 Assess and review preferences and care priorities of the dying person and their family and carers.

10.4 Understand and apply organ and tissue donation protocols, advanced planning decisions, living wills and health and lasting powers of attorney for health.

10.5 Understand and apply DNACPR (do not attempt cardiopulmonary resuscitation) decisions and verification of expected death.

10.6 Provide care for the deceased person and the bereaved respecting cultural requirements and protocols.

The chapter also covers the following areas in respect of Appendix B of the NMC Future Nurse: Standards of Proficiency for Registered Nurses, 2018:

- Assessing and managing uncontrolled symptoms and signs of distress including pain, nausea, thirst, constipation, restlessness, agitation, anxiety and depression.
- Use of infusion pumps/syringe drivers.
- Identify and support the preferences and care priorities of the dying person and their family and carers.
- Understand and apply organ and tissue donation protocols, advanced planning decisions, living wills and health and lasting powers of attorney for health.
- Recognise and apply DNACPR (do not attempt cardiopulmonary resuscitation) decisions and verification of expected death.
- Provision of care for the deceased child or adult, and their families, including bereavement support.

LEARNING OBJECTIVES

After reading this chapter, you should be able to:

- Define end of life care and identify key concepts relating to the specific care required
- Observe, assess, and manage appropriately symptoms and signs of distress at the end of life
- Discuss the care priorities of the dying person and their families, respecting their cultural or religious beliefs
- Understand the clinical skills required for the infant, child or adult at end of life

STUDENT VOICE

Providing end of life care as a student nurse is particularly frightening as knowing the best thing to do or say is difficult. From my experiences, I have learned what families truly value, and that is to be yourself, understand the family's wishes, provide autonomy, support, and time.

Helena, 3rd year, Child Nursing

To be integrally involved in the end of life care provision of one's patients is a truly privileged role that should not be underestimated. The way in which we engage with our dying patients and their families will leave a lasting impression. Be guided by the patient and their family. Our patients will only ever die once and, as such, we must embrace the process, ensuring we provide a person-centred, holistic approach. It is, after all, the final duty of care we discharge to our patients and we must always strive to get it right.

Egor, 3rd year, Adult Nursing

Caring for a patient at the end of their life is a privilege of high regard. You are presented with a duty to carry out a patient's last requests, while ensuring that they are done with compassion, respect, and empathy. The patient may be accompanied by loved ones, and it is important to provide support and comfort to all entities involved in the death of the patient. As a student nurse, I have come to acknowledge that death is a part of life and although it is an emotionally challenging time, so much can be done and given to ensure that both the patient and their family process this period knowing that true holistic care was provided throughout.

Aston, 2nd year, Adult Nursing

INTRODUCTION

Death is an inevitable process of natural life. We are born. We live. We die. However, the discussion and thought of death and dying are often met with uncomfortable, avoidant, and brief conversations, or in some instances fear and complete avoidance of the conversation and the topic itself. Evidence indicates that the final aspect of care a person receives has a profound impact on the family and subsequently their bereavement process. As a registered nurse you must be able to provide compassionate, evidence-based care to children and adults at the end of life. Sometimes there are moments of sadness and grief, and sharing in people's sadness is central to connecting with them, and caring for them. Caring during times of great joy and relief and loss may even be the reason you chose the profession. Although many health-care professionals acknowledge feelings of inadequacy around this particular provision of care and the complex topics it encompasses, many professionals would argue it is a privilege to sit at the beside of people who are approaching the end of their lives. In this chapter we will look at these complexities across the age spectrum, taking into consideration the needs of the dying person and those closest to them. End of life care is an essential aspect of your nursing care provision, ensuring that the quality of life and death is maximised to the end. Care of the body after death is often referred to as the last act of respect and dignity that the nurse can provide to the dying person. This chapter will cover evidence-based best practice in relation to end of life care and the management of distressing symptoms including pain.

Although death is inevitable, it is certainly not predictable to a given day or time. Many conditions can come with a predicted prognosis but due to many factors we are unable to confidently determine quantity of time. Now in the 21st century where science, technology and medical knowledge have advanced, we can support someone to live a much longer life than previously. However, this has led to increased awareness of quality of life and many ethical considerations in relation to 'Do Not Attempt Cardiopulmonary Resuscitation' (DNACPR) and advanced care planning decisions. Nursing students need to be aware of the many aspects leading up to a person's death, the circumstances, the context and most importantly the wishes of the deceased and their families.

Death can be expected or unexpected, traumatic, and sudden. You may experience death in all areas of practice, but some areas will have higher incidences than others. The way a death occurs impacts greatly on both the family and the medical staff attending to them. A traumatic or sudden death brings additional complications in relation to witnessing extensive trauma, resuscitation, and treatment. Families who witness this can often experience difficulties later, although research suggests that it may support the bereavement process (Johnson, 2015).

In intensive care and emergency departments, you are more likely to experience unexpected deaths from life-threatening acute conditions caused by sudden catastrophic events or existing conditions.

Death occurs within an older person's care setting through advanced progressive, incurable conditions, general frailty and coexisting conditions that mean they are at increased risk of dying within the next 12 months. Within paediatrics, there is a higher rate of death under the age of 1 year due to many factors including congenital anomalies, infection, and prematurity. Therefore, a child nursing student is more likely to experience unexpected deaths of infants within the neonatal unit.

Where a diagnosis has been established and the person has a decreased life expectancy, they are normally referred to a palliative care team. This multidisciplinary approach can provide support through plans, and decisions can be made regarding treatment options, place of care and preferred place of death together with family or carer involvement.

Terminology can be confusing when it comes to palliative and end of life care, so it is important to understand the differences.

ACTIVITY: PAUSE AND REFLECT

Think about your own answers to what the differences are between palliative and end of life care in nursing.

Now access the website below and research your answers against the Marie Curie website and make a list of the differences between palliative and end of life care. Marie Curie is the largest charitable funder of palliative and end of life research in the UK, providing care to people with terminal illness and their families.

https://www.mariecurie.org.uk/help/support/diagnosed/recent-diagnosis/palliative-care-end-of-life-care (accessed October 24, 2022).

KEY TERMS

The terms Palliative Care and End of Life Care (EoLC) will be used throughout this chapter following the NICE (2021) guidelines. These are two separate terms that overlap at times, please read the definitions of both of these topics in the list below to clarify your understanding as you read through.

End of life care: The National Institute for Health and Care Excellence define end of life as 'care that is provided in the "last year of life"; although for some conditions, end of life care may be provided for months or years' (NICE, 2019: 6).

Holistic needs: considers all aspects of the person's and family's wellbeing including a person-centred approach that meets spiritual, health and social care needs.

Palliative care: The World Health Organization (2020: 1) define palliative care as 'an approach that improves the quality of life of patients (adults and children) and their families who are facing problems associated with life-threatening illness. It prevents and relieves suffering through the early identification, correct assessment and treatment of pain and other problems, whether physical, psychosocial, or spiritual. Addressing suffering involves taking care of issues beyond physical symptoms. Palliative care uses a team approach to support patients and their caregivers. This includes addressing practical needs and providing bereavement counselling. It offers a support system to help patients live as actively as possible until death.'

Personalised care and support plan: service delivery arrangements that need to be put in place for people approaching end of life such as advanced care planning.

ANATOMY AND PHYSIOLOGY RECAP

The dying process and recognition of death

As a patient enters end of life, their body changes. It is important to be aware of these changes so that we know how to manage them. It is also important to educate the family on the changes that happen as without education both the patient and family may undergo distress. For example, a patient will not feel hungry or thirsty at end of life; the family may feel that the patient is then starving to death and may wish to intervene. Figure 12.1 summarises some of the changes that occur.

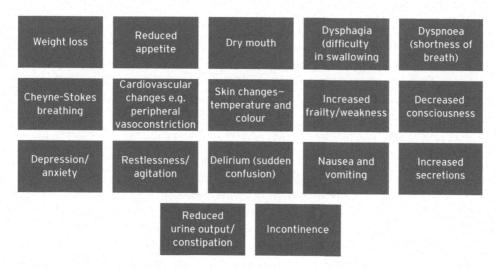

Figure 12.1   Physiological changes at the end of life

Recognition and verification of death

Recognition of dying

Delivering the best care in the last years, days (or hours) of life is everybody's business and people die in many different places: in acute care, in hospices, in their own homes, residential or nursing homes etc. From a nursing perspective management of a good death is certainly the key role of the nurse and one which reflects the skills from an acute or organised death.

As health professionals we may be called upon to decide when active treatment for an illness will cease. This can lead to a patient moving into a palliative phase of care and beyond this, end of life care. End of life presents with recognised signs and symptoms that indicate an active dying process and leads to the death of the individual. Although a recognised pattern of signs and symptoms, the process will be individual to every person with differing time frames.

The pathophysiology of dying involves all systems; when a patient is actively dying the systems will all begin to function at a slower speed producing the following changes:

- The patient will begin to lose interest in and refuse food; this is often an initial sign that the body is beginning to prepare for dying and will lead to weight loss.
- Blood will be pumped at lower pressure by the heart leading to reduced perfusion of all organs resulting in reduced and slowed function. The patient's peripheries will also become cold to the touch.

- Cognitive changes are initially seen in the form of reduced activity. Energy is being conserved and as the process of active dying progresses, the length of time sleeping increases with periods of wakefulness becoming fewer and shorter. Loss of consciousness will occur, however timing will vary with each patient.
- In contrast, periods of agitation due to reduced perfusion neurologically can also occur.
- Neurological deterioration due to reduced perfusion impacts the respiratory system. Loss of the cough and swallow reflex leads to increased secretions. Breathing may become shallow, and the breathing pattern can become variable – alternating between apnoea and hyperpnoea.
- Skin changes are progressive in the dying process. Due to the body's reduced ability to regenerate skin cells, the skin becomes thinner. In later stages, colour changes occur with skin becoming paler or mottled in appearance or dark skins may appear darker in colour.
- Urinary and gastrointestinal changes lead to reduced urinary and faecal output. This occurs due to reduced oral intake, reduced perfusion of organs, with reduced functioning and muscle control.

The individuality of the dying process should then lead us to consider the individual needs of the person. This includes their wishes within their advanced care plan (in relation to their religion/spirituality) and specific symptom management.

Verification of death

Once a patient has ceased to live, the patient must be examined by an appropriately trained practitioner to formally verify the death. It is important to note that until the verification has been completed, the patient is not yet legally deceased! Therefore, the time-of-death is the time stated by the person conducting the verification; not the moment the patient took their last breath! On some occasions, family members of the deceased will be present during the examination. Thus, the process must be done in a calm and dignified manner, often with consideration to the needs of the surrounding family members.

EXAMINATION FOR VERIFICATION OF AN EXPECTED DEATH: STEP BY STEP

- Patient identification check (via wristband if patient is in hospital).
- Observe the patient looking for signs of life (such as chest movement in respiration, or blinking of the eyes etc.).
- Call the patient's name (for example 'Hello Mr Mothukuri, can you open your eyes?').
- Assess response to painful stimuli, by squeezing the patient's trapezius muscle.
- Check for pupil response with a pen torch. Typically, the deceased will have fixed, dilated pupils which will not be responsive to light.
- Palpate a central pulse for 2 minutes (typically the carotid artery in the neck).
- Auscultate the anterior chest wall over the lung fields, listening for the presence of breath sounds. Then, auscultate over the approximate area of the heart, listening for the presence of heart sounds. Auscultation should take at least 2 minutes.
- Once this examination is complete, the practitioner will document their findings. At this point the patient is legally deceased.

CASE STUDY

Hesra

Hasra is on her first placement of her second year of the nursing programme on ward 19. During her shift Camilla was admitted to an acute medical admissions unit with a background of large intra-abdominal mass secondary to ovarian cancer which was causing obstruction. Camilla was reviewed by the gynaecology team and deemed not fit for surgical intervention. A deterioration of condition was anticipated. Camilla also presented with community-acquired pneumonia and atrial fibrillation with fast ventricular response which was treated with IV antibiotics and IV digoxin. Camilla did not have an advanced care plan and could not discuss her wishes in relation to care escalation. Next of kin was Camilla's son who had flown in from Canada to be with Camilla, however he did not hold lasting power of attorney. The clinical team made a DNACPR decision and that a palliative approach be adopted with a view to an end of life approach should further deterioration occur. This was discussed with the son who agreed the plan of escalation. Camilla was Catholic; Camilla's son expressed that she would want the priest to visit for last rites. This was arranged. Within a few days of admission to hospital Camilla deteriorated and fluids, medications, antibiotics, and taking of clinical observations were all stopped. Camilla was given morphine for pain, cyclizine for nausea and midazolam for agitation (administered subcutaneously) Camilla was made as comfortable as possible, passing away peacefully with her son at her side.

Question

In this case Camilla would have had an opportunity to discuss her wishes before acute decline. She had a known condition that was inoperable, which was at some point going to deteriorate. In such cases should the opportunity to undertake advanced care planning be offered to patients as a part of their management?

Medications considered for EoLC

During the last phases of life, a patient may experience new symptoms which they may not have had before. These can cause suffering and distress and therefore good assessment and management are required. Anticipatory prescribing allows for medications to be given to target specific causes of distress. We will discuss some of the common symptoms and their management below.

Pain

For more information on pain assessment please refer to Chapter 4. The most important aspect during end of life care is the person's symptom assessment performed by the nurse, particularly managing pain when the person has been living with an incurable illness or chronic condition towards end of life. In the terminal phase, it is important to continue any regular medication prescribed to achieve symptom control, even if the person is comatose or too weak to take oral medication. Regular medication to manage any of the symptoms mentioned in this section is usually administered via subcutaneous administration if unable to take orally. Subcutaneous infusion uses a syringe driver, which is a safer route as opposed to intravenous. This is because often cannulas may stop working, and this would mean a patient would require repeated re-cannulation. The use of these interventions will be dictated by the level of training of the nurse and the ability to care and manage these interventions accordingly from a clinical or home setting. Pain is common and associated with many of the complications of advanced malignancy and non-malignant disease processes. Pain during end of life can be very complex. Further reading is advised. You may wish to review https://www.mariecurie.org.uk/professionals/palliative-care-knowledge-zone/symptom-control/pain-control.

Pain medications follow the WHO analgesic ladder. The management of pain is dependent upon the cause of it. Non-opioid analgesics are used first such as paracetamol or NSAIDs, followed by weak opioids and then strong opioids (WHO, 1987). For more information on medications, please see Chapter 13.

Some of the strong opioids used in practice are:

- Fentanyl
- Morphine
- Diamorphine
- Oxycodone

Please be aware that the potency of opioids is not equal. It is usually measured in comparison to morphine. For example, oxycodone is three times more potent than morphine. This means that 5mg of oxycodone is approximately equivalent to 15 mg of morphine.

Nausea and vomiting

Much like pain, nausea and vomiting is also complex and the management thereof is dependent upon the cause of it. Causes may arise from a mechanical bowel problem such as constipation, which can be exacerbated by pain medication, or from a neurological cause such as a brain metastasis of a cancer. Antiemetics are medications which are used to treat nausea. They have different mechanisms of action and therefore treat different specific causes of nausea. It Is important to be aware of this because one antiemetic may not work for a patient simply because it is not treating the underlying cause of the symptoms. Further reading can be accessed here: https://www.mariecurie.org.uk/professionals/palliative-care-knowledge-zone/symptom-control/nausea-vomiting.

Some of the common antiemetics, their mechanisms of action and their sites of action associated causes are listed below:

- **Haloperidol** – dopamine antagonist targets central system. Good against chemical causes such as uremia.
- **Metoclopramide** – dopamine antagonist targeting the chemotaxic trigger zone in the brain and the gut. Also acts as a prokinetic within the upper gut.
- **Cyclizine** – histamine and acetylcholine antagonist targeting the vestibular system and the vomiting centre within the brain.
- **Ondansetron** – serotonin receptors acting on the central and gut systems. Please note that this antiemetic can be constipating.
- **Levomepromazine** – serotonin, dopamine, acetylcholine and histamine receptors. This covers many causes but can cause sedation.

Secretions

Audible breathing and respiratory tract secretions can be heard in the last hours to days of life. These rattling and unusual sounds can be frightening for the family and occur because the patient is no longer able to clear secretions and so they gather in the upper airways or oropharynx. It can be helpful to explain to families why these noises occur and explain that these are rarely distressing to the patient and that they are not choking. There is an array of treatments and management options for these symptoms, such as:

- **Non-pharmacological interventions** – changing the person's position can improve the breathing process for a short time. Ensure moving and handling techniques are adhered to (see Chapter 9).
- **Anticholinergic drugs** – help reduce any secretions the person has, aiding comfort.
- **Suction** – removing visible secretions can have an instant effect for the patient, increasing comfort for them.

Terminal agitation

Patients may become distressed or agitated at end of life and this is called terminal agitation. It is imperative that all reversible causes of agitation are considered and treated. For example, a patient may be agitated because they are experiencing pain from a full bladder in the context of urinary retention. The appropriate management of this is to help voiding of the bladder. Another cause may be discomfort from constipation and therefore a good bowel regimen treatment is required. For bowel and bladder health please refer to Chapter 8. For further reading on delirium in palliative care please see https://www.mariecurie.org.uk/professionals/palliative-care-knowledge-zone/symptom-control/delirium.

Once all reversible causes of anxiety and agitation have been considered treatments can be given to help alleviate the symptoms. Some are listed below:

- **Non-pharmacological approach** – to manage psychological distress and anxiety.
- **Anxiolytics** – low doses of anxiolytic medications are less sedating. Some common medications used are haloperidol and midazolam.
- **Sedation** – it may be appropriate to seek sedation of a patient when their symptoms are uncontrollable and causing distress. Some patients may also have expressed a wish to be sedated within their advanced care plan. Levomepromazine is often used in addition to midazolam when symptoms are severe. Phenobarbital and propofol are used with specialist advice.

PALLIATIVE CARE PLANNING

It has become apparent that the reasoning behind promoting concise care planning pathways for individual patients with palliative diseases is that it improves communication between healthcare professions, which leads to the delivery of appropriate care for patients and their families. There are many challenges in providing palliative and end of life care from a nursing care planning perspective as patients may have in place one of several care plans such as:

- Care plan
- Advanced Care Plan (ACP)
- Advanced Decision Refusing Treatment (ADRT)
- Escalation Care Plan (ECP)

For clarity definitions have been provided below:

Care planning – general care planning is to have an easily accessible document that details the planned nursing interventions for patients with progressive diseases (Alzheimer's, Parkinson's disease,

Multiple Sclerosis) not only to the nursing staff, but also to the patient and relatives. Care planning should be a dynamic and evolving process which reflects the unique individualised needs of the patient in a structured framework. Care planning forms part of the nursing process which also includes assessment, implementation, and evaluation.

Advanced care planning is an important part of palliative care and has been defined as a process of discussion and recording of wishes, values, and preferences for future care and treatment held between an individual, family members and their care providers that takes effects when the person loses capacity. An ACP is not a legally binding document/process; it can be drawn up by the individual using templates accessible via the internet or it can be created more formally by a solicitor. ACPs are usually used in the context of progressive illness and anticipated deterioration.

Escalation care planning is actioned following the recognition that a patient's physical health is declining. An ECP is an essential part of a patient's management as it ensures that patients are prevented from experiencing unnecessary treatments and distress. Each escalation of care planning is developed on an individual basis with a multidisciplinary team, patient and family involvement. Where involvement of patient and family is not possible, decisions are made in the best interests of the patient with the senior clinical/medical being the overall decision maker. An ECP should ideally start as soon as a patient is admitted into a secondary care setting. Medical teams need to be made aware of ACPs and the existence of Lasting Power or Attorney where a patient lacks capacity.

ADRT (living wills) – the only legally binding document is the ADRT, sometimes referred to as a living will. The person may want to discuss this with their doctor or nurse who knows about the persons medical history before they make their mind up. You can make ADRT if you have mental capacity to make such decisions where your decision is in a certain format that is written down (refuse a specific type of treatment sometime in the future e.g. ventilation, CPR, antibiotics), signed by you and signed by a witness. The ADRT comes with a caveat that the individual understands they are refusing life-saving or life-sustaining treatment. In some circumstances, a person may be unable to communicate their wishes, but retain capacity to make decisions regarding their care. In this case, it is imperative that the communication impairments are recognised, and the assessment is tailored to the individual's needs to maximise communication and engagement in the process.

The rules about how an advanced decision and lasting power of attorney for health and care interact can be complicated (please see the section below on law applied to palliative/EoLC).

Acknowledging a deteriorating patient within a timely manner will not only stop unnecessary interventions from happening but will also identify the appropriate needs and care for that individual person. Care plans as mentioned above will clearly detail the level of care that a patient should receive should they physically deteriorate. The plan will detail whether the patient is for resuscitation in the event of cardio/respiratory arrest, whether they should be admitted to Intensive Care or receive non-invasive ventilation of continuous positive airway pressure. In addition, the plan should clearly state if a rapid response call should be made (urgent need of review from the acute outreach team) or whether the patient should recieve ward-based care (need of clinical review but not urgent, lower level of intervention required). Where patients fail to respond to treatment the decision to use a palliative or end of life approach to care should be clearly documented. Many clinical areas use ECP forms that are placed to the front of a patient's notes which clearly detail the plan in place. It is important to continue to review each individual case-based ECP as changes happen on a daily basis.

Table 12.1 Timeline of nursing decisions from urgent to planned death

Death within a few hours/days	• The nurse should discuss with the patient and those important to them at the earliest opportunity to confirm this • Care decision tool for last days of life should be used to guide the practitioner • Continue to support, assess, communicate, and provide holistic care based on the person-centred approach • Provide care for deceased person and the bereaved respecting cultural requirements and protocols
Death not imminent (next few weeks/months/year)	• Discuss uncertain or poor prognosis with the patient and those important to them (please see communication skills section below) • Explore the patient's preferences for EoLC • Start ACP, for example preferred place of care, what is important to your patient, DNACPR, advanced decision to refuse treatment • Suggest GP adds the patient to the GP palliative care register

Death uncertain	• Check for general indicators of deteriorating health including:
	  ○ Reduced functional ability
	  ○ Weaker, spending more time in bed, drowsy, tiredness, reduced urine output, decreased interest in food and drink, difficulty swallowing oral medication
	  ○ Clinical indicators of advanced conditions
	  ○ Poor performance status, multi organ failure/cancer; heart and vascular disease; kidney and liver disease; respiratory/neurological; frailty/dementia; not responding to treatment; condition not reversible

LAW APPLIED TO PALLIATIVE / EOLC

Student nurses and professionals essentially must be aware of the legal aspects in relation to palliative/ EoLC and be very clear of its implications within a number of areas such as meeting the personal needs of the patient for care and support at the end of life and the person's capacity for independence and initiating appropriate interventions. Legal sources which are paramount for the nurse to be aware of during EoLC is their professionalism standards under the NMC Code (2018a), as registered nurses have a duty of care to act in any way they can to preserve life. This is balanced with the Mental Capacity Act (2005) underpinning principles promoting autonomy (patients making decisions for themselves) for future clinical decisions and balanced with a framework (to rebut presumptions of capacity) to work in the person's best interest. Duty to provide treatment does not allow you to override the wishes of a capable adult patient and a capable adult is entitled to refuse treatment even where this would lead to their death. Under the MCA (2005) ACP can be drawn up and treatments (lifesaving treatment like CPR or treatments using antibiotics) can be refused by the patient.

It is important that a person must have mental capacity to make an ACP (see Go Further box below for the Mental Health Capacity Act 2005 and what needs to be considered when undertaking a capacity assessment). It would be a best interest decision where relatives and friends are consulted unless the individual has appointed an attorney for welfare decisions in accordance with the procedure set down by law under the MCA 2005 when they had capacity to do so. For individuals who are un-befriended, an Independent Mental Capacity Advocate (IMCA) would need to be appointed for serious medical decisions. An IMCA supports people who cannot make or understand decisions and therefore safeguards the rights of those with nobody else to speak for them. The main benefits for the person that lacks capacity are having an independent person to review significant decisions who is articulate and knowledgeable on the person's rights, the health and social care system and care law, and receiving support from a person who is skilled at helping people who have difficulties with communication to make their own views known (UK Government, 2017). The MCA Code of Practice provides guidance for matters that should be referred to the Court of Protection if there is disagreement/conflict involving any medical decision taken.

GO FURTHER

Read the materials introducing the *Mental Capacity Act 2005* (https://www.scie.org.uk/mca/practice/assessing-capacity) and particularly *Assessing Capacity* and then answer these questions:

1   What is the MCA?
2   Which professionals are key?
3   Who can undertake assessment of capacity?
4   Four key elements need to be considered when undertaking an assessment around capacity – what are they?
5   What would you need to do if a patient lacks capacity for decisions around medication?

The content of an ACP/ECP may vary from person to person but is likely to outline thoughts around DNACPR and how they should be treated should they become acutely unwell. Often this will be related to specific conditions and presentations, their thoughts around when to cease treatment and adopt a palliative or end of life approach to their care. The ACP/ECP may also state if a patient wishes to be admitted to hospital or cared for at home although it is not legally binding and therefore can be changed if circumstances change. An ACP/ECP is important not only for the person who outlines their wishes but also for healthcare professionals looking after them. Being aware of how a person would wish to be treated allows health professionals to manage the patient according to their wishes and ensure that a clear plan of escalation is made in the event of physical deterioration.

A Lasting Power of Attorney (LPA) is a legal document that lets you (the donor) appoint one or more people (known as 'attorneys') to help you make decisions or to make decisions on your behalf (Gov.uk, 2022). There are two types of LPA:

- Health and welfare
- Property and financial affairs

If they have appointed an attorney under an LPA, the person receiving care at their home, nursing home or acute hospital setting must provide the senior clinicians with copies of the LPA agreement and ensure this document covers decisions for health and welfare as different family members may be appointed as different donors. This will be available to the clinical team within the patient's notes. It should be noted that as an ACP/ECP is not legally binding there could be circumstances where a healthcare professional does not follow the stated wishes. Such situations bring ethical dilemmas with them. As nurses we have a duty toward the patient to always do no harm and act as an advocate for the patient (NMC, 2018b). Take some time out and think about the elements of the NMC (2018a) Code of Practice that should be considered when caring for patients who hold an ACP/ECP and the types of ethical dilemmas that you may face as a nurse.

ACTIVITY: CRITICAL THINKING

1   List the key points from the NMC (2018a) that should be considered when involved with patients who present to clinical practice with an ACP/ECP/ADRT who lack capacity to make decisions.
2   Mr Goldstein is a 78-year-old Jewish man admitted with end stage cancer and has advanced stages of dementia. What additional cultural aspects need to be taken into consideration for Mr Goldstein?

Organ donation

There is an understanding during the palliative care pathway around the requirements for organ and tissue donation protocols. It is important students and professionals are aware particularly of changes in the law recently in England and Wales. In Wales, the Human Transplantation (Wales) Act 2013 initially created a soft opt-out consent to organ donation. From December 2015, changes in law now state that, unless stated otherwise, a person's consent to donation may be deemed to have been given and treated as having no objection to becoming a donor (Welsh Parliament 2013). In England, the law regarding organ donation is the same as Wales, although this came into force in May 2020. 'All adults in England are now considered to have agreed to be an organ donor when they die unless they have recorded a decision not to donate or are in one of the excluded groups'. The Organ Donation (Deemed Consent) Act 2019 amended the Human Tissue Act 2004. The organ donation law should be a conversation that could be discussed during the palliative care process, particularly with those patients who have expressed an opinion against organ donation. According to The Welsh Parliament (2013) organ donation is when healthy organs and tissues from one person are transplanted into another person. In the UK, every year over 4,000 people receive donated organs and tissues, offering them a new lease of life. The law affects everybody in England and Wales apart from excluded groups such as those under 18, people that have opted out by completing the appropriate form and registering this, and those people who lack capacity. Once your decision is made you can choose to:

- **Opt in** – this is your decision to become a donor.
- **Do nothing** – you will be treated as having no objection to being a donor and your consent will be deemed given.
- **Opt out** – this is your decision not to become a donor.

The viewpoint that strongly comes across in this chapter is that health professionals should strive to and have a medical obligation to 'first do not harm' (BMJ, 2020). This idea has certainly been tested during difficult situations like the Covid-19 pandemic through the Alpha, Delta and Omicron strains of the virus and its uncertainty. It could be argued during the pandemic, the ethical imperatives have shifted, and we must not only recognise the individual but also the clinician and the population (Fritz and Perkins, 2020). Staff in acute hospital settings for Covid-19 including nurses and students during the emergency standards would have been exposed to conflicts of interest and moral discomfort because of some of the differences of opinion about the balanced benefits and risks including complex intervention combined with varying levels of personal protective equipment and poor survival rates. This also had to be balanced with continuing to manage care for uninfected patients and other illnesses and for healthcare professionals who continued to treat them.

Despite the ethical and moral dilemmas caused during the pandemic nurses have still been at the forefront of exemplary care and compassion during EoLC decisions. This would have been compounded further by managing this without having the family and close loved ones around because of Covid-19 restrictions on visiting in hospitals. Viewpoints shared throughout national news outlets were testament to skilled professionals caring for their loved ones with genuine compassion and as a result, they were comfortable, reassured and able to make choices as long as possible and to die with dignity. This has become more relevant to student nurses in particularly settings where death may not have been commonplace or expected before the pandemic and where they may have only experienced deaths on a single or very few occasions outside the pandemic. The pandemic has without doubt placed professional skills and judgment around EoLC into sharp focus as nurses have accommodated unconventional requests from the dying person, increased use of social media and handheld devices to communicate with families, and recognised cultural and spiritual sensitivity.

Traditional nursing programmes would offer an educational/theory approach to dealing with EoLC to improve communication and skills. Exposing nursing students to end of life care simulations such as exposure to a dying patient and care of the dying patient may be one way to positively alleviate the anxieties of the experience.

ACTIVITY: COMMUNICATION SKILLS

A good attitude to the dying patient can be demonstrated and interpersonal skills such as empathy, finding the right words and supporting patient autonomy are needed. Communicating with families and managing direct questions and family dynamics have been reported as the most challenging aspect of the dying patient experience. Sensitive communication approaches include open and honest communication between staff and the person who is dying. Clear, understandable, and plain language must be used verbally and in all other forms of communication.

COMMUNICATION AND CULTURAL EXPECTATION

Aahan is a Hindu patient currently nursed on Ward 12 with end stage bowel cancer and advanced vascular dementia. Cahomine is a student nurse planning end of life care with her practice assessor Jenna. What are the cultural expectations in relation to Aahan and the family during this process? Consider the below from a cultural perspective.

BEFORE YOU MEET WITH AAHAN AND FAMILY

- A clear evaluation from the professional MDT meeting (e.g. specialist palliative care senior management/older persons mental health team) in terms of illness/disease progression and the need to engage in EoLC/palliative care discussion.

- Essential to understand and clear focus of the terms EoLC and palliative care to inform discussion with the family and preparation for death.

- Appropriate professional/non-professional who has been personally involved with the family and who has the right level of expertise, experience, knowledge and understanding to manage this sensitive area of care.

- The person breaking the news to the person/family has desirable training/education to support this sensitive area. Charities like Cruse Bereavement Support (https://www.cruse.org.uk) offer specialist training and CPD sessions on topics like loss and bereavement or breaking bad news.

- Inform the person/family of time/date options within the clinical environment/home setting as appropriate.

- The person calling the meeting must prepare well and be prepared to manage the families and their emotions on the day.

- The nurse should engage in clinical supervision or professional support to manage their own feelings, emotions and professional practice.

MEETING WITH THE PERSON AND/OR THE FAMILY

- Professional approach to appearance/language of the professional.

- Ensuring the environment is away from distractions (phones/interruptions/noise) and privacy is maintained with an appropriately decorated room and ventilation.

- Facilitation style/skills.

- Refine essential interpersonal skills. Particularly the use of silence and listening to the family's responses are extremely important and reassuring.

- Verbal communication, particularly a tone of voice that is soft, supportive, compassionate, and caring when addressing the person/family.

- Aware of powerful non-verbal cues such as body language, posture (sit forward, lean towards the person slightly and upright), eye contact, facial expressions, and gestures.

- Summarizing back to the person/family what has been said and the use of open or open directive questions.

- Providing your contact details after the meeting and times when you can be contacted in person to answer any further queries and concerns or clarify what has been said in the meeting.

- Completing documentation where necessary from a local health board/GP perspective (e.g., Clinical Online Information Network (COIN) form and relevant signatures/people informed (GP, CNS palliative care team). Signposting to 3rd sector/voluntary resources to support legal decisions such as advanced directives, living wills, lasting power of attorney for health, opt in organ donation and DNAPR orders.

Spiritual care at the end of life

Holistic spiritual care is person-centred care which includes aspects of religion, culture, and ethnicity. It encompasses the way in which a person lives their life and what is important to them at the end of their life. Spiritual care has been documented as the least understood part of end of life care which could be because of the lack of exploration of the difficulties of dealing with an emotive subject.

Spiritual care has increased significance at the end of a person's life and unmet need can result in emotional suffering. Gijsberts et al. (2019) discuss the importance of easing discomfort and how hope and empowerment are factors which need special attention at the end of life. Care given to patients is often varied and can be related to the experience of the caregiver. They advocate the enrichment of caregiver spiritual competency through education and self-reflection. This may have elements of personal spirituality, world views and religious beliefs shaped by communication skills, whether this be novice or expert.

Nurses often express feelings of inadequacy and lack of confidence when caring for the psychological needs of patients nearing death which can result in unmet needs for patients and relatives (Chapman, 2010). This can also be seen with the lack of evidence-based care, especially regarding the assessment of spiritual need. Good end of life care should be multi-directional and relational and not purely task orientated. The spirit, body and soul must be considered to enable the patient to connect with the things that are important to them, e.g. self, God, nature and others. Chapman and the National Council for Palliative Care suggest exploring how the patient and relatives understand, make sense of, or find meaning in what is happening to them. It can be helpful to identify what areas of their life give them strength and whether these are helpful to draw on at the end of life. Respectful enquiry into all spiritual or religious needs can help foster an individualised approach whilst also respecting those who are not concerned with having support (O'Callaghan et al., 2020).

Religion is a part of spirituality but if spiritual care is only viewed in terms of formal religion, then this can result in neglect of overall holistic care. It is important to pay attention to patient individual stories to ensure that pain, healing, and resolution are heard and considered. Public Health England (2019) used the 2012 Census to show how religion is distributed throughout the population of England and Wales. The Census showed that 51% of the population is Christian with 38.4% having no religion. It also demonstrated that the six biggest religions are Christianity, Islam, Hinduism, Sikhism, Judaism and Buddhism. Each of these religions has their own way of dealing with death and dying.

Education of caregivers is important to ensure that patient cues are listened to and explored – there is often a danger of misinterpreting emotional pain as physical distress or pain and then trying to medicate it. This would neglect the actual patient problem of lack of spiritual care at a time when they most need it. Family and those closest to the patient must be considered which will help when considering the needs of the patient. Cultural sensitivity is also needed throughout the whole process of end of life care. Batstone et al. (2020) believe that holistic healthcare assessments should incorporate spiritual needs and concerns and ensure that these are related to the physical and emotional pain patients are experiencing. They also feel that policies and protocols may be unhelpful and unrealistic in the current climate of excessive documentation and time constraints on staff. Chapman (2010) reflects on the poor understanding of the chaplaincy role and comments that the role could be used more, including with those patients who have no religion. Patients' information regarding their religion and religious needs should be documented. Family involvement and the need for an interpreter should also be considered at this time.

Spirituality at the end of life is a concept that is underdeveloped by the healthcare world. It seems that there is a perceived lack of confidence in the assessment and delivery of spiritual care which could result in the omission of an important section of care at the end of life. There is debate over whether policy and processes would help but the overriding observation is that the patient must have a tailored and individualised approach to their care which has resulted from a holistic enquiry.

SPECIALIST ROLES AND ORGANIZATIONS IN THE COMMUNITY FOR PALLIATIVE / EOLC

The home continues to be a desired place of care and dying (Alvariza et al., 2019). Addressing palliative care needs effectively with a person-centred focus around the dying person's, carers' and family's expressed wishes does have its challenges in a ward environment but even more so in a community setting. There has been a rapid increase in palliative home care services, and specialist palliative care nurses play a crucial role (Sarmento et al., 2017) for the reasons already mentioned in this chapter, essentially:

- **Pathophysiology** – when death will occur. Unfortunately, people are still inappropriately admitted to acute hospital for management of their physical illness (pain, respiration, anxiety) which could be managed in their own home.
- **Aspects of law** – use of advanced directives.
- **Spirituality/expressed wishes** – taken into consideration as more people are making informed decision around palliative/EoLC which should be managed around the person's own home and comfort.

According to Alvariza et al. (2019), the private home was the setting where patients have amongst the highest prevalence of palliative care needs. This does present challenges to health and social care providers and proves a challenge within the community managing the complexities of EoLC such as what team or professional coordinates the care effectively, what statutory and non statutory resources are available in general and whether these commissioned resources are available in a specific geographical area, what specialist service the person needs. Taking, for example, EoLC for a patient with severe dementia: is this managed by the community's older persons mental health team, district nursing team, general practitioner, specialist nurse, care home or social care team? As a nursing professional, let alone as a student nurse, this can be very difficult to navigate and understand, particularly when attempting to avoid unnecessary care in hospital and satisfying the family's need to have a consistent healthcare professional to liaise with to avoid any misunderstandings. There is no doubt the management of EoLC can be extremely complex, confusing, and inconsistent for families let alone the professionals involved, and therefore often requires specialist roles to bridge the gap between existing health and social care services. There are several roles within the UK that help support specialist care for people in EoLC, and therefore promote and enable quality of life and living as well as possible until the person dies.

The role of the Admiral nurse

The Admiral nurse is a specialist dementia nurse. The role of the Admiral nurse has been established in parts of the UK from around the mid-1980s to the present day and has a specific remit to support the care of the patient with dementia at any stage of their diagnosis. The term and naming of the 'Admiral nurse' was created by the family of Joseph Levy who founded the charity and subsequently had vascular dementia himself. He was known affectionately as 'Admiral Joe' because of his love of sailing. The Admiral nurse team complement each other extremely well and are very adaptive to all the patient with dementia's needs by being made up of professionals from the three fields of nursing (mental health, adult and learning disability nurses) who can then offer their unique expertise from previous roles they have undertaken such as palliative, inpatient and community specialist teams. The Admiral nurse team will sit outside traditional statutory teams like district nurses and community mental health teams and are accessible via referral criteria which may include specific information like identified diagnosis of dementia, patients who do not permanently reside in a care home, family agreement to this specialist role, specialist needs that cannot be managed by one traditional service (e.g. district nursing team) and impact on the carer or consequences to the caring role.

Admiral nurses complement and broaden the depth of skills by addressing the holistic biopsychosocial needs of the patient with dementia and their family. They use a range of psychosocial, educational, and practical approaches and are delivering person-centred and relationship-centred dementia care working collaboratively in a family-centric manner, across health and social care pathways. They provide support, expert guidance, and practical solutions to enable families/carers including the person living with dementia to maximise their wellbeing and improve the experiences of those affected by dementia. Essentially, Admiral nurses will support patients through the final phase of disease including EoLC, post bereavement and following death. Their aim is to reduce unscheduled inappropriate admissions to general hospital and to address the often complex needs this disease manifests which traditional community services may find difficult to manage. Admiral nurses will focus on the needs of the whole family, maintain relationships, improve communication, offer specialist interventions, transition and liaise with other health professionals on their behalf.

Admiral nurses are employed by the NHS and charity organizations predominantly in England and Wales. Charities as a service provider account for nearly half of all Admiral nurses and therefore the availability of this service in certain parts of the UK might be fragmented or non-existent. Admiral nurses will only cover a designated geographical area as part of their role either under a health board/ health authority or charity organization. There is also a free Admiral nurse dementia helpline on 0800 888 6678. Admiral nurses have undergone further training to support their role including an online course for registered nurses to find out more about the role, if they consider applying for a post and career as an Admiral nurse.

CASE STUDY

Tolu

Tolu is a final year student nurse working with Ahmed and they have had the following case referred. John is 69 years old and lives at home with their wife of 48 years, Betty. They have three grown up children not living locally and four grandchildren. John has just received a diagnosis of mild Alzheimer's dementia from the consultant psychiatrist in the specialist older persons mental health team following a six-month investigation into short-term memory problems and forgetfulness reported by the family. The news of this diagnosis has sent shockwaves through the family as John is otherwise physically fit and healthy with no other concerns at present. John will be followed up in OPC on a six-monthly basis and his Alzheimer's dementia reviewed. Alzheimer's dementia is a chronic condition which John could live with for 10-20 years or more, moving from mild to moderate to severe symptoms, and therefore a profound sense of loss and bereavement may be experienced by the family long before death, and indeed death might be a welcome relief. Preparation for palliative care should be considered/discussed.

Questions

1   When should professionals discuss living with dementia and palliative care options with John and why?
2   Which professional would be responsible for starting this conversation?
3   What provisions should be discussed initially with John and put in place and what provisions should follow?
4   How can voluntary/third sector organizations become involved to assist in this process?

GO FURTHER

The following is an online introductory course designed for registered nurses who wish to find out more about the role of an Admiral nurse. It is useful for health and social care professionals who wish to find out more about the complexities when supporting families with dementia. It is available via the Dementia UK website:

https://www.dementiauk.org/elearning/#/ (accessed October 24, 2022).

Community Palliative Care Nurse (CPCN)

The community specialist palliative nursing care role is highly valued by patients and families for meeting the patient on a regular basis during palliative/EoLC, during difficult times. Besides performing nursing tasks, they provide information and emotional support much like the Admiral nurse's role, although they deal with a wider range of primary diagnoses. Therefore, CPCN covers those patients living with life threatening illness such as cancer, brain tumours and respiratory diseases. CPCN play an essential role in providing EoLC in diverse environments of the private homes of patients with palliative care needs.

RECOGNITION OF DEATH: THE FOUR POST-MORTEM STAGES

It is useful for you to be aware of the post-mortem stages the body goes through after death, especially as you will be handling and caring for the deceased person immediately after death and maybe for hours and sometimes days after that. There are four stages that occur in a sequential approach: firstly pallor mortis, algor mortis, rigor mortis and finally livor mortis.

CARE OF THE BODY AFTER DEATH

Considerations

It is important to note that care for the person after death can be very different depending on the circumstances surrounding whether it was expected or unexpected, traumatic or if treatment and ventilation were withdrawn. For example, an unexpected death on the Adult ITU following resuscitation will consist of the removal of many medical adjuncts like ET tubes, IV cannulae, and catheters. Whereas with an expected death of a person with an identified condition in a hospice, all those attachments will probably have already been removed before death.

As nurses we need to be aware of the circumstances of a death before providing care for the deceased person. In certain circumstances where the cause of death may be unexplained or suspicious, minimal contact with the body is advised. All drains, lines and catheters should be left in-situ and the deceased person transferred into the care of the mortuary staff (Hospice UK, 2020).

Care of the person's body after death can be carried out in the home, or any healthcare setting. Wishes of the deceased person and their families or carers should be considered and adhered to where possible in a manner that is consistent with their beliefs, culture and religion.

Movement of a person's body after death can sometimes initiate the flow of exhaled air. This is normal but should not be mistaken for a sign of life. Family members or friends should be advised of this prior to any cares being undertaken after death. They should also be made aware of the changes to the body: colour changes, changes in body temperature and stiffening of the body.

Infants and children

Families of infants and children are encouraged to spend time with them after they have died. This has been considered beneficial in the bereavement process and aids the acceptance that the child has actually passed away. Cooling mattresses were originally introduced for families of infants to be able to spend time with them after a stillbirth. They aid in the preservation of the body allowing that extra precious time. They are now being used for older children too. Care and a sensitive approach should be taken in informing the family of changes to the body over time when using a cooling mattress.

ACTIVITY: PAUSE AND REFLECT

When caring for a patient after death there may be religious and cultural aspects that need to be considered.

In this activity explore the following:

- What religious and cultural aspects need consideration when the patient is Muslim?
- What religions require an elder or religious leader to attend at or around the time of the patient's passing?
- What religious and cultural aspects exist around washing the patient after death?

You may find some help with this activity here: https://www.mariecurie.org.uk/talkabout/articles/death-customs-of-different-faiths/260276 (accessed October 24, 2022).

When carrying out any nursing care, privacy should be maintained in respect for that person. This is just as important after death as it is in life. The NMC Code emphasises the need to 'respect that a person's right to privacy and confidentiality continues after they have died' (NMC, 2018a). Consequently, prior to commencing any after death care you should ensure that the cubicle door is closed, or the curtains drawn. Dependent on where the death has occurred, other patients or residents may be anxious or aware of the situation and should be reassured and comforted.

—— WATCH THE VIDEO ——

CARE AFTER DEATH

Watch along as you read through this step by step procedure by scanning the QR code with your smartphone camera or via https://study.sagepub.com/rowberry.

—— CARE OF THE BODY AFTER DEATH: STEP BY STEP ——

EQUIPMENT

- Identification bands x2
- Documentation – legal/organisational forms
- Property list and bag for personal possessions including valuables

- Personal protective equipment
- Bowl of warm water
- Soap/personal toiletries
- Disposable wash cloths and towels
- Personal clean clothing/shroud/hospital gown
- Oral care equipment including toothbrush
- Comb/brush
- Nail care equipment
- Clean bed linen
- Slide sheets/hoist for manual handling
- Linen skip and appropriate bags for soiled items
- Clinical/domestic waste bags
- Absorbent/continence pads or dressings
- Body bag if required (only in cases of high risk of infection or leakage of body fluids)
- Occlusive tape, gauze, dressings and bandages
- Spigots/bungs for catheters/drains/IV lines
- Disposable receiver for collecting urine

PROCEDURE

- Carry out hand hygiene prior to donning the appropriate personal protective equipment, including gloves and an apron. Adhere to the local infection prevention and control guidelines. This is essential to protect yourself from infection due to the increased risk of contact with body fluids and soiled linen.
- Just as if the person were still alive, it may be helpful to talk to the deceased person and tell them what you are going to do. This shows continuing respect for the person who has died. Many nurses report that they find this helps to support them emotionally when undertaking this care.
- Lay the person in a neutral supine position with their arms by their sides. This should be carried out by two nurses and in adherence to the local manual handling guidance (slide sheets may be useful). Depending on how long after the person has died you carry out the care, you need to consider that limbs will become stiff due to rigor mortis, so only straighten as far as you are able and inform the mortuary staff. Respecting the dignity of the person includes making them 'comfortable' and this is especially important if they are being viewed by the family.
- Ensure that the person is covered with a sheet at all times and privacy is maintained, e.g., curtains or door closed. Maintaining the dignity and privacy of the person you are caring for is paramount even after death.
- Place the head on just one pillow. This will help to keep the person supported and the mouth closed.
- Gently close the eyes by applying light pressure for about 30 seconds. This is to maintain the person's dignity and may also give some protection if the corneas are being donated. Never apply tape to close the eyes as visible marks may be left.
- Depending on whether the case has been referred to the coroner for investigation, you can begin to remove/clamp or bung any medical adjuncts, for example, IV lines, ET tubes, tracheostomy tubes or wound drains. When removing ET/tracheostomy/nasogastric tubes, you may

(Continued)

require suction equipment to manage any excess secretions. When removing wounds drains or IV lines, you may require an absorbent/occlusive dressing to be applied over the site to prevent further leakage.

- Gently drain the bladder by pressing on the lower abdomen for 30 seconds whilst collecting the urine in a disposable receiver or within the catheter bag (where the catheter is still in-situ). You can then either remove the catheter or just the bag and insert a spigot to prevent leakage as the body continues to excrete fluids after death.

- Absorbent pads or pants can be used underneath the deceased person. Any stomas should be cleaned and a new stoma bag applied. This will absorb any leakage of bodily fluids from the urethra, vagina or rectum. This will contain any leakage from the stoma as the body continues to excrete bodily fluids after death.

- If the deceased person has a surgical wound or injury, then this should be covered with an absorbent/occlusive dressing. Any clips or stitches should be left intact and not removed. This will prevent any leakage from the wound. This will minimise the risk of the wound reopening and leaking.

- Check the following before washing the deceased person: family or carers are happy for you to do so; any cultural/religious/spiritual reasons against it; or if the case has been referred to the coroner and therefore minimal contact is advised. Some family members may wish to partici-pate in this aspect of care and if so should be advised and reassured in relation to expectations, involvement and changes in the condition of the deceased person's body. This demonstrates your continued respect to the deceased person and their family.

- Using warm, soapy water, wash and dry the deceased person. Be sure to ensure you are main-taining their privacy and dignity at all times. Adhere to manual handling guidance when moving the person to wash them and to also place two clean sheets **underneath** them. Tuck in the very bottom sheet and leave the upper sheet loose until you need to wrap the person's body. Dispose of any soiled linen into the linen skip and the appropriately labelled bag. This will prevent injury to yourself or the deceased person's body and will prevent any potential spread of infection.

- Shaving a deceased person is no longer recommended. This is because the skin is still warm and there is an increased risk of bruising or marking which often does not appear until days later. There are also some religions where shaving is prohibited and some where shaving has to be undertaken by another member of that faith.

- Dress the deceased person in their personal clothing or a shroud/gown depending on the prefer-ences of the person or their family. They should NEVER be left undressed. This again demon-strates continued respect for the deceased person, but also may be aesthetically pleasing for the family if they see their loved one dressed in familiar clothing. Preferences may be detailed in the ACP.

- Clean any debris or secretions from the mouth (suction may be required). Perform oral hygiene using a toothbrush or oral sponge sticks. Any dentures should also be cleaned and then rein-serted (if able to). It is important to care for the person's oral hygiene even after death. Replacing dentures will also help to support the jaw and retain the shape of the person's face. If it becomes difficult to replace them, then send them clearly labelled with the deceased person. The funeral staff may be able to fit them securely later.

- For additional support for the jaw, you may need to use a small pillow or rolled up towel. Never bandage the person's jaw as this will leave marks on the body which can be upsetting for family members.

- Brush and tidy the hair into the preferred style (if known). A lock of hair may be offered as a memento to the family. This demonstrates dignity and respect.

- Collect any jewellery from the deceased person's body in the presence of another member of staff. It should be placed in a valuables property bag/envelope and clearly labelled. Some families may wish the jewellery to stay in-situ or it may be difficult to remove - instead secure it in place with minimal tape. Document the location of all pieces as per local policy. This is to meet legal requirements for personal property of the deceased. Again, these preferences may be detailed within the ACP. By securing the jewellery in place, you avoid the risk of the item falling off and potential loss.

- All property from the deceased person should be returned to the family. However, you need to communicate sensitively with the family in relation to items such as soiled clothing or blankets as the family may wish to keep them. This is to meet legal requirements for personal property of the deceased and to be sensitive to the preferences of the family.

- Apply identification bands to the deceased person's wrist and ankle. Toe tags are no longer used. This is to ensure the correct identification of the deceased person.

- Take the clean sheet loosely placed underneath the deceased person and begin to wrap the body. Ensure that the face and feet are covered, and all limbs are securely within the sheets. Apply tape to keep the sheet in place. This is to ensure the deceased person's body is secure and safe for transfer to the mortuary or undertakers.

- Only place the body into a body bag if leakage of body fluids is excessive, if the person was known to have had an infectious notifiable disease or it is the local policy to do so. This will reduce the risk of contamination to those handling the body for transfer.

- Complete the correct documentation such as the 'notification of death' form. You may also be required to document on this form where any property/jewellery is located on the body. This form is then normally secured to the outside of the sheet of the deceased person's body. This ensures correct identification and the legal requirements in relation to personal property of the deceased person.

ACTIVITY: COMMUNICATION SKILLS

How would you communicate and explain the care of the body after death to the family of a patient? Focus on your field of nursing.

CHAPTER SUMMARY

This chapter has outlined the importance of the knowledge needed around palliative care, end of life care and care after death. Nurses play a large part in these areas of care regardless of the speciality or area they work in. The chapter has also discussed some key specialist roles in relation to this area of nursing care; it is worth noting this list is not exhaustive, further reading will guide you to other specialist areas of practice.

ACE YOUR ASSESSMENT

1   Identify correct physiological changes at end of life.

   a   Dry mouth, weight loss, dyspnoea
   b   Pain, weight loss, hunger
   c   Dyspnoea, weight loss, confusion

2   Identify correct reasons medications are given at end of life.

   a   Pain, glucose control, thirst
   b   Pain, secretions, glucose control
   c   Pain, nausea and vomiting, terminal agitation

3   What does MCA stand for?

   a   Mood Capacity Act
   b   Mental Capacity Act
   c   Mentally Capable Act

4   What does DNACPR stand for?

   a   Do Not Attempt Cardiac Priority Response
   b   Do Not Attempt Cardio Pulmonary Resuscitation
   c   Do Not Act Circulation Pulmonary Resucitation

Answers

1   A
2   C
3   B
4   B

GO FURTHER

Marie Curie Website: https://www.mariecurie.org.uk/ (accessed October 24, 2022).

Cultural and religious care: https://www.endwithcare.org/blogs/FullPost.php?id=32 (accessed October 24, 2022).

REFERENCES

Alvariza, A., Mjörnberg, M. and Goliath, I. (2019) 'Palliative care nurses' strategies when working in private homes – A photo-elicitation study', *Journal of Clinical Nursing*, 29 (1/2): 139–51. https://doi.org/10.1111/jocn.15072

Batstone, E., Bailey, C. and Hallett, N. (2020) 'Spiritual care provision to end-of-life patients: A systematic literature review', *Journal of Clinical Nursing*, 29 (19/20): 3609–24. doi.org/10.1111/jocn.15411

BMJ (2013) '"First do no harm" revisited'. *BMJ*, 347. https://doi.org/10.1136/bmj.f6426

Chapman, S. (2010) *The Missing Piece: Meeting People's Spiritual Needs in End of Life Care*. London: National Council for Palliative Care (NCPC). http://professionals.hospiceuk.org/docs/default-source/What-we-offer/publications-documents-and-files/the-missing-piece (accessed October 24, 2022).

Fritz, Z. and Perkins, G. (2020) 'Cardiopulmonary resuscitation after hospital admission with Covid-19', *British Journal of Nursing*, 369: Article #m1387.

Gijsberts, M.J.H.E., Liefbroer, A.I., Otten, R. and Olsman, E. (2019) 'Spiritual care in palliative care: A systematic review of the recent European literature medical sciences', *Medical Sciences*, 7 (2). doi.org/10.3390/medsci7020025

Gov.uk (n.d.) *Make, Register or End a Lasting Power of Attorney*. https://www.gov.uk/power-of-attorney/make-lasting-power (accessed December 2022).

Holloway, M., Adamson, S., McSherry, W. and Swinton, J. (2011) 'Spiritual care at the end of life: A systematic review of the literature', Department of Health. http://assets.publishing.service.gov.uk/government/uploads/system/uploads/attachment_data/file/215798/dh_123804.pdf (accessed October 24, 2022).

Hospice UK (n.d.) *Hospice UK Innovation Hub*. https://www.hospiceuk.org/innovation-hub (accessed December 10, 2022).

Johnson S. (2015) 'Paraneoplastic syndromes in palliative care: A literature review from a nursing perspective', *Journal of Palliative Care*, 31 (3): 177–88.

Marie Curie (2022) 'What is palliative care', mariecurie.org.uk, August 10. https://www.mariecurie.org.uk/help/support/diagnosed/recent-diagnosis/palliative-care-end-of-life-care (accessed October 24, 2022).

National Institute for Health and Care Excellence (NICE) (2019) *End of Life Care for Adults: Service Delivery* (NG 142), NICE. https://www.nice.org.uk/guidance/ng142/resources/end-of-life-care-for-adults-service-delivery-pdf-66141776457925 (accessed October 24, 2022).

National Institute for Health and Care Excellence (2021) *End of Life Care for Adults: Quality Standards* (QS13), NICE. https://www.nice.org.uk/guidance/qs13 (accessed October 24, 2022).

Nursing and Midwifery Council (2018a). *The Code*. London: NMC. https://www.nmc.org.uk/globalassets/sitedocuments/nmc-publications/nmc-code.pdf (accessed October 7, 2022).

Nursing and Midwifery Council (NMC) (2018b) *Future Nurse: Standards of Proficiency for Registered Nurses*. NMC, May 17. https://www.nmc.org.uk/standards/standards-for-nurses/standards-of-proficiency-for-registered-nurses/ (accessed October 24, 2022).

O'Callaghan, C.C., Georgousopoulou, E., Seah, D., Clayton, J.M., Kissane, D. and Michael, N. (2020) 'Spirituality and religiosity in a palliative medicine population: Mixed-methods study', *BMJ Supportive & Palliative Care*, 12 (3): 316–23. https://spcare.bmj.com/content/early/2020/06/04/bmjspcare-2020-002261 (accessed October 24, 2022).

Office of National Statistics (ONS) (2012) 'Census 2011: Religion in England and Wales 2011', ons.gov.uk. www.ons.gov.uk/ons/rel/census/2011-census/key-statistics-for-local-authorities-in-england-and-wales/rpt-religion.html (accessed October 24, 2022).

Public Health England (2016) *Faith at End of Life: A Resource for Professionals, Providers and Commissioners Working in Communities*. London: Public Health England. https://assets.publishing.service.gov.uk/government/uploads/system/uploads/attachment_data/file/496231/Faith_at_end_of_life_-_a_resource.pdf (accessed October 24, 2022).

Sarmento, V.P., Gysels, M., Higginson, I.J. and Gomes, B. (2017) 'Home palliative care works: But how? A meta-ethnography of the experiences of patients and family caregivers', *Supportive and Palliative Care*, 7 (4). doi.org/10.1136/bmjspcare-2016-001141

UK Government (2004) *The Human Tissue Act 2004*. London: HMSO. https://www.legislation.gov.uk/ukpga/2004/30/contents (accessed October 24, 2022).

UK Government (2005) *Mental Capacity Act 2005*. London: HMSO. https://www.legislation.gov.uk/ukpga/2005/9/contents (accessed October 24, 2022).

UK Government (2019) *The Organ Donation (Deemed Consent) Act 2019*. https://www.legislation.gov.uk/ukpga/2019/7/contents/enacted (accessed October 24, 2022).

Welsh Parliament (2013) *Human Transplantation (Wales)*. https://www.legislation.gov.uk/anaw/2013/5/contents (accessed October 24, 2022).

World Health Organization (WHO) (2020) 'Palliative care', who.int, August 5. https://www.who.int/news-room/fact-sheets/detail/palliative-care (accessed October 24, 2022).

MEDICATION ADMINISTRATION

13

NICOLA HENWOOD

NMC STANDARDS COVERED IN THIS CHAPTER

ANNEXE B NURSING PROCEDURES

11   Procedural competencies required for best practice, evidence-based medicines administration and optimisation

11.1   Carry out initial and continued assessments of people receiving care and their ability to self-administer their own medications

11.2   Recognise the various procedural routes under which medicines can be prescribed, supplied, dispensed and administered; and the laws, policies, regulations and guidance that underpin them

11.3   Use the principles of safe remote prescribing and directions to administer medicines

11.4   Undertake accurate drug calculations for a range of medications

11.5   Undertake accurate checks, including transcription and titration, of any direction to supply or administer a medicinal product

11.6   Exercise professional accountability in ensuring the safe administration of medicines to those receiving care

11.7   Administer injections using intramuscular, subcutaneous, intradermal and intravenous routes and manage injection equipment

11.8   Administer medications using a range of routes

11.9   Administer and monitor medications using vascular access devices and enteral equipment

11.10   Recognise and respond to adverse or abnormal reactions to medications

11.11   Undertake safe storage, transportation and disposal of medicinal products.

LEARNING OBJECTIVES

After reading this chapter, you should be able to:

- Appraise and differentiate the relevant legislation surrounding medication administration
- Identify the safest approaches to storing, preparing and administering medication
- Explain and apply best practice when administering medication through all routes
- Appraise your current knowledge and abilities in relation to medicines administration

STUDENT VOICE

I don't think I will ever forget my first drugs round! It was nerve wracking to see the documentation and so many types of medication that I needed to find my way through. Looking back there was so much that I didn't know I would *need* to know! It was one of the things that made me feel like I was stepping into the shoes of a qualified nurse.

Freya, 3rd year, Adult Nursing

INTRODUCTION

Administering medication is often a daunting task for a student nurse. This physical act of dispensing prescribed medication can feel like your first steps to being a 'real nurse'. However, handing medication to a patient is one of the final steps. Prior to this there have been careful, often unseen processes. Being a competent registered nurse involves a good working knowledge of the legal considerations as well as practical considerations to minimise opportunities for error. After administering medication, the nurse needs to be vigilant for any signs of complications as well as completing accurate documentation and disposal of potentially hazardous waste. The nurse needs to be able to provide competent communication with the patient and/or their families and carers. Communication is vital to ensure that all who are involved understand what is happening and informed consent can be obtained. This ensures *patient focus*, instead of *task focus*.

Nursing is a science, based on evidence. Put simply, when the evidence changes, so do the recommendations. There is an earlier chapter in this book on evidence-based practice that covers this in greater detail. A competent nurse will never finish learning and will always be open to changes in practice. Within the domain of medication administration, this can be new medications or changes to existing recommendations. This includes how the medication should be given, as well as changes to storage and preparation. Initially, this can feel incredibly overwhelming. You are not expected to know each and every drug, but you will be expected to know what you are giving, what it is for and be able to administer it in a safe manner. You may find that your placement areas each have common medications for the specialty. Becoming familiar with commonly prescribed medication is helpful.

The *British National Formulary* is a reference book for drugs in the UK. It has handy information about medications. This includes dosage, indications, contraindications, side-effects and costs. You will often find brightly coloured copies of this book in any environment where medication is commonly prescribed or administered. It is updated and re-published twice per year, March and September, so it is important to make sure you have a recent copy. The BNF is also available electronically and as an app for smart devices which are much more pocket friendly. Child nursing students may prefer to use the BNF for Children, which notes the dosages suitable from neonates to teens. When researching medications, it is important that your sources are reputable. The BNF is *the* go-to book for medications.

When you build your understanding about medication, you will become aware medicines can also be significantly problematic. Medication is administered to improve the quality of life, a person's ability to function, or to eradicate illness, but can often cause unwanted side effects. There can be unintended harm, or even death. It is estimated that 238 million drug errors occur each year in England alone (Elliott et al., 2021). Your role in safe storage, handling, preparation and administration of medication can help to reduce harm that is caused through errors.

This chapter aims to equip you with some of the legal and procedural considerations before introducing you to the physical skills of medication administration. It is hoped that this chapter, combined with your theory and practice placements, will create a firm foundation to build your nursing journey on.

DRUGS AND THE LAW

What is medication?

Medication and medicines are often used interchangeably, but what is the difference between a drug and a medication? Outside the world of healthcare, the term drug is often used to refer to illicit substances. Simply put, a drug is a chemical substance that changes the functioning of living things and the organisms that infect them, such as bacteria, viruses and parasites. As such, you may think that the terms drug and medication may be used interchangeably. However, a *medication* (or *medicine*) may have no *drugs* within it; such as paediatric rehydration solution. A drug needs to be formulated into a preparation for it to be administered. An example may be a tablet, injection or suppository. Once the drug is in a prepared form, it can be considered a medicine.

As a student nurse, you will practice the skills to ensure safe handling, storage and administration of drugs. In the United Kingdom, drugs and medicines are classified into categories, based on their function and potential harms. All medications are regulated by the Medicines and Healthcare products Regulatory Agency (MHRA). A drug is recognised as a *medication* if it fits into either of the criteria below:

- Substances presented as having properties for treating or preventing disease
- Substances that can restore, correct or modify physiological functions by exerting a pharmacological, immunological or metabolic action, or making a medical diagnosis. (European Parliament, 2001)

Whilst this is a legal definition of a medication, it is worth considering what patient perceptions are. As discussed at the introduction of this section, there can be confusion about drugs and medication. Some people may not consider their drug to be 'significant' enough to mention, particularly if it is not prescribed. This can often be the case with widely available medications such as antacids or nicotine replacement. This perception can be especially true if the medication is not taken in tablet form. Medication that is topically applied, such as preparations for skin conditions, can often be overlooked by patients.

Medications or drugs may be omitted by a patient or their family when they provide a drug history. Patients may not disclose if they fear being judged by the professionals. There may be a perceived sense of shame from using certain medications, such as those used for treating impotence or a mental health condition. Patients may fear judgement from practitioners, especially with herbal or complementary preparations. Finally, they may be using drugs that are illegal for use in the UK such as cannabis or ecstasy. This is important because it may be clinically relevant to know if a patient is using them. Patients should feel able to discuss any drugs or preparations that that are using, as it may interact with additional drugs being prescribed. As a registered nurse, you are expected to work within *The Code* (NMC, 2018b). *The Code* stipulates that nurses must avoid making assumptions and recognise individual choice (1.3) as well as respect the contribution that people can make to their own health and wellbeing (2.2). Whilst you may hold private opinions about the choice patients are making, this must not impact your role as their nurse.

ACTIVITY: PAUSE AND REFLECT

Miss Key has a number of physical and mental health conditions. A family friend advised her to visit a Traditional Chinese Medicine Clinic locally, in the hopes that it may help to improve her health. For the last three months she has been taking additional herbal remedies. On admission she did not tell you this, but you noticed them on her bedside table as you were taking her vital signs. She put them out of sight quickly and told you they were 'nothing'.

- Why is it important to know about supplements and additional remedies?
- Why would patients conceal medications they are using?
- What would you do to encourage Miss Key to disclose this information?

Regulation

Laws and regulations exist to protect individuals and groups from direct and indirect harm from medication. The manufacture, licensing, sale and advertising of medication is strictly controlled to ensure a safe product. Where there is potential for harm, restrictions exist to make sure that people are only able to access the drugs that are most appropriate for themselves.

How are drugs classified?

Within the UK, all drugs and medicinal products are classified by the MHRA and advised by ministers. Cases are presented with evidence of harm or benefit and classified accordingly. The Acts of Parliament below will provide background to why they came into effect and the impact of the Acts on members of the public and registered professionals. These are important for you to be aware of, as you will be handling medication that can carry criminal charges if mishandled or abused.

Making medicines safer - The Medicines Act (1968)

In the 1950s there was a global increase in birth defects, later found to have been caused by the drug Thalidomide (Shah, 2001). Thalidomide was marketed as a suitable treatment for morning sickness. It had not been tested in humans and there was no evidence that it was safe to use in pregnancy. It was also available over the counter. The Medicines Act (1968) was part of the response by the UK government to improve the safety of medications, preventing untested or unsafe medication being available. The Medicines Act covers medications for human and animal use in England and Wales. It governs the processes around manufacture, supply, and administration of medicines. This Act also governs the promotion and sales of medicines.

This Act meant that manufacturers subjected their products for peer-review to be approved or withdrawn from the market. This included 39,000 current medications and any new medications after the Act was passed. Out of 39,000 medications in use prior to the Act, only 5,000 were given full licenses (Royal Pharmaceutical Society, 2014).

To prevent harm, The Medicines Act states that responsibility for the safety of medications should lie with Ministers, who were advised by a Medicines Commission. Any new medications are checked for safety, quality, and efficacy by the licensing authority, now known as the MHRA (Medicines and Healthcare Products Regulatory Agency). The purpose of the regulations is to have precise standards of safety. Whilst medications are not without risks, this robust approach seeks to achieve an optimum and fully informed risk-to-benefit ratio to ensure correct information is provided to health professionals and individuals needing to take medication.

It is this Act that defines medications into separate categories:

Table 13.1   Categories of medication in The Medicines Act

Category	Explanation	Example
POM – Prescription only medication	Access to these drugs is restricted. They can only be supplied by a pharmacist after being prescribed appropriately. There is a potential for these medications to cause physical harm or addiction. The prescriber should weigh any harm against potential benefit and provide monitoring if appropriate.	Examples include antibiotics, antipsychotics and opioid analgesia.
P – Pharmacy medication	Access to these drugs is restricted. Pharmacy medicines can only be obtained from a pharmacist, but can be purchased without a prescription. These drugs are usually recommended for the treatment of minor ailments or injuries, or health promotion. Increasingly, drug manufacturers are seeking to reclassify their medications from POM to P.	Drugs suitable for managing acute or chronic conditions, as well as so-called 'lifestyle drugs' such as sildenafil for erectile dysfunction and orlistat for obesity.
GSL – General sales list	This is sometimes referred to as 'over the counter' or OTC medication. General sales list medicines can be bought from any venue without a prescription. Drugs within this list are helpful for common, easily recognized ailments which usually last around 2-3 days. When taken according to the manufacturing instructions, they are not likely to cause harm. These are predominantly for oral administration, but also include medications such as pessaries for thrush, and topical solutions for the treatment of verrucae.	This would include drugs such as: antacids, antihistamines and analgesia like paracetamol.

The Medicines Act defines each category of drug. Should a person be in possession of POM without a prescription, this can be illegal if the POM is *also* a controlled drug (see Misuse of Drugs Act 1971 for more). There are exemptions to this act to permit healthcare professionals to supply and administer medication in accordance with a PGD (Patient Group Direction), discussed further in this chapter.

GO FURTHER

Safer manufacture, sale and access: The Human Medicines Regulations (2012) https://www. legislation.gov.uk/uksi/2012/1916/contents (accessed October 25, 2022).

Within the regulations, a human medicine is described as a

Substance or combination of substances presented as having properties of preventing or treating disease in human beings, that may be used by or administered to human beings with a view to restoring, correcting or modifying a physiological function by exerting a pharmacological, immunological or metabolic action, or making a medical diagnosis.

These regulations are concerned with the manufacture, import, distribution, sale and supply of human medicines. This also includes their labelling, advertising, and pharmacovigilance. Pharmacovigilance is also known as drug safety. This is the monitoring of drugs after they have been licensed to identify previously unreported adverse effects. The Human Medicines Regulations have enforcement powers for the authorisation and supervision of medicinal products for human use. Within this regulation, there are named professionals who can use a PGD; it also outlines how a PGD should be constructed.

GO FURTHER

Preventing misuse: Misuse of Drugs Act 1971. https://www.legislation.gov.uk/ukpga/1971/38/contents (accessed October 25, 2022).

This Act replaced previous Acts relating to Dangerous Drugs. It seeks to prevent the misuse of controlled drugs. Regulations within the Act govern safe storage, destruction and supply to known addicts.

Controlled drugs are Classified A, B or C. It also includes any drug subject to temporary control. Temporary controls can be applied for up to 12 months if the drug isn't already classified and there is evidence to suggest that it should be applied, because of its harm or potential for abuse. This amendment was made in 2011, when the rise of novel psychoactive substances meant legal, or not-yet-illegal, substances were causing widespread harm. By marketing these substances as bath-salts, room deodorisers or 'research chemicals', so-called 'Head shops' were able to sell them without the rigourous testing or checking that would be required under the Medicines Act. Whilst under Temporary Control, testing can be undertaken to ensure the quality and safety of the product. Its manufacture, possession, and supply become unlawful.

As a result of the Misuse of Drugs Act, controlled drugs have penalties for unlawful supply, intent to supply, import, export or production. This Act also prevents unlawful possession, as having these drugs without an appropriate reason is a criminal offence. The police have powers to stop, detain and search people if they have a reasonable suspicion that they are in illegal possession of a controlled drug.

KEY TERMS

Class A: Examples include: Cocaine, MDMA, Diamorphine, Hydrocodone, Methadone.

Class B: Examples include: Amphetamine, Cannabis, Codeine, Ketamine.

Class C: Examples include: Diazepam, Lorazepam, Tramadol, Zopiclone.

As indicated in the box above, some of the drugs listed are medicinal drugs, which would also be covered by the Medicines Act. Possession of these POMs with an appropriate prescription is not an offence.

The classifications relate to penalties that can be applied for possession, supply, and production. Classifications are reviewed in line with emerging evidence by the Advisory Council on the Misuse of Drugs (ACMD).

In the UK, there is an ongoing attempt to balance the 'war on drugs' with a harm reduction approach to individuals who use substances. The harm reduction approach is to help those who use drugs to do so in the safest possible way. Multiple initiatives have attempted to mitigate the harm from legal and illegal drugs. Schemes include drug testing facilities in night clubs and festivals or needle exchanges and take home naloxone schemes to reduce the risk of a fatal opioid overdose. A recent amendment to the Human Medicines Act Regulations (2015) means that a wider range of people can carry naloxone including the family and friends of people at risk, professionals, and volunteer programmes. As we will see in the box below, however, some countries are taking a new approach to tackling illegal drugs.

ACTIVITY: PAUSE AND REFLECT

Drug reform in Portugal

In some countries, drug use is no longer being treated as a criminal issue, but a health and social issue. In Portugal, for example, if you are found to be in possession of substances you are referred to the 'Commissions for the Dissuasion of Drug Abuse (CDT)' instead of the criminal justice system.

The CDT provides timely health and social care interventions such as housing and support to reduce or stop the substance use. This has had an improvement in health outcomes, such as a reduction in new HIV and Hepatitis B diagnoses. It has also created an opportunity to reroute funds from criminal justice and prosecution into prevention (Pombo and Félix da Costa, 2016). Some of the most impressive findings have seen a 32% decrease in heroin users, and those that continued, adopted safer practices such as smoking rather than injecting (Pombo and Félix da Costa, 2016). Funding for treatment centres has increased so there are additional services, but an overall reduction in the numbers of people using substances has also reduced the number of people requiring these services (Silvestri, 2014). Those who are seeking support are also shown to be more engaged with services that offer them, which may account for the effectiveness of the interventions (Pombo and Félix da Costa, 2016).

Do you consider drug use to be an individual problem, or a public health issue?

Before reading this, what were your perceptions about people who use illegal drugs?

When you were reading about this approach, what were your initial thoughts?

So how does the evidence from Portugal relate to your medication administration chapter? It is important to acknowledge our own stigma and bias around all forms of drugs, as well as the people who use them.

Global approaches inform our practice when the evidence suggests a change may be helpful. When patients use illegal drugs, you may be able to advise of harm reduction approaches or ways that families of substance users can support their loved ones. There is a direct impact too, such as drug testing facilities that are able to provide updates about concerning substances that they test. In the UK, The Loop is a non-government organisation that will routinely provide drug testing at events such as festivals. Other specialist projects have been commissioned across the UK allowing people to test small samples of drugs they have used or are planning to use. In Wales, the Wedi Nos project can alert health services of suspicious or of-concern substances, which may inform the care and treatment they receive if people require medical intervention (www.wedinos.org). There are also ongoing trials to investigate the therapeutic uses of currently illegal substances, such as using small doses of psilocybin (magic mushrooms) to treat depression.

WHO CAN PRESCRIBE AND HOW?

Traditionally, the role of prescribing was solely in the realm of medical doctors and dentists. In the 1980s, The Cumberlege Report (Rogers, 1986) recognised that patients in the community experienced delays in treatment because Community Nursing Teams would need to request a GP to prescribe appropriate medication. By the early 90s, legislation was amended to allow specific nurses to gain qualifications to enable them to prescribe from a specific Nurse Prescribers Formulary. This was a reduced formulary, with a specific focus on medications commonly required by patients accessing health support in the community. As professional and public trust in these roles has grown, so has the level of autonomy of these practitioners.

Today, nurses and other healthcare professionals are able to train as non-medical prescribers and prescribe from an almost complete formulary. This is no longer limited to the community environment. The initial steps into nurse prescribing were made by community nurses, but their reach has expanded to include specialist services such as sexual health and contraception, and management of long- term conditions such as respiratory, dermatology and drug and alcohol teams. These prescribing practitioners are equally valued in primary care such as GP surgeries and acute care such as Emergency Departments.

The number of NMC registered prescribers is increasing annually, but more slowly than hoped (Graham-Clarke et al., 2018). In 2017, 11% of NMC registrants had a recognised prescriber qualification, which had increased to 13% by 2021 (NMC, 2021). In view of this, strategic plans have been created to enable more nurses to access the training required. Nurse training has been modernised and updated to fit with the New Standards for Nursing and Midwifery Education (Nursing and Midwifery Council, 2018b). Part of this modernisation was to ensure that newly qualified nurses are better prepared to undertake prescriber training, instead of the previous requirement for them to have been on the register for two to three years. It was recognised that being on the register for a specific length of time didn't guarantee that a nurse was suitably ready to undertake the additional training.

Your university is delivering a course that has been approved as meeting the threshold set by the NMC in the *Future Nurse: Standards of Proficiency for Registered Nurses* (2018a). Nurse training programmes were overhauled to ensure a greater standard of skills in assessment, diagnosis, care planning, pharmacology and leadership. The Future Nurse Standards are the foundation of a safe prescriber, but in addition to completion of your course, you will also need to demonstrate that you are a safe and effective clinician and that a nurse prescriber is required in your work area.

Table 13.2 Nurse prescribers

Prescriber type	Current number of registrants	Prescribing ability
Community Practitioner Nurse Prescriber	41,000	Nurse Prescribers formulary
Independent Prescriber & Supplementary Prescriber	50,000	Full British National Formulary (BNF) within scope of practice

In Nursing there are three main types of prescriber. Community Practitioner Nurse Prescribers, Independent Prescribers and Supplementary Prescribers.

- **Community Practitioner Nurse Prescriber:** A nurse who has undertaken additional training in order to prescribe from the Nurse Prescribers Formulary. This is a reduced list but commonly contains analgesics, contraceptives, laxatives, nicotine replacement, medicated dressings, and catheter equipment.
- **Independent Prescriber:** A prescribing healthcare professional who is responsible and accountable for the assessment of patients with undiagnosed or diagnosed conditions. They are also responsible for decisions about the clinical management required, including prescribing.
- **Supplementary Prescriber:** A prescriber who forms a voluntary partnership between a doctor or dentist, to prescribe within an agreed patient-specific clinical management plan with the patient's agreement.

(The Royal Pharmaceutical Society, 2021)

Previously, all non-medical prescribers were governed by their respective professional bodies. In 2019, this was replaced with the *Competency Framework for all Prescribers* (RPS, 2021). This change aims to create parity between all types of prescribers. As a result, nurse prescribers are now held to the same standard as medical or other non-medical prescribers (RPS, 2021). Patient outcomes from non-medical prescribers are largely similar to medical prescribers, and there are marginally better outcomes in the management of hypertension, high cholesterol and blood sugar levels (Weeks et al., 2016).

HOW ARE MEDICATIONS PROVIDED TO PATIENTS?

Medicines are administered to patients in accordance with a prescription, Patient Specific Direction (PSD) or Patient Group Direction (PGD). Each approach has specific and strict procedures surrounding them, in order to maintain patient safety:

- **Prescription:** A written instruction by a qualified prescriber for a medicine to be dispensed to a named patient. Traditionally these were handwritten but more recently there has been an increase in electronic prescriptions in primary care and inpatient settings.
- **PSD:** An instruction from a prescriber for a medicine to be supplied or administered to a named patient after the prescriber has assessed that patient on an individual basis, e.g. written directions in a patient's notes or inpatient chart. The most common example of this is the hospital prescription form ('TTO') detailing the medicines to be dispensed for a patient to take home on discharge.
- **PGD:** A written direction that allows the supply and/or administration of a specified medicine or medicines, by named authorised health professionals, to a well-defined group of patients requiring treatment of a specific condition (RPS and RCN, 2019), for example:
  o   Seasonal and other types of vaccination.
  o   In well-established services where assessment and treatment follow a clearly predictable pattern (e.g., immunisation clinics, contraception and sexual health services).

The supply and administration of medicines under PGDs should be reserved for situations where this offers advantages to patient care without impacting patient safety.

Hard copies of inpatient medication administration records are less likely to be used today, as many areas move towards using electronic prescriptions and record keeping. There are a number of benefits to this approach, such as statistically significant reduction in medication errors and an increase in quality of documentation (Mills et al., 2017). Electronic documentation removes any potential difficulty with handwriting and often has built-in safety features such as the patient's allergy status or warnings of possible drug interactions. Additionally, electronic prescriptions cannot be misplaced. As an electronic document, they can be accessed by staff without needing to be in the same room as the patient, saving time when other departments such as pharmacy or the medical team require access to the document.

However, electronic documents can be a barrier for nursing students trying to spend time familiarising themselves with medication as they can be more inaccessible than hard copies. If you are hoping to expand your drug knowledge during your placement opportunities, is important to have a plan of how you will achieve this. During your theory and practical placements you will be introduced to medications, but you will need to complete additional private study to deepen and develop this knowledge.

CASE STUDY

Sam, first year mental health nursing student

Sam is on a community placement with a registered nurse and is visiting a patient at home to provide morning medication. This is the first time Sam has met the patient. The registered nurse asks Sam about the medication on the chart.

Sam is unfamiliar with one of the medications listed. They are concerned about seeming unprofessional or inexperienced in front of their new colleague, and don't want to worry the patient by asking questions.

The registered nurse is ultimately responsible for the decision about administering or withholding a medication, but it is important that you think about wider considerations as a student too.

Questions

Consider how you would handle this situation before you find yourself in it. What do you think Sam could say to their colleague? How can Sam gain familiarity with this medication?

Verbal orders

Verbal orders should only be accepted in exceptional situations where patient care would be compromised by a delay. The prescriber should amend the chart as soon as possible, within a maximum of 24 hours (RPS and RCN, 2019). The changes should also be communicated in an appropriate secure electronic method to confirm the verbal instruction.

Verbal orders have a high rate of error due to many opportunities for misinterpretation to occur. As prescribers will no longer need to be in possession of the physical chart, the frequency of verbal orders should reduce. There should be a local protocol surrounding verbal orders; usually this will include:

- Two nurses independently receive the order.
- Both nurses repeat the intended medication and the dose back to the doctor.
- The name of the prescriber as well as the name and dose of the medication to be written down in the medical notes and nursing notes. This should be countersigned by both nurses who received the order.
- As it is an exceptional circumstance, an incident form should also be completed.

Drug calculations

Undertake accurate drug calculations for a range of medications: Discussion

Errors can occur at any stage of the process, but miscalculation is one of the most prevalent medicines administration errors (Wright and Shepherd, 2017). It occurs in all fields of nursing, and in all locations. It is imperative that all nurses understand how to minimise the potential for medication errors, as the impact can be fatal. It is recommended that all medicines that require calculations should be double checked, where practical to do so (RPS and RCN, 2019).

Most frequently, errors tend to be related to confusion about the units (micrograms, grams etc.), selecting the wrong equipment (syringe that measures millilitres instead of international units), or errors during calculation that result in an inaccurate dose or rate of delivery (RPS and RCN, 2019). A good understanding of the units that are used in medicine dosage is a good foundation to build from. Those most commonly used are listed in the table below.

Table 13.3   Units of measurement used in medicine dosage

Unit	Abbreviation	Description	Example
Grams	g	These measure the weight of the drug.	1g paracetamol
Milligrams	mg		600mg sodium valporate
Micrograms	Not recommended		25 micrograms levothyroxine
Nanograms	Not recommended		500 nanograms alfacalcidol
Litres	L (upper case)	These measure the volume of a solution.	1L sodium chloride
Millilitre	ml		10ml algenic acid
Standardised unit*	U or IU (recommended to be written as 'units' in full)	A unit is a measure of a specific therapeutic effect of a drug. This has been standardised so they can be prescribed in unit dosages.	7 units insulin
Millimols*	mmol	A standardised number of molecules of a substance.	Potassium chloride 30mmol in glucose 5% 1L
Ratio	e.g. 1:1000	Relationship between two quantities 1:1000	1:1000 adrenaline (1g adrenaline:1000ml solution)
Percentage	%	An amount out of a possible 100	Glucose 5% (5 parts glucose, 95 parts water).

Millimols, Units and International units are not converted to any other units. They should be calculated and administered within their same systems.

Source: Adapted from (Wright and Shepherd, 2017)

Nurses need to be competent at converting weights between units. Most frequent weights are noted in the table above, however patient weight may also need to be considered (typically measured in kilograms, kg). Calculations can be more complex if they are titrated to patient specific features such as weight. This can often be expressed as (dose)/kg. This is commonly seen in paediatrics.

Typically, medication doses are not unusual to the form they are available, particularly with oral medication. If your calculations suggest that you need to give a patient 15x1mg tablets, it seems likely that your calculations may contain an error, or that another dose may be available (1x10mg, 1x5mg, perhaps). Similarly, if your calculations suggest that you need to give ¾ of a tablet or 0.21 of a capsule, it is likely that there may be an error in the prescription or the calculation.

UNDERTAKE ACCURATE DRUG CALCULATIONS FOR A RANGE OF MEDICATIONS: STEP BY STEP

The best way to begin your calculations, is to start with PEACE - **P**lan, **E**stimate, **A**pproach, **C**alculate, **E**valuate (RNC, 2019).

- **Plan** - Consider what you are trying to achieve.
- **Estimate** - Use 'easier' or whole numbers to estimate what your final answer is likely to be.
- **Approach** - What method are you going to use to solve the problem? Do you need to follow a formula? Do you need a calculator? Do you need to convert any units? The nursing formula will be discussed below.
- **Calculate** - Perform the calculation. If using a calculator, be mindful of the numbers you are entering and ensure they are correct.
- **Evaluate** - Check the outcome. Is it similar to your estimate? If not, return to your initial step and check your workings. Double check all calculations with another member of staff.

When approaching the calculation, two common methods are:

Simple addition – Check the dose that the medication is available in (25 micrograms) and add this number to itself until it matches the required dose (75 micrograms). For this example, 25 micrograms + 25 micrograms + 25 micrograms = 75 micrograms = 3x25 microgram tablets. This method will only work for exact numbers, and is usually most suitable for oral medication. It can be a helpful way to make your estimations however.

The nursing formula – If the dose is not straightforward, you may need to make some calculations to ensure you administer the correct number amount. In order to do this, you can apply what is commonly called the nursing formula.

Ensure that all your units are the same before you begin your calculations (e.g. all in mg). If you try to make calculations in mixed units, your calculation will be incorrect.

What you want / What you've got = What you need

Next, insert the figures you have into the calculation above. What you want (the prescribed dose: 75 microgram) / What you have got (the dose available, 25 microgram) = 3 (3x25 microgram tablets).

Liquids

If you are trying to calculate liquid doses, they are often expressed as dose per volume, for example 5mg/ml. This denotes that there is 5mg of the active drug in each 1ml of fluid. In order to find out how many ml are needed, you will need to use the following formula:

1   Ensure the units for 'what you have got' and 'what you want' are the same.
2   Insert your figures into the following formula

   (What it's in/What you've got) x What you want = What you need

   e.g. (1ml/5mg) x 75mg = 15ml

IV infusions

IV infusions of medication can be administered via a gravity line, or through an electronic infusion controller. This is to ensure that it is administered at an appropriate speed. If delivered too quickly or too slowly, the medication may produce undesirable side effects, or may not be effective. Precision calculations are important to ensure the optimisation of IV medication.

If delivered through an electronic infusion or pump, the flow rate needs to be calculated. This is programmed into the pump and allows precise control.

1   Ensure your liquid volume is in ml and your time is in hours as your result will be expressed as ml/hr.
2   Insert your figures into the following calculation:

Volume (ml) / Time (hours) = Flow rate (ml/hr)

e.g. 100ml / 0.5 hours = 200ml/hr

If the medication is being delivered via a gravity line (no electronic pump), the drop rate needs to be calculated. The drop rate relates to the number of drops per minute through the chamber and is a way of setting the speed of an infusion. The following calculation should be used:

Drop factor x Volume / 60 x Time (hours) = Drop rate (drops per minute)

Drop factor is the number of drops that make 1ml. This is determined by the giving sets that are used and cannot be changed. It is noted on the packaging.
    Volume of the infusion to be administered.
    Time (in hours) that the infusion should be given over.
    Once this is calculated, the nurse adjusts the giving set to match the calculated drop rate.

ACTIVITY: PAUSE AND REFLECT

This section stresses the importance of competent maths skills. Mathematic ability isn't a genetic component; it is a skill. Like all skills, it can be learned and improved through practice and repetition. What is your current response to drug calculations? Usually, we avoid the things we are least likely to be good at or are worried about. Flex your maths skills and begin practising them in your clinical environments as soon as you are able to. Most universities also have an electronic medication administration or maths package that you can regularly access. These are particularly helpful as they help refine the skill of extracting the relevant information from products (the dose, the rate, etc.) as well as the calculation.

In practice, the two nurse check is to reduce the risk of medication calculation errors. However, this is less likely to be effective if the person is simply checking your sums: they need to work out the calculation independently and compare their answer with yours independently. Invite your colleague to check in a quiet area without distraction. Ask for their calculation, then to compare this with yours.

You will also be expected to check the calculations of those around you. It isn't about being able to pass a medication test in a classroom, it's about being confident in your skills to reduce your chance of error and being able to spot a mistake in a colleague's calculation, too.

STORAGE AND HANDLING OF MEDICATION

Undertake safe storage, transportation and disposal of medicinal products

All staff who handle medication need to be competent, appropriately trained and authorised to do so. If appropriate, medications and other substances should be stored in a manner that limits or prevents access to those who are not authorised. Professional guidance on this by The Royal Pharmaceutical Society (2019) highlights specific examples as outlined in Table 13.4.

Table 13.4   Storage of medication

Medicines should be stored in locked rooms or cupboards	To restrict unauthorised access
Medicines should be grouped by route of administration	To avoid drug administration error
Medicines with similar names should be clearly differentiated (in line with national risk circulars)	To avoid drug administration error
Where indicated, medicines stored in temperature controlled environments (e.g. fridge)	To prevent degradation
Environmental consideration when storing heavy medications such as large volumes of liquid or cylinders of gas	To prevent injury related to manual handling or fall

The safety considerations outlined above are important. The environment can contribute to the likelihood of an injury or error. Working in line with published guidance helps nurses to recognise, and take steps to minimise the risks. Due to the rotational nature of your student journey, you will be exposed to a variety of clinical environments. It may be appropriate to share good practice from previous areas, or to be curious about why things are different in each new area. There is no singular format or clinical room blueprint that would suit all areas, but small changes can make big improvements.

Storage of controlled drugs

It is important that all drugs are stored safely and securely, but additional legal requirements are in place for the safe storage of controlled drugs in clinical settings. There will be some differences, but the minimum standard ensures that controlled drugs are double checked and signed into the clinical environment. There will be a regular auditing of the stock, which is also checked by two registrants each time medication is signed out of their securely locked area. A controlled drug register accounts for controlled medication that is received, administered to patients, or wasted. Discrepancies should be reported urgently.

TECHNICAL SKILL

At this point of the chapter you should be aware of the safeguards in place to ensure that medication is safe to use, produced and stored appropriately, and has been prescribed appropriately. The final steps are to administer the medication to the patient. The Five Rights (Federico, 2014) outline the essentials of good practice which should be adhered to at each episode of medicine administration and with every patient.

The Five Rights of medication administration

1   **Patient** – Check the name on the prescription and then ask the patient to tell you their name. If they are unable to provide this, it can be confirmed by their wristband in an inpatient setting.
2   **Medicine** – Check the prescription and check the label on the medication to ensure it is what you think it is.

3   **Route** – Does the route match the route prescribed? Is it an appropriate route for the patient? This can change dependent on the patient's condition and may need to be reconsidered if it is no longer appropriate.

4   **Time** – When is it due to be given? What is the frequency of the dose? When was it last given? Ensure the medication hasn't also been administered as a one-off dose or 'as required' (also known as PRN).

5   **Dose** – Calculate the appropriate dose (if needed). Is it an appropriate dose for the patient and the condition?

Additional steps have been proposed to this process (Martyn, et al. 2019), some of which include:

1   **Documentation** – Be sure to document immediately after the medication has been administered. This should include your signature and any other specific information that is needed.

2   **Reason** – Confirming the reason for the medication and questioning if it is still required. This is an important part of antibiotics stewardship and issues related to poly pharmacy.

3   **Response** – Has it had the right response? Review the patient to ensure it has had the desired effect and that they are not experiencing any unpleasant side effects.

These steps should be adhered to for every patient at every administration opportunity in order to minimise risk.

Medication given, withheld or denied

In order to account for the administration, the healthcare employee must observe the patient taking the medicine before recording their signature. If the medicine or fluid is given as an intermittent or continuous infusion, the administration chart should be signed immediately after the infusion has commenced.

ACTIVITY: PAUSE AND REFLECT

Take some time to plan how you can maximise learning opportunity in your placement. Often, students carry a small notebook with them and write down terms to look up later. On the first medication rounds, focus on the task you are doing. In subsequent weeks aim to highlight 1-2 medications that are frequently used.

Name of drug	What is it used for?	Typical dose	Cautions or contraindications	Common side effects

Self-administration

Where it is suitable, patients should be encouraged to self-administer medication. If they are in a hospital, this encourages independence with medication when they return to their home. If they are in a care home or are a long-term inpatient, it helps to maintain their independence and maintain active participation in their own health and treatment.

When in an inpatient setting, all patients' own medications should be stored securely (RPS, 2017a) and at the earliest opportunity, staff should aim to encourage and support self-administration, where appropriate (RPS, 2017a) Each area will have specific risk assessments and local policies to ensure the suitability and safety of individual patients, as well as the safety of others within the clinical area.

Considerations:

- Is the patient willing and able to safely self-administer medication?
- Are they currently well enough?
- Is the patient confused, forgetful or disorientated?
- Has the patient got a history of drug or alcohol abuse?
- Is the patient at risk of using medications for self-harm or suicide?
- Has the patient got the dexterity to open the storage locker and the packaging of the medications?
- Does the patient know what their medication is for, the dose, the instructions for safe use and the side effects?

(Lister et al., 2020)

CASE STUDY

Salma

Salma is a 51-year-old patient who has been an inpatient at an acute hospital for three days. She is waiting for surgery and likely to remain in hospital for at least the next ten days. Before admission, she was independent with her medication and had been taking them regularly for her long-term conditions for over ten years. Her wife speaks with you at visiting time and lets you know that Salma would like to take her own medication for the rest of her time as an inpatient. She told her wife that she is often in pain between medication rounds, so would prefer to self-administer.

Questions

You speak with Salma who confirms what her wife told you. What information do you need to consider about Salma to decide if this is suitable for her? If it is not suitable, what else can be done to address Salma's concerns?

ADMINISTERING MEDICATIONS USING A RANGE OF ROUTES: DISCUSSION

The route by which a medication is being administered (e.g. oral, intravenous or topical) and the formulation (e.g. liquid, capsule, or tablet) influences how the medication is available to the body. This is known as bioavailability. Bioavailability of IV medication is higher than oral or other routes, due to it being immediately in systemic circulation. This is seen in the rapid relief of pain with an IV opioid, compared to the 15–45 minutes of an oral tablet. If the medication is absorbed well through the gastrointestinal mucosa the IV and oral dose is the same, however this isn't usually the case. As a result, most oral doses are higher than doses given parenterally (administered in a way that does not involve the alimentary canal) (Shepherd and Shepherd, 2020).

KEY TERMS

EPMA: Electronic prescription and medicines administration

PGD: Patient Group Directive

POM: Prescription Only Medication

Topical: medication that is applied to the skin

Oral administration

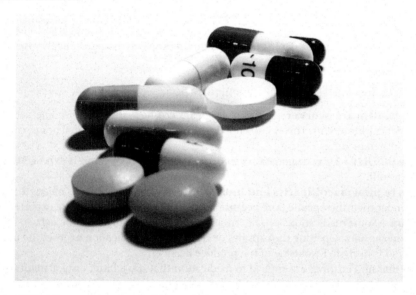

Figure 13.1   Tablet, capsule, and wafer preparations

Source: WordPress.org/e-MagineArt.com (CC BY 2.0)

The oral route is the most frequently used, most convenient and most cost effective route of medication administration (Lister et al., 2020). Preparations can be in a variety of forms, including tablet, capsule, powder (for suspension) and liquid. Wafer preparations are also available for some medications to assist with rapid administration, without needing to be swallowed. This is helpful for the migraine medication rizatriptan, as migraine sufferers can also have nausea (Shepherd and Shepherd, 2020). Olanzipine wafers are also available for treatment of schizophrenia. Wafer preparations can help when providing essential medication to someone who may be resistive to treatment when acutely unwell as they melt quickly and are absorbed through the membranes in the mouth (Shepherd and Shepherd, 2020).

Splitting and crushing of tablets

Some medication is able to be safely crushed or split, but not all. This may be considered because of swallowing difficulties or to obtain a smaller dose, such as cutting a 5mg tablet in half to have a 2.5mg dose. Crushing or splitting medication can cause undesirable effects or an increase in side effects, changes to the absorption of the medication, or harm to those in the environment. If a solid tablet is scored in the middle, this is usually an indicator that it can be safely cut. You are likely to get the most accurate cut by using a pill cutter. A pharmacist is able to advise on suitability for adjusting specific medications but you may also want to consult local guidelines. The NEWT guidelines have been produced by Wrexham Hospital Pharmacy to provide guidance for administration of medication to patients with enteral feeding tubes or those with swallowing difficulties (Wrexham Maelor Hospital Pharmacy Department, 2019). Covert administration of medication, such as crushing medication into food, should not be standard practice. This should not occur unless they have been assessed and deemed to be lacking capacity to make decisions about their health at that time, and that administering the medication covertly is in their best interest. Consent can be provided by parents of children under the age of 18, or Gillick competency can be used if the child is able to understand and consent to treatment. It should be assumed that all adults have capacity, unless deemed otherwise. It is important to understand that capacity is a fluid and changeable state, rather than fixed. Decisions around capacity should include staff who have a very good understanding of the Mental Capacity Act and Deprivation of Liberty Safeguards (DoLS) to make sure that capacity is appropriately assessed.

What are the issues with modifying oral medication?

- **Risk to healthcare workers** – When drugs are crushed, they can become aerosolised and inhaled by healthcare staff. This is known to be problematic with hormonal drugs, corticosteroids and chemotherapy drugs.
- **Drug instability** – Drug degradation can occur when the medication is exposed to light when crushed or split.
- **Changes in pharmacokinetics and bioavailability** – Put simply, this means that the patient may be under their therapeutic dose because it has not been absorbed in the expected area.
- **Irritation** – Some medications can be irritating to the oesophagus or stomach, so are coated or enclosed in capsules. Opening the capsules or crushing the medication exposes the irritant to the patient, and is likely to be outside of the produce licence.
- **Taste** – Films and coatings are applied to medication that has a bitter taste. Patients may decline to take a medication if it is bitter or unpleasant to taste.

(RPS, 2019)

Release

Medication can have specific coatings to adjust the way in which it as available for absorption within the body. Immediate release is most common. This kind of medication will dissolve in the acidic stomach environment and be immediately available for absorption. Enteric coating is a specific coating to prevent the medication being dissolved in the acidic stomach, usually becoming available in the intestinal tract (Long and Yisheng, 2009). The coating is to prevent irritation or to create a delay until it has reached a specific site in the GI tract, such as when treating Crohn's Disease.

Extended-release products release a drug over a longer period of time – usually over 12 to 24 hours. The aim is to produce a constant plasma drug concentration over the period that the drug is released. It can often be identified by these abbreviations after the product name:

CR Controlled Release

ER Extended Release

LA Long Acting

SR Slow Release

XL Extra Long

XR Extended Release

These types of medication should never be crushed, split or modified as this has the potential for a large bolus dose being delivered rather than a controlled release over the intended timescale, resulting in a potentially toxic dose of medication and an increased risk of adverse effects. It will also result in under dosing later in the timescale, reducing clinical effectiveness of the prescribed medication (RPS, 2011).

Alternatives to crushing or splitting medication

If the medication is not suitable to be modified in any way, it may be more appropriate to request the medication in a different dose. A pharmacist can help you to identify if it is available as a liquid suspension or via an alternative route, such as injection.

Alternative oral route - enteral tubes

Percutaneous Endoscopy Gastronomy (PEG), Nasogastric (NG) and Nasojejunal (NJ) tubes are commonly used enteral tubes. These may be used short or long term. Formulations for this route should be carefully considered, as not all oral formulations are licensed to be administered in this way and some are inappropriate (Boyd, 2013).

Advice should be sought from a pharmacist, or by consulting specialist guidelines such as NEWT Guidelines (www.newtguidelines.com).

Topical and transdermal

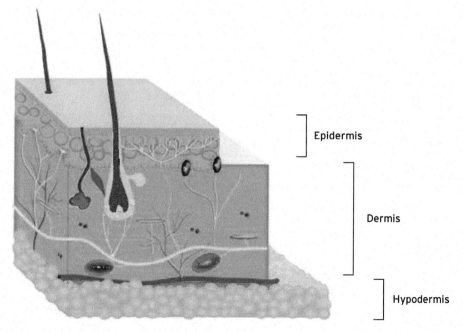

Figure 13.2   Skin layers

Anatomy and physiology recap

The skin is the largest organ of the body. It has a number of functions, including protecting the body from pathogens and helping to regulate temperature. The skin is made up of three distinct layers, as seen in Figure 13.2. The epidermis is the outermost layer of skin. This is a protective, waterproof barrier. The dermis is the middle layer. It contains hair follicles, nerves and blood vessels. The subcutaneous or hypodermis is the innermost layer, and is known as the fatty layer. This cushions muscles and bones as well as connecting the skin to muscles and bones via connective tissue. Blood vessels become larger within this layer, leading to faster absorption.

Discussion

Topical medication is applied to skin and absorbed through the derma or mucous membranes. There are a wide range of formulations, including drops, creams, patches, gels, foams, pastes and powders. Topical formulations tend to have a localised effect, such as antifungal cream, whilst transdermal preparations have systemic effects such as testosterone gel or nicotine patches. As these preparations are designed to penetrate the skin, it is necessary to wear gloves if you are applying these for a patient. Patches deliver a specific controlled dose over a specified period of time. This can vary from one day for nicotine patches, to seven days for the contraceptive patch. They need to be applied to hairless areas of skin, to ensure adhesion of the entire patch to the skin. Where possible, patient education and self-administration are encouraged, particularly if the patient will need to continue to use the medication at home without support.

It is important that the purpose of the medication is known, to ensure appropriate considerations can be made, for example if the medication is suitable for use on broken skin. If the preparation isn't designed to be used on damaged skin it can cause irritation to skin tissue or be absorbed too quickly (Potter et al., 2017). Additionally, it may be beneficial for the patient to have the application as part of their usual hygiene routine (e.g. just after a shower).

TOPICAL MEDICATION: STEP BY STEP

EQUIPMENT

- Appropriate PPE
- Medication
- Applicator if recommended
- Any recommended aftercare (e.g. dressing)

PROCEDURE

- Explain the procedure and gain consent. Where possible, fully informed consent should be sought to gain co-operation and build trust. This may not be possible in emergency situations, or when a patient does not have capacity to consent, such as a child without Gillick competence or someone with impaired mental capacity. Family and carers should be involved where possible.
- Check the prescription and gather supplies.
- Communicate what you are doing to the patient as you are doing it.
- Maintain privacy and dignity by closing doors or bedside curtains. Assist the patient into a comfortable position if assistance is needed and expose the area required. Use towels or sheets for modesty, if required. Be sensitive to the needs of the individual patient you are treating.

- Perform hand hygiene and don PPE as appropriate. Glove use is likely to be required as the medication is designed to penetrate the skin, and the nurse will need to be protected from this.

- Perform the Five Rights of medication administration (Federico, 2014).

- Assess the condition of the skin. Check the skin in the area you are planning to apply the medication, remove the previous patch and wash and dry skin if required, then apply as directed. Skin should be observed for changes to skin colour, tone or texture. Compare to the skin in other, untreated areas of the body. It is important to follow prescriber instructions, such as using a specific length of cream or gel, to ensure consistent dosage (Pastore et al., 2015; Lister et al., 2020).

- Record administration and document its effect if appropriate.

Important considerations

Patches can result in irritant and/or allergic contact dermatitis from the drug and the agents within the patch (Pastore et al., 2015). This is more likely if application is repeatedly on the same site. It is advised that the position of a patch is changed regularly to reduce risk of irritation (Jevon et al., 2010). Clinicians should be vigilant for irritation and act accordingly (see adverse drug reactions).

Table 13.5   Irritant or allergic reaction?

Feature	Irritant	Allergic
Location	Defined border - only where contact was made with irritant	Initially at site of exposure, then spreading
Symptoms	Burning, itching, pain	Itching is the dominant symptom
Surface appearance	Erythema, blisters, pustules, bleeding, crusting, scaling; irritated skin	Irritated skin; oedema, blistering
Onset	Usually rapid	Usually delayed (12-72 hours)

(Novak-Bili et al., 2018)

Nasal spray/drops: Discussion

Nasal drops and sprays can be used for local or systemic effect. The mucous membranes are highly vascular, so it is a suitable route for rapid absorption. They can be particularly useful for patients who are unable to take oral medication.

NASAL SPRAY/DROPS: STEP BY STEP

EQUIPMENT

- Medication
- Tissues

(Continued)

PROCEDURE

- Explain the procedure and gain consent. Where possible, fully informed consent should be sought to gain co-operation and build trust. This may not be possible in emergency situations, or when a patient does not have capacity to consent, such as a child without Gillick competence or someone with impaired mental capacity. Family and carers should be involved where possible.

- Check the prescription and gather supplies.

- Prepare the patient. Outline the posture they will need to adopt. If possible, the patient should sit down or lay on their back, with their neck hyperextended. Ensure that they are aware that it is preferred that they remain in this position for 2–3 minutes after administration to aid absorption. Encourage them to clear their nose into a tissue before administration.

- Ensure the appropriate hand hygiene and the Five Rights of medication administration (Federico, 2014) have been completed.

- Communicate what you are doing to the patient as you are doing it.

- Insert nozzle or dropper into nostril and apply specified amount.

- Retain position. Encourage patient to stay in position for 2–3 mins.

- Record administration appropriately.

Ottic drops

WATCH THE VIDEO

ADMINISTERING EAR DROPS

Watch along as you read through this step by step procedure by scanning the QR code with your smartphone camera or via https://study.sagepub.com/rowberry.

This is very helpful in demonstrating the slight upward extension of the patient's ear.

OTTIC DROPS: STEP BY STEP

EQUIPMENT

- Medication
- Tissues or cotton wool for excess drops

PROCEDURE

- Explain the procedure and gain consent. Where possible fully informed consent should be sought to gain co-operation and build trust. This may not be possible in emergency situations, or when a patient does not have capacity to consent, such as a child without Gillick competence or someone with impaired mental capacity. Family and carers should be involved where possible.

- Check the prescription and gather supplies.

- Prepare the patient. Outline the posture they will need to adopt; they may be more comfortable lying on one side with their affected ear exposed. Ensure that they are aware that it is preferred that they remain in this position for 2–3 minutes after administration to aid absorption.

- Ensure the appropriate hand hygiene and the Five Rights of medication administration (Federico, 2014) have been completed.

- Communicate what you are doing to the patient as you are doing it. Extend the pinna upwards with forefinger and thumb to increase the volume of ear canal (Lister et al., 2020). Avoid touching the dropper to the ear canal, to prevent contamination (Jevon et al., 2010).

- Insert nozzle or dropper into ear canal and apply specified amount.

- Retain position. Encourage patient to stay in position for a few minutes.

- Record administration appropriately.

Optic drops

WATCH THE VIDEO

ADMINISTERING EYE DROPS

Watch along as you read through this step by step procedure by scanning the QR code with your smartphone camera or via https://study.sagepub.com/rowberry.

OPTIC DROPS: STEP BY STEP

EQUIPMENT

- PPE including gloves
- Medication
- Saline and cotton wool for cleaning if appropriate

(Continued)

PROCEDURE

- Explain the procedure and gain consent. Where possible, fully informed consent should be sought to gain co-operation and build trust. This may not be possible in emergency situations, or when a patient does not have capacity to consent, such as a child without Gillick competence or someone with impaired mental capacity. Family and carers should be involved where possible.

- Check the prescription and gather supplies.

- Prepare the patient. Outline the posture they will need to adopt; they may be more comfortable sitting in a chair or lying in bed. Check if the patient has contact lenses, which may need to be removed. Compare the prescription with the patient's expectations, for example if they are expecting one or both eyes to be treated.

- Ensure the appropriate hand hygiene and the Five Rights of medication administration (Federico, 2014) have been completed. Don PPE if required.

- Communicate what you are doing to the patient as you are doing it. If the eye needs to be cleaned prior to drops being administered, use balls of saline-soaked cotton wool in a single sweeping motion from inside to outside (Jevon et al., 2010).

- Prepare the eye and administer. Gently pull the lower lid down with a downward motion on the under eye/cheek area. Ensure that the dropper does not become contaminated by touching the eye (Jevon et al., 2010), but refrain from dropping from a height, as this can be painful (Lister et al., 2020). Encourage the patient to blink between drops if more than one is required.

- Assist the patient into a comfortable position. Remove and discard PPE.

- Record administration appropriately.

CASE STUDY

Toyo

Toyo is 18 years old and needs eye drops for an eye infection. His carer is struggling to administer drops to him. Toyo is autistic, and has sensory difficulties as a result of this. He finds it overwhelming to have close contact and has previously told you he feels like he can 'hear, smell and see things much better than other people'. Toyo explains to you that he can smell his carer's breath when they get close to him, and that pulling down his eyelid feels like his skin is burning. Toyo has declined to have any more treatment and begins to cry when you enter the room with his medication. You explain that without the drops, his infection may last longer or get worse. He wants to feel better and asks you if there is anything that may help to make it easier, or even if he could do it himself. Your colleagues are in disagreement about Toyo being able to administer this medication with support because of his autism.

Questions

1   An estimated 1:57 children are diagnosed with autism. What is your current level of knowledge about autism? What do you think could help Toyo to have his medication?
2   Toyo has been able to pinpoint and verbalise the specific difficulties he is having with the procedure. Consider how you would be able to manage this situation with someone who was not able to communicate in this way.

Rectal

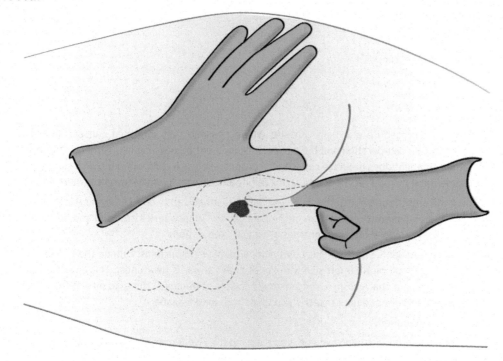

Figure 13.3 Rectal administration

Source: Wikimedia Commons/British Columbia Institute of Technology (BCIT) (CC BY 4.0)

This route of administration is understandably unpopular with patients, and likely to be indicated only when there is a lack of consciousness, or nausea and vomiting prevents oral preparations being administered. It is also useful for if patients are at risk of aspiration from when experiencing seizures. Many antipyretics, anti-inflammatory drugs, antiemetic and anticonvulsive drugs are available as rectal suppository formulations. The active drug can be administered in two forms; suppository or an enema. A suppository is a small and solid preparation. It has a blunt end and a tapered tip, similar in shape to a bullet. An enema is a liquid formulation. The distal end of the rectum is sensitive to pain, touch and temperature, but above it is only sensitive to stretch, so the medication should not cause any pain once it has been carefully situated (Lowry, 2016). A suggestion to overcome the embarrassment associated with this route is to teach self-administration, where appropriate (Hanning et al., 2020).

ADMINISTERING RECTAL MEDICATION: STEP BY STEP

EQUIPMENT

- Appropriate personal protective equipment
- Clinical waste bag
- Absorbent pad in case of discharge

(Continued)

- Gauze swabs or tissues
- Bedpan, or access to a toilet if required
- Prescription chart
- Medication as prescribed
- Lubricant

PREPARE THE PATIENT

- Explain the procedure and gain consent. Where possible fully informed consent should be sought to gain co-operation and build trust. This may not be possible in emergency situations, or when a patient does not have capacity to consent, such as a child without Gillick competence or someone with impaired mental capacity. Family and carers should be involved where possible.
- Check the prescription and gather supplies. Set up the medication on a clean and stable surface. The next step depends on the form of the medication. Suppositories are solid and designed to melt at body temperature while enemas are liquid preparations.
- Prepare the patient. Ensure privacy and dignity by drawing curtains. Outline the posture they will need to adopt: on their left side with knees drawn towards their chest. This enables gravity assisted flow into the rectum. Use blankets or towels to minimise the exposure of the patient. Place an absorbent pad underneath the patient in case of leakage.
- Don PPE as required.
- Ensure the appropriate hand hygiene is applied and the Five Rights of medication administration (Federico, 2014) have been completed.
- Communicate what you are doing to the patient as you are doing it. Communicate with your patient throughout, explaining the actions you will be taking prior to carrying them out. Be sure that the patient can hear you, as they will be facing away from you.
- Inspect the area. The perianal area should be observed for signs of irritation, infection, infestation, bleeding or structures such as skin tags and haemorrhoids. These are not contraindications, but you may need to seek advice before continuing (Lowry, 2012). If these are noted or absent, it should be documented in the notes.
- Administer medication in line with recommendations below.
- Record administration appropriately, as well as the medication effect if necessary.

IF THE MEDICATION IS IN A SOLID FORM (SUPPOSITORY)

- Apply lubricant onto the tapered end of the suppository. Manufacturers usually recommend inserting this end first (Lowry, 2012).
- Ask the patient to relax and take long slow breaths to help them.
- Part the buttocks and gently insert the suppository into the anus with a gloved index finger. It should be inserted tapered end first (Lowry, 2012), 2-4cm in depth (Shepherd and Shepherd, 2020) in order to reach the distal rectum, just above the internal anal sphincter and the anorectal ring (Schellack, 2011).
- Wipe excess lubrication away from the anus for the comfort of the patient.
- Place all used equipment in a clinical waste bag, remove PPE and wash hands.
- Encourage the patient to retain the suppository for at least 20 minutes, if comfortable, for absorption. When leaving the patient, ensure that they are comfortable and have the call bell in reach in case it is required.
- Document that you have administered the medication and its result.

IF THE MEDICATION IS IN A LIQUID FORM (ENEMA)

- Apply lubricant onto the tip and length of the enema nozzle.
- Part the buttocks with one hand and hold the nozzle of the enema with the other. Gently insert the tip into the anal canal.
- Slowly squeeze the bag or pack until empty. While still squeezing (which helps to avoid any re-entry of contents due to a vacuum effect in the enema) gently withdraw the nozzle.
- Following administration, dispose of used equipment and perform hand hygiene. Check the patient is in a dignified and comfortable position with a call bell in reach before you leave them.
- Document that you have administered the medication and its result.

It is important to note that there are two main types of enema; evacuant and retention. An evacuant should be held in place as long as possible and will likely have a rapid effect. A retention enema should be kept in place to absorb through the mucous membranes, usually at least 30 minutes.

Vaginal

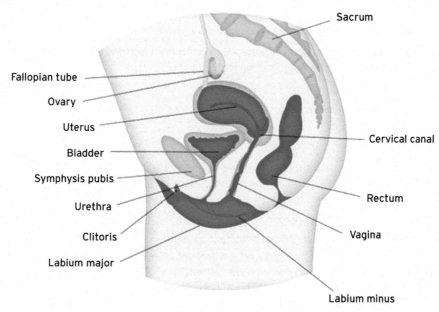

Figure 13.4 Vaginal anatomy

Anatomy and physiology recap

The vagina is an elastic, muscular, flexible canal. This curved organ is typically 8–12cm from the vulva to the cervix. It is comprised of the entrance, a transition zone and a wider forniceal zone (upper portion) (Minkin and Mirkin, 2021). When standing, the vagina is a largely horizontal tube, rather than the vertical depiction often seen in medical illustrations (Alexander et al., 2004), making retention of medicines likely. The initial quarter of the vagina receives sensory input from peripheral nerves, but the remaining ¾ of the vagina is a largely insensitive area (Alexander et al., 2004; Minkin and Mirkin, 2021). Nerves detect stretch, but are not sensitive to localised sensation, as demonstrated by tampon users not feeling them once in-situ. External genitalia can naturally vary in shape, size and colour, but it is important to be observant for signs of female genital mutilation. As a healthcare professional, you have a duty to notify police if you become aware of this due to the Female Genital Mutilation Act 2003.

Discussion

Vaginal medication is available in a variety of forms including gels, pessaries (sometimes referred to as vaginal suppositories), foam and devices such as hormonal rings. This route of administration has traditionally been seen as a method of local action, such as combatting vaginal thrush, but there is a growing interest in vaginal administration for systemic use (Minkin and Mirkin, 2021). This route has a steady absorption rate through vaginal epithelium into the systemic circulation. Additionally, it is not metabolised by the liver, so smaller doses can be used, which often reduces the impact of unwanted side effects (Alexander et al., 2004).

———— VAGINAL ADMINISTRATION: STEP BY STEP ————

EQUIPMENT

- Personal protective equipment including non sterile gloves
- Medication (and any equipment recommended by the manufacturer, e.g. warm water to clean external genitals before use or lubrication for pessary)
- Sanitary pad
- Bedsheets/cover for privacy

PROCEDURE

- Introduce yourself and explain the procedure and what it is for. Let the patient know that they need clothing removed from their lower half. Ensure good communication of your actions throughout, as the patient is unable to see what you are doing during this intimate procedure.
- Explain the procedure in an appropriate way that the patient will understand and gain consent.
- Outline the posture they will need to adopt and assist if necessary. The position is a modified lithotomy - on their back with knees bent and relaxed outwards. If the patient is unable to get into this position, a left lateral position is also acceptable (Potter et al., 2017). This enables good visualisation of the external genitalia. This will help to identify any tissue damage or structural anomalies, or evidence of infection.
- Ensure privacy and dignity by drawing curtains and using blankets or towels to minimise the exposure of the patient.
- Ensure the appropriate hand hygiene, and Five Rights of medication administration (Federico, 2014) have been completed.
- Insert medication in line with manufacturer guidelines, using its included applicator, if appropriate. It is important to ensure medication is deposited in the correct area of the vagina. Overall, the lower portion is more appropriate for localised response, whereas high vaginal application is more likely to result in systemic exposure (Alexander et al., 2004). High vaginal administration is typically the length of an entire index finger (Lister et al., 2020).

- Ensure patient comfort by wiping the vulva or providing wipes to remove any excess lubrication. Advise the patient if they may experience any discharge and provide a sanitary pad.

SELF-ADMINISTRATION

- If appropriate, patients are able to self-administer. Ensure that you provide clear, unambiguous guidance to ensure insertion into the vagina rather than being held within labial folds or inserted into the anus mistakenly (Potter et al., 2017). Use of a model or a diagram may be helpful to describe each step.
- Following administration, dispose of used equipment and perform hand hygiene. Check the patient is in a dignified and comfortable position before you leave.
- Document the medication that has been administered and any relevant observations.

Pulmonary/inhaled

Medications can be inhaled to deliver medication directly to the lungs. This approach works rapidly, requires lower doses than systemic administration and has fewer adverse effects (Braido et al., 2016). The most common devices for this are Pressurised Metered-Dose Inhalers (pMDIs), Dry-Powder Inhalers (DPIs), Soft Mist Inhalers (SMI) and liquids for nebulisation.

Pressurised metered-dose inhalers

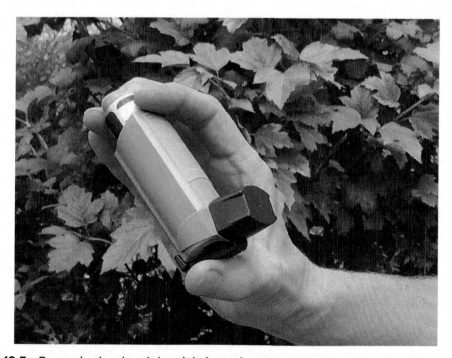

Figure 13.5   Pressurised metered-dose inhaler and spacer

Source: Shutterstock/Fahroni

These devices deliver a single precise and pressurised dose when the canister is pressed. They require a level of dexterity from the patient, as they need to coordinate their breathing and pressing the canister. pMDIs can be used with a spacer if they find this difficult. The spacer elongates the time that the medication is available to be inhaled, by containing it in a space.

Dry powder inhalers

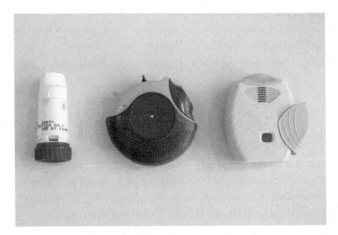

Figure 13.6   Dry powder inhaler

Source: Wikimedia Commons/BrettMontgomery(CC BY-SA 4.0)

The dose does not need to be coordinated manually, as these inhalers are activated by the patient's sharp intake of breath whilst the inhaler is in their mouth. A dose is prepared by twisting or otherwise preparing the device, prior to being put in the mouth.

Soft mist inhalers

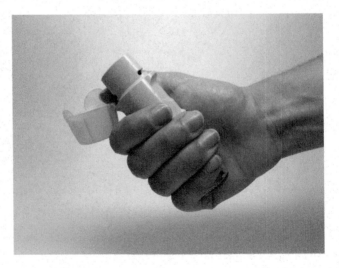

Figure 13.7   Soft mist inhaler

Source: WordPress.org/NIAID (CC BY 2.0)

These newer inhaler devices deliver fine mist at a slower speed. This reduces the importance of coordinating actuation and inhalation, because the mist is available for deep inhalation for longer than its aerosolised competitors (pMDIs) (Iwanaga, 2019).

Nebuliser

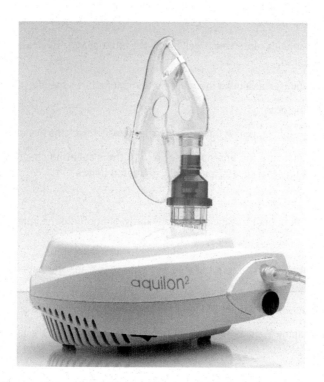

Figure 13.8 Nebuliser machine, mask, tubing, dosing chamber

Source: Wikimedia Commons/Trainer2a (CC BY-SA 3.0)

A nebuliser is a device that forces air through liquid medication to turn it into a fine mist for inhalation through a face mask. It is usually used in emergency situations, in treatment of severe lung conditions and if the patient is unable to use an inhaler.

INHALED MEDICATION ADMINISTRATION: STEP BY STEP

PREPARE THE PATIENT

Patient education is paramount for this method of administration. Patients and their families/carers will need to know how to care for the equipment as well as how and when to use it. Research suggests that patients overestimate their confidence in their inhaler technique, so routine checking and education can help patients to manage their pulmonary conditions more competently (Litt et al., 2020). The patient's posture and breathing pattern can help to deliver more of the medication

(Continued)

directly to the lungs, so an upright seated position is recommended to encourage full lung expansion. If the inhaler contains steroids, the patient should be advised to rinse their mouth after administration to reduce the risk of oral thrush. Prior to administration, ensure hand hygiene, appropriate PPE and the Five Rights of medication administration checks are completed (Federico, 2014).

ADMINISTRATION

1   Prepare the inhaler device

- Remove the inhaler cap, shake it well to mix the product and attach a suitable spacer to the pMDI, if required.

- If using a nebuliser, assemble the machine to manufacturer specifications.

2   Prepare or load the dose

- Inhaler – if the inhaler is new, it may need to be primed. Check the manufacturer instructions.

- Nebuliser – measure the appropriate dose into the dispensing chamber. Do not combine medications together unless specifically instructed to mix.

3   Exhale

- Encourage the patient to exhale fully and gently, but not into the inhaler.

4   Adjust position

- Whilst maintaining the upright seated position, encourage the patient to tilt the chin up slightly.

- Inhaler – instruct the patient to insert the mouthpiece and create a seal with their lips.

- Nebuliser – apply the mask with a secure and comfortable fit to the face.

5   Inhale

- pMDI – the canister is depressed completely at the start of a slow inhalation.

- SMI – the inhaler is activated by pressing a button on the chamber at the start of a slow inhalation.

- DPI – this device is activated by a quick, deep inhalation.

- Nebuliser – the machine is turned to the 'on' position and the patient should take slow and steady breaths until the nebulised medication is completed (approximately 4ml/10 min (Lister et al., 2020).

6   Remove the inhaler

- pMDI, SMI, or DPI – once the dose is administered, remove the device and encourage the patient to hold their breath for up to 10 seconds, if they are able to.

- Nebuliser – switch off the nebuliser and remove the mask.

7   Repeat if required

- Wait for a few seconds then repeat if necessary.

Source: Based on *Seven Steps to Using an Inhaler Device* (Scullion and Fletcher, 2019).

- Document the medication that has been administered and any relevant observations.

GO FURTHER

Good inhaler technique can prevent flare ups and help patients to manage their chronic conditions. All nurses are encouraged to routinely check patients' inhaler technique and provide education where beneficial. Visit https://www.asthma.org.uk/advice/inhaler-videos/ to see demonstrations of specific inhaler techniques to support your skills.

Good communication with patients can also allow you to understand why patients may be reluctant to use their inhaler, such as if they are fasting for Ramadan. Nurses can demonstrate cultural competence by being sympathetic to this concern, and checking with reputable authorities such as The British Islamic Medical Association (https://www.britishima.org).

Injections and infusions

Administering injections using intramuscular, subcutaneous, intradermal and intravenous routes and managing injection equipment: Discussion

A safe injection is one that:

- does not harm the recipient
- does not expose the provider to any avoidable risk
- does not result in any waste that is dangerous for other people. (WHO, 2003)

Injections are usually administered for rapid absorption, to bypass the stomach and GI system, or when accurate doses of medication are required. However, injections can be painful and invasive, particularly if they need to be administered repeatedly (Shepherd, 2018). If the medication can be delivered by another route, this should be considered in order to minimise discomfort and risk to the patient. The physical skill of administering an injection is important, as the correct technique can minimise the risk of injury to the patient.

Needle fear affects 33%–63% of children and 14%–38% of adults (Taddio et al., 2012; Deacon and Abramowitz, 2016). This can be from poor previous experiences or an expectation of pain (Jenkins, 2014). It is important to consider the psychological impact of this intervention, especially in young patients, those with learning or cognition difficulties or those with a pre-existing needle fear. If the nurse is able to provide clear and appropriate communication, this may improve the patient's needle fear for future interventions.

Injections are suitable for administering small volumes over a short period of time. Sometimes the volume needs to be larger to administer a larger dose, to dilute the medication or to administer it over a longer period of time. This is known as an infusion and will be covered later in the chapter.

ACTIVITY: PAUSE AND REFLECT

Your approach and communication skills may help patients to feel more comfortable with an injection. Often adult patients can be engaged in small talk as a method to distract away from the task in hand. Asking the patient to take a few deep breaths or to relax their muscle intentionally can also

(Continued)

be helpful. In young patients, their family can be involved to distract, however there is some sugges-tion that combining a comforting family member with a distracting TV show can be more successful (Bellieni et al., 2006).

Consider your most recent placement area. Do you recall any patients who were cautious, upset or worried about having an injection?

How did the staff deal with patients who were nervous? What communication and distraction techniques could you add to your own skill set? Consider how you could adapt these techniques to make them suitable for patients who are particularly vulnerable, such as those with learning or cognitive difficulties?

Skin preparation

Swabbing the skin prior to injection is common in many areas, but the subject of much controversy. It is argued that using a single use 70% alcohol wipe on skin before an injection is unnecessary, as it does not eliminate skin flora because of the limited contact time (usually less than 30 seconds). In addition, most bacteria in skin flora is likely to be non-pathogenic and introduced in a lower than minimal infectious amount. The consensus from The World Health Organization (WHO, 2010) and UK Department of Health (Salisbury et al., 2013) is that skin should be visibly clean prior to injection.

Which site?

Most commonly, injections are given intradermal (just below the level of the dermis), subcutaneous (into the adipose tissue below the dermis and epidermis), intramuscular (into the muscle fascia), or intravenous (into the vein). Each route has specific benefits and cautions to be aware of.

Administering injections using intradermal, subcutaneous, intramuscular, and intravenous routes and managing injection equipment

Intradermal injections

Intradermal injections have a local rather than a systemic effect (Jevon et al., 2010). They are usually for local anaesthetic or diagnostic purposes, such as allergy or TB testing. This method is used as the injection into the dermis is absorbed slowly, because of the skin layer's limited blood supply. The inner forearm or the upper back are typically used as they are hairless sites, making observation of reactions more reliable.

INTRADERMAL: STEP BY STEP

EQUIPMENT

- PPE
- Medication

- Needle (25 or 27G)
- 1ml syringe
- Alcohol swab
- Sharps bin

PREPARE THE PATIENT

- 'Hello, my name is...' and discussion with patient about the procedure to ensure informed consent is obtained.
- Ensure the appropriate hand hygiene, preparation of medication and pre-administration checks have been completed.
- Gather appropriate equipment and draw up appropriately.
- Ensure patient dignity is maintained by drawing curtains and minimal adjustments to clothing. Ensure modesty is preserved with a separate item of clothing, towel or sheet if appropriate. Consider the suitability of distraction techniques.
- Check the intended site to make sure that the area is visibly clean. Additional cleaning is only required if the area is visibly dirty. Routine disinfection is not required.

ADMINISTRATION

- When the patient is ready, visualise the area you intend to use to ensure suitability. Communicate with your patient as each action is performed.
- Pull the skin taut with non-dominant hand to stretch the skin.
- Insert the needle (bevel facing up) at a 5-15 degree angle until the bevel is just under the epidermis. There is no need to aspirate, as this is a largely avascular site (Potter et al., 2017).
- Administer the injection slowly - a wheal or bubble will be apparent at the skin surface. This is often referred to as a 'bleb'. Do not use more than 0.1ml unless confirmed (Love, 2006), but up to 0.5ml is typical (Jevon et al., 2010).
- Once completed, remove the needle at the same angle it was inserted.
- Dispose of the sharps immediately. Do not resheath a used needle to reduce the risk of a needlestick injury. Remember that gloves are not protection against needlestick injuries so are not routinely recommended for injections (WHO, 2010).
- Perform hand hygiene, observe the patient for any signs of adverse drug reactions and document appropriately.

CAUTIONS

Do not use an area that has existing skin damage or is hairy as it will be difficult to visualise any resulting reaction. Lighter skin tends to show irritation as redness, whereas darker skin can appear more purple.

Advise the patient to avoid touching and massaging the area as it can affect the results (Love, 2006).

Subcutaneous injections

WATCH THE VIDEO

SUBCUTANEOUS INJECTION

Watch along as you read through this step by step procedure by scanning the QR code with your smartphone camera or via https://study.sagepub.com/rowberry.

When you watch the video, take note of the speed and control by the nurse as they administer this injection.

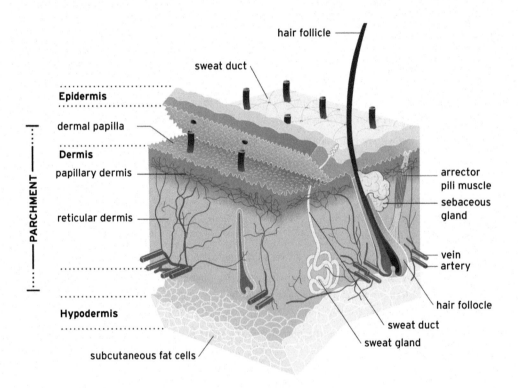

Figure 13.9 Skin layers

Source: Wikimedia Commons/Sean P Doherty (CC BY 4.0)

Subcutaneous injections are used for small volumes of medication (less than 2ml) needing slow and continuous absorption. The subcutaneous layer has a relatively reduced blood flow, which results in a slower absorption rate (Jevon et al., 2010). Medications that are commonly administered via the subcutaneous route include insulin and low molecular weight heparin.

Injections into this layer penetrate the dermis and deposit into the fat (adipose tissue) and connective tissue below. Typical sites are the lateral aspect of the upper arm, umbilical region of the abdomen and the lateral thigh below the greater trochanter (rather than mid thigh). The lower abdomen typically has the thickest layer of subcutaneous tissue.

It is important to choose a suitable site for your patient, as there is variability between the thickness of the subcutaneous layer. If the subcutaneous layer is thin, the injection could go into muscle just under the epidermis, resulting in faster absorption (Lister et al., 2020). If this occurs, it can cause significant unwanted side effects. If, for example, insulin was injected into the muscle, the resulting rapid absorption could cause a hypoglycaemic episode in patients with diabetes.

SUBCUTANEOUS: STEP BY STEP

EQUIPMENT

- 25G needle (orange) and appropriate syringe **or** prefilled syringe/device
- PPE as indicated
- Sterile gauze
- Clinically clean tray

PROCEDURE

- Introduce yourself to the patient and explain the procedure. Gain consent and ensure the environment is suitable for maintaining privacy and dignity. Perform appropriate checks as you prepare the medication and check the Five Rights of medication administration.
- Prepare the patient.
- Assist the patient, if necessary, into an appropriate and comfortable position, then expose the injection site.
- Assess the skin for suitability. It should be free from inflammation, oedema, infection and lesions to prevent trauma, infections and ensure effectiveness of administration (Lister et al., 2020).
- Assess the thickness of the subcutaneous layer – decide if pinching a skin fold may be necessary.
- Hold syringe in dominant hand. If the needle is less than 6mm (often seen with insulin pens) it can be given at a 90 degree angle in adults. Otherwise, administer into the skin at a 45 degree angle. Use a swift motion to reduce discomfort for the patient.
- Administer the medication at a constant rate, then withdraw swiftly at the same angle of entry (Jevon et al., 2010).
- Apply gentle pressure with sterile gauze, do not rub or massage as this can cause damage to underlying tissue (Potter et al., 2017).

CAUTIONS

Patient education may be required if the patient will need to continue the medication for a longer period, such as a person with diabetes requiring insulin. This will include information about preparation and administration of the injection, as well as wider aspects of safe storage, handwashing and safe disposal of equipment (Potter et al., 2017). If a patient is able to continue to self-administer, under the supervision of a nurse, this should be encouraged (RPS, 2017). Physical and cognitive

(Continued)

disabilities may make self-administration more challenging, but this does not mean it cannot be done. All patients should be supported to acquire the skills if they seek to. Learning disability nurses and occupational therapists are valuable team members who can support you to create bespoke, patient focused solutions.

Intramuscular injections

WATCH THE VIDEO

INTRAMUSCULAR INJECTION

Watch along as you read through this step by step procedure by scanning the QR code with your smartphone camera or via https://study.sagepub.com/rowberry.

As you are watching, notice the depth that the needle is inserted and how slowly the volume is administered.

Intramuscular (IM) injections are given into larger skeletal muscles and provide a route that rapidly absorbs medication. The muscle is usually less sensitive than subcutaneous, so viscous (thick, oily) liquids are more appropriately administered via this route. Four muscle sites are recommended for IM administration (see Figure 13.10).

The dorsogluteal is no longer recommended due to its increased risk of injury to the sciatic nerve (Small, 2004) and potential for a build-up of drugs (Malkin, 2008). This method also needs the buttock to be visualised for accurate placement, and so becomes additionally undignified for the patient.

It is important that the most appropriate site is chosen for administration. This will be based on the drug that is being administered (consider the viscosity), the volume of fluid and the patient's body type. Thick liquids and larger volumes should be administered into larger muscles, to minimise discomfort. If the patient has poor muscle density or tone, it is advised that you use the larger muscles to reduce the risk of accidental injury. It is important that you consider the drug you are administering as well as the patient you will be giving it to; consider muscle tone and density, their age, and the amount of adipose tissue (fat) that they have. The deltoid is the smallest of the recommended muscles, and so the maximum injectable volume should not exceed 1ml (Cocoman and Murray, 2008). Larger muscles are more suitable for larger volumes. Vastus lateralis and rectus femoris can be used for larger volumes up to 5ml. Wherever possible, ventrogluteal is the recommended site of administration as there are no major nerves that could be impacted and the muscle is sufficiently thick (Cocoman and Murray, 2008). This site should tolerate up to 3ml.

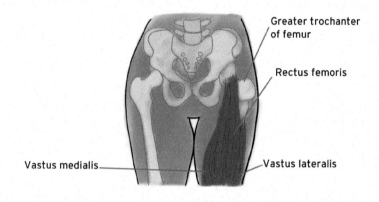

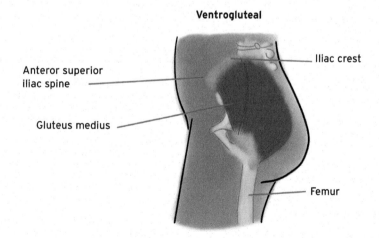

Figure 13.10   Muscle sites for IM administration

INTRAMUSCULAR: STEP BY STEP

EQUIPMENT

- Medication and dilutant if necessary
- Drawing up needle
- Administration needle
- Cotton ball
- Clean and stable surface
- Sharps bin

PROCEDURE

- 'Hello, my name is...' and discussion with patient about the procedure to ensure informed consent is obtained.
- Prepare the patient.
- Ensure the appropriate hand hygiene, preparation of medication and pre-administration checks have been completed.
- When drawing up the medication, you should consider the appropriate site for the drug you are administering, and the patient you are administering it to. Your needle selection will need to be considered.
- Ensure patient dignity is maintained by drawing curtains and minimal adjustments to clothing. Ensure modesty is preserved with a separate item of clothing, towel or sheet if appropriate. Consider the suitability of distraction techniques.
- Check the intended site to make sure that the area is visibly clean. Additional cleaning is only required if the area is visibly dirty. Routine disinfection is not required.
- Hold the needle in your dominant hand and use your non-dominant hand to hold the skin taut (see z-track video – link below). This technique reduces the chance for medication to backtrack and leak out of the insertion point.
- Insert the needle with a swift, dart-like movement at a 90 degree angle to the limb.
- Depress the plunger at a rate of 1ml/10 seconds for patient comfort (Lister et al., 2020). Once completed, remove the needle at the same angle it was inserted.
- Dispose of the sharps immediately. Do not resheath a used needle to reduce the risk of a needlestick injury. Remember that gloves are not protection against needlestick injuries so are not routinely recommended for injections (WHO, 2010).
- Perform hand hygiene, observe the patient for any signs of adverse drug reactions and document appropriately.

— WATCH THE VIDEO —

Z-TRACK

Watch along as you read through this step by step procedure by scanning the QR code with your smartphone camera or via https://study.sagepub.com/rowberry.

It can be difficult to visualise this skill, so take your time to understand what is happening when the pressure is applied.

Intravenous injections

Intravenous (IV) medication is administered through a patent venous cannula in a vein. Typical medication via this route includes contrast media, antibiotics, fluids, analgesia and blood products. Medication can be administered as a bolus or an infusion. A bolus is usually a small volume via syringe. Infusions tend to be mixtures of medication and diluents that are administered over a longer period of time. This may be to reduce the irritant nature of a medication, or to provide the dose at a slower or more controlled rate. Infusions can be intermittent, such as a number of minutes, or continuous, such as a 24 hour infusion.

Table 13.6   Risks of IV infusions

Overinfusion	Fluids can be administered too quickly. This can lead to congestive cardiac failure or electrolyte imbalances.
Infiltration and extravasation	Infiltration - inadvertent administration to surrounding tissues. Extravasation - visicant inadvertantly administered to surrounding tissue (significant irritant). This can cause blisters, tissue damage and necrosis.
Irritation and infection	Phlebitis - inflammation of the vein through irritation. Cellulitis - infection in lower dermis and subcutaneous tissues. Aseptic technique at insertion and when the cannula is being used can minimise this risk.
Systemic complications	Sepsis, emboli, air or mechanical (due to fragments) thrombus.
Rapid systemic circulation and inability to withdraw/ recall	Can be problematic in the case of allergic reactions.

Healthcare professionals undertaking IV administration are required to undergo additional training and must be deemed competent before undertaking this aspect of medicine administration (All Wales Medicines Strategy Group, 2015).

Venous access devices need to be in-situ for this medication to be administered. This is sometimes referred to as a vascular access device, cannula or venflon. They should be inserted, assessed and removed with aseptic non-touch technique (see Chapter 11). If they are unused for 24 hours or more they should be removed to reduce the risk of infection. There is no evidence to support that routine removal at 72 hours reduces the risk of infection (Webster et al., 2019).

Check for patency

Before using the cannula, it should be checked for patency and any signs of infection. A Visual Infusion Phlebitis score can be calculated to assist clinical decision-making.

Table 13.7   A Visual Infusion Phlebitis score

Appearance	Score	Action
Appears healthy	0	No sign of phlebitis. Continue to observe cannula at least daily.
One of the following is evident: Slight pain or redness* at IV site	1	Possible first signs of phlebitis. Observe cannula.
Pain and redness* at IV site	2	Early stage phlebitis. Remove cannula and site new cannula.
Pain, redness* and swelling evident	3	Medium stage phlebitis. Remove cannula and site new cannula.
Pain, redness*, swelling and palpable venous cord	4	Advanced phlebitis or start of thrombophlebitis. Remove cannula and site a new cannula. Consider treatment of phlebitis.
All of the above and pyrexia	5	Advanced thrombophlebitis. Remove and site a new cannula. Initiate treatment of thrombophlebitis.

*It is important to be aware that redness is typically seen in light skin. In darker skin, this may present as purple or darker discolouration. It is best practice to compare the site with other areas of skin to look for discolouration. The absence of redness on dark skin does not indicate the absence of phlebitis.

Preparation of IV bolus and infusion

IV medication may be supplied ready for administration, requiring dilution or reconstitution. This specific area of preparation should be undertaken with aseptic non-touch technique, to maintain the sterility of the infusion.

The medication and any dilutants should be checked to ensure they are in date and free from any particulates (Lister et al., 2020). When reconstituting, care should be taken to ensure powders are fully dissolved and fully incorporated into dilutants. This is best achieved through slow inversions, rather than shaking the containers (Potter et al., 2017).

Ensure appropriate calculations are undertaken and checked with a second registrant. A bolus will be delivered from the syringe into the patient, but an infusion or fluids needs to be delivered through a giving set (compatible with a pump or gravity flow). This should be primed to remove the air from the tubing, to ensure optimum medication delivery and prevent the risk of introducing air into a patient's vein.

IV PUSH ADMINISTRATION: STEP BY STEP

EQUIPMENT

- PPE
- Medication
- Dilutant
- Clinically clean tray
- Sterile syringe and needle
- Flushing solution as per local policy
- 2% chlorhexidine skin preparation
- Dressings trolley
- Dressings pack
- Sharps bin

PREPARE THE MEDICATION

- Draw up medication and flush in line with local guidance. Place in clinically clean receptacle.
- Collect the required equipment on the bottom shelf of a clean dressings trolley.
- Perform hand hygiene.
- Open dressings pack with ANTT and place on top of the trolley.

PROCEDURE

- Visually inspect the cannula for signs of damage of phlebitis.
- If there is another infusion running, check it is at the appropriate rate and that it is compatible with the bolus medication.
- Perform hand hygiene.
- Place a sterile field under the patient's limb.
- Clean the patient's skin and the device with 2% chlorhexidine.
- If required, stop any infusion. Flush the cannula with 0.9% sodium chloride to check patency and prevent mixing of previous infusion and bolus.
- Inject the drug at a steady and recommended pace. Observe for adverse signs at the insertion site or pain reported by the patient.
- Once completed, remove and immediately dispose of any sharps. Do not resheath a used needle to reduce the risk of a needlestick injury.
- Flush with 0.9% sodium chloride and recommence infusion, if necessary.
- Perform hand hygiene, observe the patient for any signs of adverse drug reactions and document appropriately.

IV INFUSION: STEP BY STEP

EQUIPMENT

- PPE
- Medication
- Dilutant (if required)
- Giving set
- Pump (if required)
- Drip stand
- Clinically clean tray
- Sterile syringe and needle
- Flushing solution as per local policy
- 2% chlorhexidine skin preparation
- Dressings trolley
- Dressings pack
- Sharps bin

PREPARE THE MEDICATION

- Draw up medication and flush in line with local guidance. Place in clinically clean receptacle.
- Collect the required equipment on the bottom shelf of a clean dressings trolley.
- Perform hand hygiene.
- Open dressings pack using ANTT and place on top of the trolley.

PROCEDURE

- Visually inspect the cannula for signs of damage of phlebitis.
- Check that there are no other infusions running, or that the last infusion has ended, to prevent overloading the vein.
- Perform hand hygiene.
- Place a sterile field under the patient's limb.
- Clean the patient's skin and the device with 2% chlorhexidine.
- Flush the cannula with 0.9% sodium chloride to check patency and prevent mixing of previous infusion.
- Attach the primed line to the patient. Ensure the flow or drip rate is correct. Observe for adverse signs at the insertion site or pain reported by the patient.
- Once the infusion is complete, remove and flush with 0.9% sodium chloride.
- Perform hand hygiene, observe the patient for any signs of adverse drug reactions and document appropriately.

WATCH THE VIDEO

BOLUS INJECTION

Watch along as you read through this step by step procedure by scanning the QR code with your smartphone camera or via https://study.sagepub.com/rowberry.

The cannula in this video has a clamp along the line that also needs to be released. You may use different equipment in your clinical areas so remember to spend time looking at your patient, not just the task.

WHEN THINGS GO WRONG

All errors and near misses should be reported in line with local policy to help protect the patient, and to explore the contributing factors to reduce the chances of it happening again.

Medication calculation errors

Accurate calculations ensure patients receive the dose of medication they have been prescribed. Errors with medication administration tend to be either a calculation or concept error (Fleming et al., 2014). Calculation errors are the most frequently cited error (Wright and Shepherd, 2017). Due to the often weight-based dosages, children under the age of 5 are impacted by a disproportionately higher level of error than the rest of the patient population (Wright and Shepherd, 2017). When calculations are needed, The Royal Pharmaceutical Society and The Royal College of Nursing (RPS and RCN, 2019) recommends that they are double checked by a second person. Local policy will dictate the minimum standard, but you should use your professional accountability to seek out second-checks, if needed. Typically, the two-check standard applies to:

- high risk medicine administered via the IV or subcutaneous route
- controlled drugs
- cytotoxic agents
- where the recipient is a child, young person or neonate
- when calculation of dosage is required (including dose adjustments for infusions already in progress)
- when an IV administration is made up or an IV or subcutaneous infusion is commenced or the rate of infusion is changed.

(All Wales Medicines Strategy Group, 2015)

ACTIVITY: PAUSE AND REFLECT

SMART plans

You have decided you need to brush up on your maths skills? This is excellent. To make your practice into a regular habit, make your plan SMART:

- **Specific** - What exactly would you like to focus on? Where is your difficulty? What would you like to be able to do easily?
- **Measurable** - How would you know if you were getting better at it? A timed test perhaps?
- **Achievable** - Be sure that your intention is within your capability. Don't be too ambitious, think about what you would like to achieve and set your sights on improvement.
- **Relevant** - Make sure that you study a mix of basic numeracy and medicines-specific practice to help you to improve in the areas you are weaker in.
- **Timely** - When are you going to review you progress and readjust your SMART goal?

Previous plan: I'm going to get really quick at calculations.
   New plan: I'm going to improve my confidence with calculations through practise. I will download a maths program onto my phone and set a weekly alarm to do a 30-minute practice every Thursday evening.

Accuracy in calculations is important, but you also need to be able to extract the correct information to be able to insert it into a formula. Several reasons have been identified for why medication errors occur. Most commonly they are:

- Misidentification of a medicine
- Misidentification of a patient
- Lack of knowledge about a drug
- Poor quality documentation including prescriptions
- Inexperienced staff, especially when working alongside other inexperienced staff
- High workload and stress/fatigue
- Lack of equipment
- Interruptions or distractions

(Keers et al., 2013)

It is your individual responsibility to keep your knowledge and skills up to date. As a nurse you need to take part in appropriate and regular learning activities to maintain and develop your competence and improve your performance (NMC, 2018b). If you are not confident about your maths skills, it is important that you use your university's resources to improve this. Many courses will have a specific learning programme or pathway available to you. There are also a multitude of targeted resources available online or from your library.

   If an error is made, it is important to report it as soon as possible, as well as take necessary steps to reduce or prevent harm. Nurses have a professional duty of candour built into The Code (NMC, 2018b), which states that they should be open and transparent when mistakes have been made.

This is both with the employer and the patient. It is important that local policies are followed, including incident forms. This helps to determine why the error occurred and highlights opportunities to prevent it reoccurring in the future.

Adverse drug reaction

Medicines are rigourously evaluated to assess their safety, but no medicine is entirely risk free. Nurses should be aware of any potential problems that patients may experience when taking any medication, and know how and when to report these.

An Adverse Drug Reaction (ADR) is harm directly caused by the medicine at normal doses, during normal use. Largely, this falls into the following types:

- **Type A – Augmented reaction.** This is where the drug is given at the usual dose but the intended effect, or known side effects, are at an increased level. This is the most common ADR. For example, bleeding with warfarin (exaggerated intended effect) or dry mouth with tricyclic antidepressants (exaggerated known side effect).
- **Type B – Bizarre reaction.** These are novel responses that are not expected from the actions of the drug. These are less common, but often more serious. This includes anaphylaxis with penicillin.
- **Type C – Continuing reactions – persisting for a long time.** An example of this is osteoporosis with oral steroids.
- **Type D – Delayed.** These become apparent after some time of using the medication. Because of the delayed timing, it is more difficult to detect.
- **Type E – End of use reactions.** ADRs associated with the withdrawal of medication. This is common.

(MHRA, n.d.)

ADRs are more likely to occur if a patient is taking more than one medication, if they have comorbidities (such as renal disease), or if they have any known allergies. Preventing ADRs and detecting them is known as pharmacovigilance. It important for detecting issues that may be occurring within specific patient populations that may not have been captured during safety testing. Disruptions to, and by, the menstrual cycle are typically much more likely to be captured after approval, as seen with recent Covid-19 vaccination, antipsychotics, cardiac drugs, and antibiotics (Zopf et al., 2008; MHRA, 2022).

When ADRs are detected they should be reported and managed in line with your local policies. If appropriate it should also be reported to the Yellow Card Scheme (RPS and RCN, 2019). The Yellow Card Scheme was set up in 1964 by the MHRA to create a centralised database to report side effects of medication. Health professionals and patients are able to provide this information. This approach helps create an early warning that a product may need additional testing. As a result of Yellow Card reporting, medications have had additional scrutiny, been reclassified from the General Sales List to a Pharmacy Only Medication or required changes to the treatment regime.

An extension of the safety around new medications is the Black Triangle Scheme. New medications, or those that have recently changed for a significantly new indication or population (e.g. previously just adults but broadened suitability for children) feature a black triangle next to their name in the BNF and Nurse Prescribers' Formulary for two years. This indicates it is under closer surveillance after marking to ensure its suitability and the incidence of any rare adverse effects

Side effects, allergic and anaphylactic reactions

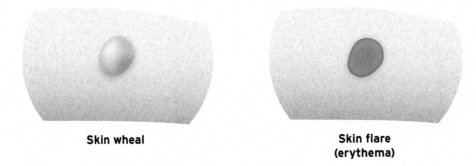

Skin wheal

Skin flare
(erythema)

Figure 13.11 Skin reactions in allergy

Side effects are known effects from a medication. They can cause unpleasant symptoms such as GI upset, skin rashes, and itching. They can be found in the patient information leaflet inside the medication, but are also listed in *The BNF*. Steps can be taken to manage the side effect, such as prescribing additional drugs to combat the side effect (e.g. opiates and laxatives) or providing lifestyle advice to minimise the effect (e.g. standing up slowly to prevent dizziness). If side effects are reducing a patient's quality of life or adherence to prescribed medications, a review should be encouraged in case a suitable alternative can be offered.

An allergic reaction is an immune response triggered by an allergen. Antibodies release histamine in response, resulting in swelling, inflammation and itchiness. On white skin, swelling can appear red, raised, with an orange peel texture. In darker skin tones hives can look darker or purple. Other symptoms include sneezing and GI upset. Typically, an allergic reaction can be managed by removing the allergen and administering antihistamines. Prominent skin features such as facial swelling and generalised urticaria, without airway/breathing/circulation problems, can be misdiagnosed as anaphylaxis (Johnston et al., 2003).

Anaphylaxis is a potentially life threatening allergic reaction and a medical emergency. It develops suddenly and progresses rapidly. Anaphylaxis may have some of the features of an allergic reaction, such as swelling, but also airway/breathing/circulation difficulties.

Table 13.8 Signs of anaphylaxis

Airway Problem	Airway swelling (throat and tongue) Difficulty swallowing or breathing A feeling of narrowing in the throat Hoarse voice Stridor (high pitched inspiratory noise)
Breathing Problem	Increased work of breathing Wheeze and/or cough Fatigue from effort of breathing Hypoxaemia (SpO2 <94%) – this can cause confusion and/or central cyanosis Respiratory arrest
Circulation Problem	Signs of shock: Pale and clammy Tachycardia Hypotension Dizziness Decreased conscious level or loss of consciousness Arrhythmia Cardiac arrest

Source: Adapted from Resuscitation Council UK (2021)

The Resuscitation Council (2021) recommend the following for someone suspected of having an anaphylactic reaction:

- Recognition that they are seriously unwell
- An early call for help (resuscitation team or ambulance)
- Initial assessment and treatment based on an ABCDE approach
- Prompt treatment with intramuscular adrenaline
- Investigation and specialist follow-up in an allergy clinic

The treatment for anaphylaxis is IM adrenaline. It should be give IM into the anterolateral thigh and repeated after 5 minutes if problems persist (Resuscitation Council UK, 2021).

CASE STUDY

Tomas and Jacob, parent and son

Tomas has brought his son, Jacob, to a busy Emergency Department after three days of increasing pain in the head. Jacob is given an oral dose of amoxicillin for a suspected dental abscess. Whilst the medical team make the decisions about the next steps in managing his care, Tomas alerts staff that Jacob has developed a raised itchy rash on his side. It seems that this is Jacob's first allergic reaction. Once the emerging situation is managed, Tomas asked you questions about the allergy. He is upset and worried – he tells you that he is frightened that Jacob may be allergic to other things.

Questions

How would you help Tomas to manage this serious new medical information? What information or support would you be able to provide?

CHAPTER SUMMARY

Your role within medicines administration is very important. It is hoped that this chapter has introduced you to your roles and responsibilities, as well as technical skills such as calculations and the acts of administration. As with all skills, practice is important. Revisit the information within this chapter and ensure you attempt the activities.

ACE YOUR ASSESSMENT

Complete the questions below. Remember to use *The BNF* to support you if you are unsure.

Q1   Your patient is due to be administered oral medications, but they have been vomiting and continue to feel nauseous. Do you:

   a   Administer the dose and record if the patient vomits
   b   Contact pharmacy to check if the medication can be crushed
   c   Contact a member of the medical team for the medication to be charted to an alternative route
   d   Withhold the dose

(Continued)

Q2   What is the skin checked for when applying topical medication (choose two):

   a   Irritation
   b   Broken skin
   c   Freckles
   d   Pulse

Q3   A patient admitted for exacerbation of their pulmonary disease demonstrates a poor inhaler technique but explains that this is how they have been doing it for years. What do you do?

   a   Consider the patient to be the expert. They have had the condition for a long time and probably know what they are doing
   b   Tell them they are wrong and refer to a respiratory nurse
   c   Make a complaint about their practice nurse as they must have a poor teaching technique
   d   Begin an open discussion with the patient and provide education about the correct technique with supporting resources

Q4   What is a z-track and why is it used?

   a   An electronic device for delivery of medication through an NG tube
   b   An applicator for topical medication to prevent absorption through the palms
   c   A maneuver performed whilst administering an injection to prevent bleeding
   d   The reporting system for unexpected side effects

Answers

1   C
2   A & B
3   D
4   C

GO FURTHER

- The Nursing Times – Drug Calculations in Practice. This online series has been written to help build confidence and ability in maths related to medicines administration https://www.nursing-times.net/clinical-archive/medicine-management/how-to-calculate-drug-doses-and-infusion-rates-accurately-16-10-2017/ (accessed October 25, 2022).

- Betsi Cadwaladr University Health Board. (2015) 'The NEWT Guidelines for administration of medication to patients with enteral feeding tubes or swallowing difficulties'. https://www.newt-guidelines.com/index.html (accessed October 25, 2022).

- Brown Skin Matters – A community-built collection of skin conditions on non-white skin. This includes examples of dermatitis and urticaria. https://brownskinmatters.com/ (accessed October 25, 2022).

- Barber, P. (ed.) (2013) *Medicine Management for Nurses: Case Book.* Maidenhead: Open University Press.

- NICE (2015) *Medicines Optimisation: The Safe and Effective Use of Medicines to Enable the Best Possible Outcomes.* https://www.nice.org.uk/guidance/ng5 (accessed October 25, 2022). This discusses safe and effective use of medicines to the greatest possible benefit by encouraging medicines reconciliation, medication review and the use of patient decision aids.

REFERENCES

Alexander, N., Baker, E., Kaptein, M., Karck, U., Miller, L. and Zampaglione, E. (2004) 'Why consider vaginal drug administration', *Fertility and Sterility*, 82 (1): 1–12.

All Wales Medicines Strategy Group (2015) *All Wales Policy for Medicines Administration, Recording, Review, Storage and Disposal.* https://cavuhb.nhs.wales/files/policies-procedures-and-guidelines/patient-safety-and-quality/a-patient-safety/ff-allwalespolicyformedicinesadministration-recording-review-storageanddisposal-pdf/ (accessed October 25, 2022).

Bellieni, C., Cordelli, D., Raffaelli, M., Ricci, B., Morgese, G. and Buonocore, G. (2006) 'Analgesic effects of watching TV during venepuncture', *Archives of Diseases in Childhood*, 91 (12): 1015–17.

Boyd, C. (2013) *Medicine Management Skills for Nurses: Student Survival Skills.* Oxford: John Wiley & Sons.

Braido, F., Chrystyn, H., Baiardini, I., Bosnic-Anticevich, S., van der Molen, T., Dandurand, R.J. [...] and Price, D. (2016) 'Trying, but failing – the role of inhaler technique and mode of delivery in respiratory medication adherence', *Journal of Allergy and Clinical Immunology in Practice*, 4 (5): 823–32.

Cocoman, A. and Murray, J. (2008) 'Intramuscular injections: A review of best practice for mental health nurses', *Journal of Psychiatric and Mental Health Nursing*, 15 (5): 424–34.

Deacon, B. and Abramowitz, J. (2016) 'Fear of needles and vasovagal reactions among phlebotomy patients', *Journal of Anxiety Disorders*, 20 (7): 946–60.

Elliott, R., Camacho, E. and Jankovic, D. (2021) 'Economic analysis of the prevalence and clinical and economic burden of medication error in England', *BMJ Quality & Safety*, 30: 96–105.

European Parliament (2001) 'Directive 2001/83/EC of the European Parliament and of the council of 6 November 2001 on the community code relating to medicinal products for human use', *Official Journal L,* 311: 67–128. https://www.ema.europa.eu/en/documents/regulatory-procedural-guideline/directive-2001/83/ec-european-parliament-council-6-november-2001-community-code-relating-medicinal-products-human-use_en.pdf (accessed October 25, 2022).

Federico, F. (2014) *The Five Rights of Medication Administration.* Institute for Healthcare Improvement. https://www.ihi.org/resources/pages/improvementstories/fiverightsofmedicationadministration.aspx#:~:text=The%20Five%20Rights%20of%20Medication%20Administration%20by%20Frank,dose%2C%20the%20right%20route%2C%20and%20the%20right%20time (accessed January 30, 2023).

Fleming, S., Brady, A. and Malone, A. (2014) 'An evaluation of the drug calculation skills of registered nurses', *Nurse Education in Practice*, 14 (1): 55–61.

Graham-Clarke, E., Rushton, A., Noblet, T. and Marriott, J. (2018) 'Facilitators and barriers to non-medical prescribing: A systematic review and thematic synthesis', *PLOS One*, 13 (4). doi.org/10.1371/journal.pone.0196471

Hanning, S., Walker, E., Sutcliffe, E. and Tuleu, C. (2020) 'The rectal route of medicine administration for children: Let's get to the bottom of it!', *European Journal of Pharmaceutics and Biopharmaceutics*, 157: 25–7.

Iwanaga, T.T. (2019) 'The Respimat® Soft Mist Inhaler: Implications of drug delivery characteristics for patients', *Clinical Drug Investigations*, 39: 1021–30.

Jenkins, K. (2014) 'II. Needle phobia: A psychological perspective', *British Journal of Anaesthesia*, 113 (1), 4–6.

Jevon, P., Payne, L., Higgins, D. and Endacott, R. (2010) *Medicines Management: A Guide for Nurses.* Oxford: John Wiley & Sons.

Johnston, S., Unsworth, J. and Gompels, M. (2003) 'Adrenaline given outside the context of life threatening allergic reactions', *British Medical Journal*, 326 (7389): 589–90.

Keers, R., Williams, S., Cooke, J. and Ashcroft, D. (2013) 'Causes of medication administration errors in hospitals: A systematic review of quantitative and qualitative evidence', *Drug Safety: An International Journal of Medical Toxicity and Drug Experiences*, 36 (11): 1045–67.

Lister, S., Hofland, J. and Grafton, H. (2020) *The Royal Marsden Manual of Clinical Nursing Procedures* (10th edition). Oxford: John Wiley & Sons.

Litt, H.K., Press, V.G., Hull, A., Siros, M., Luna, V. and Volerman, A. (2020) 'Association between inhaler technique and confidence among hospitalized children with asthma', *Respirology Medicine*, 174: Article #106191.

Long, M. and Yisheng, C. (2009) 'Dissolution testing of solid products', in Y. Qiu, Y. Chen, G. Zhang, L. Liu and W. Porter (eds), *Developing Solid Oral Dosage Forms*. Kidlington: Elsevier. pp. 319–40.

Love, G. (2006) 'Administering an intradermal injection', *Nursing 2022*, 36 (6): 20.

Lowry, M. (2016) 'Rectal drug administration in adults: How, when, why', *Nursing Times*, 112 (18): 12–14.

Malkin, B. (2008) 'Are techniques used for intramuscular injection based on research evidence?', *Nursing Times*, 104 (50): 48–51.

Martyn, J., Paliadelis, P. and Perry, C. (2019) 'The safe administration of medication: Nursing behaviours beyond the five-rights', *Nurse Education Practice*, 37: 109–14.

Medicines and Healthcare Products Regulatory Agency (MHRA) (n.d.) *Guidance on Adverse Drug Reactions*. https://assets.publishing.service.gov.uk/government/uploads/system/uploads/attachment_data/file/949130/Guidance_on_adverse_drug_reactions.pdf (accessed October 25, 2022).

Medicines and Healthcare Products Regulatory Agency (2022) 'Coronavirus vaccine – weekly summary of yellow card reporting', gov.uk, October 7. https://www.gov.uk/government/publications/coronavirus-covid-19-vaccine-adverse-reactions/coronavirus-vaccine-summary-of-yellow-card-reporting (accessed October 25, 2022).

Mills, P., Weidmann, A.E. and Stewart, D. (2017) 'Hospital electronic prescribing system implementation impact on discharge information communication and prescribing errors: A before and after study', *European Journal of Clinical Pharmacology*, 73 (10): 1279–86.

Minkin, M.J. and Mirkin, S. (2021) 'Celebrating the vagina: The vagina as effective route of drug delivery', *Contemporary OB/GYN*, 66 (9): 1–4.

National Institute for Health and Care Excellence (NICE) (2022). *Approved List for Prescribing by Community Practitioner Nurse Prescribers* (NPF). nice.org.uk. https://bnf.nice.org.uk/nurse-prescribers-formulary/ (accessed October 25, 2022).

Novak-Bilić, G., Vučić, M., Japundžić, M.-Š. J., Stanić-Duktaj, S. and Lugović-Mihić, L. (2018) 'Irritant and allergic contact dermatitis – skin lesion characteristics', *Acta Clinica Croatica*, 57 (4): 713–20. doi.org/10.20471/acc.2018.57.04.13

Nursing and Midwifery Council (NMC) (2018a) *Future Nurse: Standards of Proficiency for Registered Nurses*. London: NMC. https://www.nmc.org.uk/standards/standards-for-nurses/standards-of-proficiency-for-registered-nurses/ (accessed October 25, 2022).

Nursing and Midwifery Council (2018b) *The Code: Professional Standards of Practice and Behaviour for Nurses, Midwives and Nursing Associates*. London: NMC. https://www.nmc.org.uk/globalassets/sitedocuments/nmc-publications/nmc-code.pdf (accessed October 25, 2022).

Nursing and Midwifery Council (2018c) 'Part 1: Standards framework for nursing and midwifery education', in: *Realising Professionalism: Standards for Education and Training*. London: NMC. https://www.nmc.org.uk/standards-for-education-and-training/standards-framework-for-nursing-and-midwifery-education/ (accessed October 25, 2022).

Pastore, M., Kalia, Y.N., Horstmann, M. and Roberts, M.S. (2015) 'Transdermal patches: History, development and pharmacology', *British Journal of Pharmacology*, 172 (9): 2179–209. doi.org/10.1111/bph.13059

Pombo, S. and Félix da Costa, N. (2016) 'Heroin addiction patterns of treatment-seeking patients, 1992-2013: Comparison between pre-and post-drug policy reform in Portugal', *Heroin Addiction and Related Clinical Problems*, 18 (6): 51–60.

Potter, P.A., Perry, A.G., Hall, A.M., Stockert, P.A. and Ostendorf, W.R. (eds) (2017) *Fundamentals of Nursing* (9th edition). Kidlington: Elsevier.

Resuscitation Council UK (2021) *Emergency Treatment of Anaphylaxis: Guidelines for Healthcare Professionals*. London: Resuscitation Council UK. https://www.resus.org.uk/sites/default/files/2021-05/Emergency%20Treatment%20of%20Anaphylaxis%20May%202021_0.pdf (accessed October 25, 2022).

Rogers, R. (ed.) (1986) *Neighbourhood Nursing - A Focus for Care (The Cumberlege Report)*. London: King's Fund Centre. https://archive.kingsfund.org.uk/concern/published_works/000003610?locale =en#?cv=0&xywh=162,298,1740,994 (accessed October 25, 2022).

Royal College of Nursing (RCN) (2019) 'Tackling number problems'. https://www.rcn.org.uk/clinical-topics/safety-in-numbers/dosage-for-solid-medicines (accessed January 30, 2023).

Royal Pharmaceutical Society (RPS) (2011) *Pharmaceutical Issues when Crushing, Opening or Splitting Oral Dosage Forms*. https://filestore.medicineslearningportal.org/docs/RPS%20 pharmaceuticalissuesdosageforms.pdf (accessed October 25, 2022).

Royal Pharmaceutical Society (2014) 'The evolution of pharmacy, Theme E, Level 3 Thalidomide and its aftermath', RPS. https://web.archive.org/web/20170325030100/https:// www.rpharms.com/museum-pdfs/e3a-thalidomide-and-its-aftermath-2011.pdf (accessed October 25, 2022).

Royal Pharmaceutical Society (2017a) *Professional Guidance on the Safe and Secure Handling of Medicines*. London: RPS. https://www.rpharms.com/recognition/setting-professional-standards/ safe-and-secure-handling-of-medicines/professional-guidance-on-the-safe-and-secure-handling-of-medicines (accessed October 25, 2022).

Royal Pharmaceutical Society (2017b) *Professional Standards for Hospital Pharmacy*. London: RPS. https://www.rpharms.com/recognition/setting-professional-standards/hospital-pharmacy-professional-standards (accessed October 25, 2022).

Royal Pharmaceutical Society (2021) *A Competency Framework for all Prescribers*. London: RPS. https:// www.rpharms.com/resources/frameworks/prescribing-competency-framework/competency-framework (accessed October 25, 2022).

Royal Pharmaceutical Society and Royal College of Nursing (RCN) (2019) *Professional Guidance on the Administration of Medicines in Healthcare Settings*. London: RPS.

Salisbury, D., Ramsay, M. and Noakes, K. (eds) (2013) *Immunisation against Infectious Disease: Green Book*. UK Department of Health. https://assets.publishing.service.gov.uk/government/uploads/ system/uploads/attachment_data/file/147832/Green-Book-updated-140313.pdf (accessed October 25, 2022).

Schellack, G. (2011) 'Drug dosage forms and the routes of drug administration', *Professional Nursing Today*, 15 (6): 10–16.

Scullion, J. and Fletcher, M. (2019) *UKIG Inhaler Standards and Competency Document*. United Kingdom Inhaler Group. https://www.ukinhalergroup.co.uk/uploads/s4vjR3GZ/InhalerStandardsMASTER. docx2019V10final.pdf (accessed October 25, 2022).

Shah, R. (2001) 'Thalidomide, drug safety and early drug regulation in the UK', *Adverse Drug Reactions Toxicology Review*, 20 (4): 199–255.

Shepherd, E. (2018) 'Injection technique 1: Administering drugs via the intramuscular route', *Nursing Times*, 114 (8): 23–5.

Shepherd, M. and Shepherd, E. (2020) 'Medicines administration 1: Understanding routes of administration', *Nursing Times*, 116 (6): 42–4.

Silvestri, A. (2014) *Gateways from Crime to Health: The Portuguese Drug Commissions*. Winston Churchill Memorial Trust and Prison Reform Trust. https://www.sicad.pt/BK/Dissuasao/Documents/AS%20report%20GATEWAYS%20FROM%20CRIME%20TO%20HEALTH.pdf (accessed October 25, 2022).

Small, S.P. (2004) 'Preventing sciatic nerve injury from intramuscular injections: Literature review', *Journal of Advanced Nursing*, 47 (3): 287–96. doi: 10.1111/j.1365-2648.2004.03092.x. PMID: 15238123.

Taddio, A., Ipp, M., Thivakaran, S., Jamal, A., Parikh, C., Smart, S., Sovran, J., Stevens, D. and Katz, D. (2012) 'Survey of the prevalence of immunization non-compliance due to needle fears in children and adults', *Vaccine*, 30 (32): 4807–12.

Webster, J., Osborne, S. and Rickard, C. (2019) 'Clinically-indicated replacement versus routine replacement of peripheral venous catheters', *Cochrane Database of Systematic Reviews*, 23 (1): Article #CD007798.

Weeks, G., George, J., Maclure, K. and Stewart, D. (2016) 'Non-medical prescribing versus medical prescribing for acute and chronic disease management in primary and secondary care', *Cochrane Database of Systematic Reviews*, 11 (11): Article #CD011227.

World Health Organization (WHO) (2003) *Aide-memoire for a National Strategy for the Safe and Appropriate Use of Injections*. https://apps.who.int/iris/handle/10665/66696 (accessed October 25, 2022).

World Health Organization (2010) *WHO Best Practices for Injection and Related Procedures Toolkit*. https://www.who.int/publications/i/item/9789241599252 (accessed October 25, 2022).

Wrexham Maelor Hospital Pharmacy Department (2019) *The NEWT Guidelines*. www.newtguidelines.com/AdminOfTablets.html (accessed October 25, 2022).

Wright, K. and Shepherd, E. (2017) 'How to calculate drug doses and infusion rates accurately', *Nursing Times*, 113 (10): 31–4.

Zopf, Y., Rabe, C., Neubert, A., Gaßmann, K. G., Rascher, W., Hahn, E.G., Brune, K. and Dormann, H. (2008) 'Women encounter ADRs more often than men do', *European Journal of Clinical Pharmacology*, 64: 999–1004.

INDEX

Figures are indicated by *f*; tables by *t*

ABCDE assessment 260, 292, 301, 423
abdominal distension 91
abdominal guarding 90
abdominal masses, palpable 91
abdominal regions and quadrants 89f
abdominal tenderness 90
abduction 254
absorption 174
accidents and their procedures 265f
active listening 57
Activities of Daily Living (ADLs) 80
acute kidney injury (AKI) 215, 220
adduction 254
adenosine triphosphate 287
admiral nurses 365–6
adolescents
    abdominal pain, case study 91–2
    asthma attack, case study 300–1
    nutritional needs 176
    urostomy, case study 234
advanced care planning (ACP) 354, 355, 358, 360, 371
    and mental capacity 359
advanced decision refusing treatment (ADRT, living wills) 358
Advanced Trauma Life Support 267
adverse drug reactions (ADRs) 421
Advisory Council on the Misuse of Drugs (ACMD) 381
aesthetic knowledge 16
'affirmed experience' 16
airborne transmission 328
airway devices 302–4
    and pressure damage 162
airway suctioning 305–9
    end of life care 357
    suction pressure and catheter size 306t
alarm parameters 42
allergic reactions 422
    case study 423
Alvariza, A. 365
alveoli 284, 285, 286f, 287
Alzheimer's disease
    and incontinence, case study 245
    and palliative care, case study 366
Amsterdam Declaration 120
anaemia 322, 323
analytical study design 5
anaphylaxis 422–3, 422t
angle of Louis/sternal angle 102, 103
anterior axillary line 102, 103

antibiotics 292, 319, 324, 415
    improper use 223, 317
anticholinergic drugs 357
anti-embolic stockings, and pressure damage 161
antiemetics 356
antihistamines 204, 422
anuria 215
anxiety
    and bladder/bowel conditions 244
    and emotional support, nursing in action 24, 25
    and heart rate 110
    terminal agitation 357
anxiolytics 357
Apfel Score 202
apnoea 287, 354 *see also* sleep apnoea
Arjo 252
Arjo MaxiSlide 271f
arms assessment 80–1
arrhythmias 110
arterial blood gas (ABG) analysis 291
arterial leg ulcers 154t
aseptic non touch technique (ANTT) 166, 167, 192, 317, 344–5
aspiration pneumonia 200
assessment 29–47
    clinical reasoning and decision making 30–3
    ethical dilemmas in 35–6
    ethical dilemmas, case study 35
    gathering patient information 33–5
    in ICU settings 40–6
    Nursing Process 30, 30f
    remote/virtual 33, 38–9
assessment tools 34–5
    incorrect or inaccurate use 34–5
asthma 6, 83, 84, 290, 298, 302
    case study 300–1
    severity 301t
Attend-anywhere 38
attributable risk 8
    calculating 9f
autism 398

Babbel, S. 123
bacteria 315, 316, 316f
    clinically significant 319, 320f
    common commensals and their locations 319, 319t
    differentiation by Gram staining 318–19
    differentiation by shape 318

on hands 331, 333
   infection type and severity 317, 318t
bad news breaking 62–5, 363
   definition 62
   incidents seen as 63
   lower level in a modern healthcare system 63
   potential outcomes of not engaging 65t
   SPIKES 63–4
Baile, W. F. 63–4
barrier creams 164
bathing 142–3
Batstone, E. 364
bed rails 257–8
   risk assessment 257
bedsheets, and pressure damage 162
bedtime fading 126
bedtime routine 126–7
Bender, E. 131
bias 5
bilirubin in urine 220
bioavailability 390, 392
Bisoprolol 110
Black Triangle Scheme 421
bladder 212
   drainage after death 330
   normal elimination 213, 215
bladder cancer 8, 220, 223, 234
bladder health 210–11, 246
   anatomy and physiology 212–13, 213f
   catheterisation and urinary drainage 223–34
   continence 213–16
   psychological health and mental health issues
       241–6
   stomas and stoma care 211, 213, 234, 235, 237–8
   urinary assessment 217–23
bladder scanning 224
blood and body fluid spillages 342
blood in urine 219
blood pressure 110–12, 111f
   Korotkoff sounds 111–12, 111f
blood products 192, 415
blood urea nitrogen/creatinine ratio 190
BMI (Body Mass Index) 174, 177
body image, and stomas 237, 238
bolus feeding 182–3
bones 253
Boole, G. 19
Boolean Operators (AND/OR/NOT) 19–20
bowel cancer 220, 362
bowel elimination 216
bowel health 210–11, 246
   anatomy and physiology 211–12, 212f
   Bristol stool assessment tool 216–17, 216f
   continence 213–14, 216
   psychological health and mental health
       issues 241–6
   rectal examination and manual evacuation
       240–1
   stomas and stoma care 211, 213, 234–8
   suppositories and enemas 238–40

bowel ischaemia 90
bowel obstruction 90
bowel sounds 91
breastfeeding 172, 175
breathing patterns 83
breathlessness (dyspnoea) 288
   assessing 288–90
   causes 289t
Bristol stool assessment tool 216–17, 216f
British National Formulary (BNF) 376, 422
British Nutrition Foundation 176
British Thoracic Society guidelines 298
bronchodilators 292, 301
   nebulisers vs. inhalers 302
'burn-out' syndrome 46
burns 154t

cancer 11, 321, 361
   eating and drinking assistance 179
   malignant wounds and fungating tumours 154t
   see also specific cancers
Cancer Research UK 20
candida/Candida albicans 145, 324
cannabis 37, 380
cannulation 105–6
capsules 391, 391f
carbon dioxide 284, 285, 286–7, 290, 293
cardiovascular auscultation 84–8, 85f
   case study 88
   clinical findings 86
   oedema 87
   valve pathologies 86
care bundles and assessment tools 44–5, 45t
care environment, safe management 340
care planning 357–8
Carper, B. 15–16, 25
case control studies 7–8
   vs cohort studies 9–10, 10f
case studies 11
CASP tool 21
catheter passports 225
catheters
   and bladder drainage 225
   indwelling 226
   sizes 226–7
   suprapubic 226
catheterisation 223–34
   and after death care 369
   bladder scanning 224
   care planning 232–3
   catheter sample of urine (CSU) 231–2
   clinical indications for 223
   female 227–9, 227f
   intermittent 225
   male 229–31, 229f
   and moisture lesions 164
   post insertion 232–3
   and pressure damage 162
   removal of catheter 233
   UTI detection in catheter users 222–3

cervical cancer 14–15, 321
chair method (for babies' sleep) 126
chair use, and pressure damage 162–3
Chapman, S. 364
Chemoreceptor Trigger Zone 202
chest auscultation 81–4
    findings 83–4
    special considerations 83
chest symmetry 83
children
    airway suctioning 306
    assessment for dehydration associated with
        diarrhoea 190t
    bedtime routine 126
    breathlessness 289, 290
    care of the body after death 367–8
    chest auscultation 83
    dehydration 190
    diarrhoeal illness 323
    estimation of fluid deficit 190t
    medication calculation errors 419
    moving and handling 254–5, 257
    nebulisers vs. inhalers for asthma 302
    non-verbal communication 55
    nutritional needs 176
    oropharyngeal (OP) airways 303
    oxygen therapy 296
    pain assessment 76, 76f
    past medical history 74
    personal care 140
    recommended fluid intake 196–7, 197t
    tube feeding 182, 183, 185–6
    vomiting 201
Children Acts (1989, 2004) 255
chronic obstructive pulmonary disease (COPD) 44,
    84, 107, 290, 295
    case study 291–2
cilia 298
circumduction 254
Class A drugs 380
Class B drugs 380
Class C drugs 380
cleaning 337–8, 340
clinical experience 16
clinical reasoning
    definition 30
    5 rights 31
    in the Nursing Process 32f
clinical reasoning cycle 31f
clinical skills and their application to practice
    23–25
Clostridioides difficile (C. difficile) formerly
    Clostridium difficile 317, 320f
Code of Practice on the Prevention and Control of
    Infections 329
cohort studies 8–10
    vs. case control studies 9–10, 10f
collective involvement in healthcare 16–17
colloids 192
colonisation 316

colostomy 235
    changing/emptying bag 235–7
colostrum 175
comfort 119, 123, 132
commensals 315
    common commensals and location 319, 319t
    functions 317
common cold (Rhinovirus) 316, 321
communication 51–67
    active listening 57
    barriers to, in healthcare 52–3, 65–6
    breaking bad news 62–5
    and care of the body after death 371
    case study 56
    developing rapport and relationships 53–4
    and drug administration 376
    and ECG preparation 104
    empathy in 54
    and end of life care 362–3
    and handovers 60–2
    and handovers, case study 59–60
    of health information 55
    how and with whom 58–60, 58t
    and IV fluid administration 195
    and monitoring fluid intake 198
    and nasogastric feeding tubes 187
    and personal care 139–40, 141
    and safety and patient satisfaction 58
    verbal and non-verbal 55–6, 55t
    what it is 52
communication difficulties
    and advanced decision refusing treatment 358
    and bladder/bowel health 245
    and handover communication 60
    and pain assessment 76–7
    and personal care 141
    and remote consultations 39, 40
    see also language barriers
community palliative care nurse (CPCN) 367
community practitioner nurse prescribers (CPNPs) 383
compassion 54, 121, 140, 144, 362
Competency Framework for all Prescribers 383
compliance (lungs, airways) 285, 287
confidence interval 7, 8
confidentiality
    and after death care 368
    in handovers 61
    in remote practice 37
confounding variables 5
consciousness assessment
    AVPU (Alert-Voice-Pain-Unresponsiveness) score 109
    Glasgow Coma Scale 261
consent/informed consent 35
    for airway suctioning 305
    and animal products 192
    for medication administration 376, 392, 394,
        396, 397, 398, 400
    for moving and handling 257
    and organ donation 361
    and personal care 140

for tube feeding 182, 183
constipation 24, 91, 216, 243, 246, 356, 357
continence 211, 213–16
   and mental health 244–5
   tips for promotion and management 245–6
   see also incontinence
continuous feeding 182–3
Continuous Positive Airway Pressure (CPAP)
    machine
   and palliative care planning 358
   and pressure damage 161
   for sleep apnoea 129, 129*f*
control groups 6
controlled before and after studies 7
controlled drugs 380–1
   storage 388
controlled trial without randomisation 7
cooling mattresses 367–8
co-ordination testing 98, 100, 101
corticosteroids 301
Covid-19 pandemic 314, 315, 321, 329
   'burn-out' syndrome 46
   and end of life care 361–2
   and limits on non-verbal communication 56
   and remote consultations 36, 37, 39–40
crackles (chest) 84
cranial nerves examination 92–4, 93*f*
   anatomy and physiology 92–3
critical illness 40–1
critical practice, pillars of 17
Crohn's disease 90, 237, 242, 392
Cruse Bereavement Support 363
crystalloids 192
cultural and religious factors
   and bladder/bowel conditions 242
   and body language 56
   and breathless self-assessment 290
   and colloid/blood products 192
   and diet and fluid intake 172, 177
   and end of life care 361, 362–3, 364, 368, 370
   and ethical dilemmas 36
   and hand hygiene 334
   ICU patient, case study 46
   and inhalers 407
   and personal care 141
   and personal care, case study 141
   and shaving 147
   and urine colour 217
Cumberlege Report (1986) 382
cyanosis 289
cyclizine 204, 355, 356

Data Protection Laws 37
death 351–2
   care of the body after 367–71
   four post-mortem stages 367
   timeline of nursing decision from urgent to
      planned 359*t*
   verification 354
decision making

clinical reasoning and 30–3
   ethical dilemmas in assessment and 35–6
decontamination 339–40, 339*t*
defaecation 211
dehydration 179, 188–91
   factors contributing to 189*t*
   and heart rate 110
   older adults 176
   and osmotic pressure 175
   responding to and managing 189–91
   and risk of falls 260
   signs and symptoms 189*t*
   see also intravenous (IV) fluid therapy
Della-Monica, C. 125
dementia 24, 216, 245, 257, 310
   Admiral nurses 365–6
   and end of life care 361, 362, 365–6
   eating and drinking assistance 179
   and remote consultations 40
   see also Alzheimer's disease
denture care 146
   deceased persons 370
Department of Health 121
Department of Health and Social Care 156
dependent patients
   hair care 152
   moving and handling 257
depression
   and bladder/bowel conditions 237, 243–4
   and poor sleep 124
   and psilocybin 382
Deprivation of Liberty Safeguards (DoLs) 120,
      121, 257, 392
dermatones 96–8, 97*f*, 99
dermis 138
descriptive phenomenology 11
descriptive study design 11
deterioration, identifying signs 106–16
   'baseline' considerations 107
   blood pressure 110–12, 111*f*
   consciousness level (AVPU score) 109
   heart rate 109–10
   NEWS2 107, 108*f*
   NEWS2 calculation 114–15, 115*f*
   NEWS2 escalation of care 115–16, 116*f*
   oxygen saturations 112–13
   respiratory rate 109
   temperature 113
diabetes 139, 165, 199, 219, 411
   and ketones in urine 220
   and urination increase 220
diabetic foot ulceration 154*t*
diagnostic test terms 13–15
diamorphine 356, 380
diarrhoea 201, 220, 329
   degree of associated dehydration in children 190*t*
   giardiasis 323
diastole 86
diffusion 285–6, 287, 288
digestion 174

digestive system 173f, 174
dignified care 121, 132
    case study 124
dignity 120–3
    and after death care 369, 370
    as merit 120
    of all human beings (Menschenwürde) 120
    of morality 120
    and personal care 140, 141
    of personality 120
disinfectant wipes 338
disinfection 338–9
diuresis 211
do not attempt cardiopulmonary resuscitation
        (DNACPR) 351, 355, 360
documentation 59
    aid for fallen patients 263–4
    and end of life care 363, 371
    digital/electronic 33, 59, 383–4
    hardcopy 33, 59
    medication administration 389
    prescriptions 383–4
    pressure damage assessment 160
    remote consultations 37–8
DRE (digital rectal examination) 211, 240–1
dressing 144
    deceased persons 370
DRF (digital removal of faeces) 211, 240–1
droplet transmission 328
drug calculations 385–7
    errors 385, 419–21
    IV infusions 386–7
    liquids 386
    PEACE 386
    units of measurement 385t
drug history (DHx, Meds) 74–5
drug toxicity 220
drugs
    classification 378–80, 378t
    harms reduction approach 381
    vs. medication 377
    recreational 75
    reform in Portugal 381
    regulation 378–82
dry powder inhalers 404, 404f
dying
    physiological changes 353, 353f
    recognition of 353–4
dyspnoea 288, 290 see also breathlessness
dysuria 211

Early Warning Systems 107 see also NEW2
ecstasy 378
Edgar, A. 120
elderly patients see older adults
electrocardiogram (ECG) 101–4
    ambulatory 102
    how to perform 101–3
    morphology 102
    procedure 103

resting 101
    stress/exercise 101
    12-lead 102
electrolyte imbalance 195, 215
elimination 211
    bladder 213, 215
    bowel 216
Ellis, P. 17
emails 53
embarrassment
    as communication barrier 52, 66
    and personal care 140
emotional pain 123
    at end of life 363–4
empathy 54
    vs. sympathy 54
empirical knowledge 16
empowering others 17
end of life care 349–72
    anatomy and physiology 353–7, 353f
    care of the body after death 367–71
    case studies 355, 366
    communication and cultural e
        xpectation 362–3
    definition 352
    law applied to 359–62
    medications considered 355–7
    palliative care planning 357–9
    recognition of death 367
    specialist roles and organizations in the
        community 363–7
    spiritual care 363–4
    vs. palliative care 352
endogenous infections 316
enemas 238, 401
    administering 239–40
enteric coating 392
enuresis 211
environment
    as communication barrier 52–3, 66
    ICU assessment 42
    and sleep 125, 131
epidermis 137
EPMA (electronic prescription and medication
        administration) 391
Epworth sleepiness scale 129, 130t
equipment, safe management 337–40
    cleaning 337–8
    decontamination 339–40, 339t
    disinfection 338–9
    'single use' medical devices 340
    sterilisation 339
erythema 157, 159, 162, 238, 422f
escalation care planning (ECP) 358, 360
Escherichia coli (E.coli) 320f
ethical committees 6
ethical knowledge 16
ethics
    and advanced care plans/ethical care plans 360
    case studies 6, 35

dilemmas in assessment and decision
    making 35–6
  shift during Covid-19 361
ethnography 10
eversion 254
evidence-based practice 4–23, 25
  appraising evidence 21–3
  beyond scientific research 15–17
  hierarchy of evidence 4, 4f
  researching evidence 18–21
  study design 5–12
  understanding common test terms 13–15
evidence sources 16–17
exogenous infections 316
expert committees 12
extended-release products 392–3
extension 99, 254
external rotation 254
extracellular fluid (ECF) 174–5
eye 149f
eye care 148–50

facemasks (medical/surgical) 335
facemasks (oxygen therapy)
  simple 293, 294f, 296t
  reservoir (non-rebreathe) 294, 295f, 296t
  Venturi 294
facial hair 148
falls 258–70
  case studies 259, 265–6
  conditions leading to 258–60
  consequences 260–3
  emergency care following injury 264–6, 265f
  helping a patient to stand 264
  HoverJack use 268–70
  minimal aid for fallen patient 263–4
  patient becoming violent and aggressive 266–7
false negatives 13, 13f
false positives 13, 13f
Farrel, C. 17
Fawcett, T. 72
febrile 322, 323
feeding devices 182
feeding methods via NG/NJ/PEG 182–3
Female Genital Mutilations Act (2003) 402
fentanyl 356
'first do not harm' 361
flexion 99, 254
flora 315–16
  function in the body 317
  skin 331, 333, 408
  normal distribution in the body 317f
  see also commensals
Flucloxacillin 187–8
fluid intake and output
  case study 199
  recording fluid balance 195–9
  recommended daily intake 196–7, 196t, 197t, 215
fluid retention (oedema) 87, 161, 199–200
  case study 199–200

management 199
  signs and symptoms 199
fluids 174–5
foot care 150–1
fractional exhaled nitric oxide (FENO) 302
fractures 262–3, 266
  categories 263
  patterns 263
full body assessment 79–101
  cardiovascular auscultation 84–8, 85f
  chest auscultation 81–4
  cranial nerves examination 92–4, 93f
  gait assessment 80–1
  neurological examination 95–101, 95f, 97f, 98f
  gastrointestinal examination 88–92, 89f
fungi 315, 316f, 323–5

gait 80
  assessment 80
gall bladder 212
gas transport 287
gastrointestinal examination 88–92, 89f
  case study 91–2
  findings 90–1
General Practitioner (GP) surgeries, remote care 36
giardiasis 323
Gijsberts, M. J. H. E. 363
Gilbert, H. 17
Gillick Competency 392
Glaister, A. 17
Glaser, B. G. 11
Glasgow Coma Scale 261
gloves 335–6
  sterile vs. non-sterile 166, 336
  torn/contaminated 337
glucose in urine 219
Glynn, H. 242
graduated crying (Ferber method) 126
Gram staining 318–19
grounded theory 11

haemofiltration 215
haemoglobin 46, 112, 217, 287, 291
hair care 143, 152–3
  deceased persons 370
haloperidol 356, 357
hand care 150–1
hand hygiene 330–4
  after death care 369
  community perspective 334
  equality and diversity considerations 334
  five moments 331–2
  three levels 332–3t
hand washing 330, 332, 334, 345
handovers 60–2, 62t
  case study 59–60
  SBAR format 61, 62, 62t
Hare, R. D. 10
Hartmann's solution 192
head injuries 261

head trauma 266
Health and Social Care Act (2008) 329
Health and Social Care Act Regulations (2014) 252
health care associated infections (HCAIs) 314–15, 316, 319, 331
  minimising incidence 343
hearing impairments 37, 40, 53, 60, 66, 141
heart 85f see also cardiovascular auscultation
heart rate 109–10
heart sounds, identifying 87
Heat and Moisture Exchange (HME) filters 298
heel pressure ulcers 139, 163
Heidegger, M. 11
hepatitis 321–2, 342
hepatitis A 321
hepatitis B 321–2, 342, 381
hepatitis C 322
hepatitis D 322
hepatitis E 322
herbal/complementary preparations 377, 378
hidden curriculum 1
hierarchy of evidence 4, 4f
history of presenting complaint (HPC, HxPC) 73–4
history taking 72–9
  drug history (DHx, Meds) 74–5
  format 72
  history of presenting complaint (HPC, HxPC) 73–4
  pain assessment 75–7, 76f
  past medical history (PMHx) 74
  presenting complaint (PC) 73
  psychiatric/mental health history 77
  social history (SH, SHx) 75
  suicide/self-harm signs 77–9, 78f
holistic needs 352
Holton, G. J. 10
Hombali, A. 130
homelessness 40
HoverJack use 268–70
Human Medicines Act Regulations (2015) 381
Human Tissue Act (2004) 361
Human Transplant (Wales) Act (2013) 361
humidification 298
Husserl, E. 11
hydration 172, 177, 205
  assisting patients with drinking 179–81
  fluids 174–5
  intravenous (IV) fluid therapy 191–5
  nausea and vomiting 200–205
  recording fluid intake and output 195–9
  and stool quality 217
  see also dehydration
hydrolysis 175
hydrostatic pressure 175
hygiene 136, 139–53, 167, 316
  assessment of needs 140
  bathing 142–3
  communication 139–40, 141
  dignity and privacy 140
  dressing 144

eye care 148–50
hair care 143, 152–3
management of needs 139–41
nail, hand and foot care 150–1
oral care 144–7
risk assessment 140
shaving 147–8
spiritual and cultural preferences, case study 141
see also hand hygiene; respiratory and cough hygiene
hypercapnia 83, 114, 288
hypercapnic respiratory failure 112, 291, 293, 295
hyperkalaemia 220
hyperpnoea 354
hyperreflexia 99
hypodermis 138
hyponatremia 220
hypoxaemia 288, 290, 291
hypoxia 288, 290, 301, 305, 306

I-Am-A-STAR 77
ICU settings
  assessment of patients 40–1
  case study 46
  colleagues 46
  environmental assessments and safety checks 42
  family/friends 45–6
  holistic, individualised approach to assessment 44–6
  risk assessment 45
  systems-based assessment 42–4, 42–3t
  unexpected deaths 351
ileostomy 235, 238
illegal drugs 380–2
immune system 125, 316, 321, 322
incidence 7
incontinence 211, 213–14
  and Alzheimer's disease, case study 245
  and catheterisation 164, 224, 224
  and depression and anxiety 244
  factors increasing risk 214
  and learning disability 244
  and moisture lesions 163–4
  older adults 210
  support without catheter 224–5
  types 214
  and urine output measurement 197
independent mental capacity advocates (IMCAs) 359–60
independent prescribers 383
indirect transmission 328
individual involvement in healthcare 17
infants/babies
  airway suctioning 306
  amount of sleep needed 126
  breastfeeding 175
  breathlessness signs 290
  care of the body after death 367–8
  chest auscultation 83
  moving and handling 254–5

oral intake reduction, case study 199
oropharyngeal (OP) airways 303
recommended fluid intake 196–7, 197t
sleep routine 126
tube feeding 182, 183, 185–6, 187
unexpected deaths 352
vomiting 201
weaning 176
infection/inflammation
and bladder/bowel health 220
and increased heart rate 110
infection prevention and management 313–46
advice for visitors, case study 344
aseptic non touch techniques (ANTT) 166, 167,
192, 317, 344–5
blood and body fluid spillages 342
chain of infection 327, 327f
hand hygiene 330–4
health care associated infections (HCAIs) 314–15,
316, 319, 331, 343
infection risk, definitions 329–30
microbiology 315–25, 316f, 317f, 318f, 319t, 320t
occupational safety: prevention and exposure
management 343
patient assessment for infection risk 329–30
personal protective equipment (PPE) 140, 211,
335–7, 342
physical and biochemical barriers 317f
respiratory and cough hygiene 334–7
risk 329–30
routes of transmission 327–8
safe disposal of sharps 342–3
safe management of care equipment 337–40
safe management of care environment 340
safe management of linen, 341–2
signs and symptoms of infection 326f
standard infection control precautions (SICP) 328
virulence 325–6, 326f
inflammatory bowel disease (IBD) 90, 242, 243
and suicidality 244
influenza 334
informed consent see consent
ingestion 174
inhaled/pulmonary medication 403–7
injections and infusions 407–19
skin preparation 408
insensible fluid loss 175, 197
insomnia 124, 127–8
case study 124
intensivists 41
intercostal space 102, 103
internal (medial) rotation 254
interpretive (hermeneutic) phenomenology 11
interrupted time series studies 7
intervention 5
intervention groups 6
intimate examinations, remote 38–9
intracellular fluid (ICF) 174
intradermal injections 408–9
intramuscular injections 412–15

muscle sites 413f
Z-track 415
intravenous (IV) fluid therapy 191–5
5 Rs 191
types of fluids 191–2
intravenous (IV) medication 415–19
bolus injection 419
flow rate and drop rate 386–7
intravenous (IV) infusion 418–9
preparation of bolus and infusion 416
push administration 417, 419
risks of infusions 415t
Visual Infusion Phlebitis score 416t
intussusception 201
inversion 254
irritant/allergic reactions 395, 395t
ischaemia 158

jargon or abbreviations 55, 65
jaundice 90
Jehovah's Witnesses 46
Jewish people 360
joints 253

Keenan, P. 244
KENHUB 96
keratinocytes 137
ketones in urine 220, 221
kidneys 212
knowing, patterns of 15–16
Korotkoff sounds 111–12, 111f

language barriers
and advice on infection 344
and 'dip stick' test 220
and non-verbal communication 55
and remote consultations 39, 40
large intestine 212, 217
Lasting Power of Attorney (LPA) 358, 360
for health and welfare 359, 360
for property and financial affairs 360
learning/cognitive disability
and advice on infection 344
and communication 198
and incontinence 244
and legs assessment 81
and needle fear 407, 408
and non-verbal communication 55
and past medical history 74
and personal care 140
and remote consultations 39, 40
and self-injection 411–12
and sleep deprivation 128
see also communication difficulties
leukocytes in urine 219
Levett-Jones, T. 31
levomepromazine 356, 357
Levy, Joseph 365
ligaments 253–4, 262
linen, safe management 341–2

clean 341
   infectious linen 341
   used 341
listening 54
   active 57
liver 212
local evidence 17
longitudinal studies 9
The Loop 381–2
loss of appetite, hypothetical scenario 24
lower limb neurological testing 100–1
lumbar flexion 81
lung cancer 9, 309
lungs 284, 286*f*
lymphatic system 213

making a difference 17
malaria 322–3
malignant wounds and fungating tumours 154*t*
malnutrition 179
   and risk of falls 259–60
Malnutrition Universal Screening Tool (MUST)
   177, 178
Mansel, B. 77
Manual Handling Operation Regulations Act
   (1992) 255
Marie Curie 352
medial malleolus 102, 103
medical records and remote consultations 37–8
Medical Research Council Dyspnoea scale 288, 290*t*
medication administration 375–424
   administration routes 390–419
   adverse drug reaction (ADR) 421
   calculation errors 385, 419–21
   drug calculations 386–7
   enteral tubes 187–8, 393
   Five Rights 388–9
   given, withheld or denied 389
   injections and infusions 407–19
   medication vs. drugs 377
   nasal sprays/drops 395–6
   optic drops 397–8
   oral 391–2
   ottic drops 396–7
   provision to patients 383–4
   pulmonary/inhaled 403–7
   rectal (per rectum) 240, 399–401, 399*f*
   self-administration 390, 403
   regulation 378–82
   side effects, allergic and anaphylactic
      reactions 422–3
   storage and handling 387–8, 388*t*
   topical and transdermal 393–5, 393*f*
   vaginal 401–3, 401*f*
   what medication is 377–8
   who can prescribe and how 382–3
   see also enemas; suppositories
medications
   analgesic 123, 356
   and decline in mobility 272*t*

and end of life care 355–7
and heart rate 110
nausea and vomiting, causing 202
nausea and vomiting, managing 204
and polyuria 216
and urine colour 217–18
and wound healing 165
Medicine and Healthcare Products Regulatory
   Agency (MHRA) 377, 378, 379, 421
Medicines Act (1968) 378–80, 381
   categories of medication 379*t*
melanocytes 137
Mental Capacity Act (MCA, 2005) 182, 257,
   359, 360, 392
   Code of Practice 360
mental health
   and bowel/bladder health 241–6
   and falls 265–6
   psychiatric/mental health history 77
   and risk of falling 259
   and sleep disorders 130
mental state examination (MSE) 259
meta-analysis 5
meta-ethnography 10–11
meta-synthesis 10–11
metoclopramide 356
microbiology 315–25
   main groups of microorganisms 316*f*
micturition 211, 213, 215
mid-axillary line 102, 103
midazolam 355, 357
migraine 321
mindfulness 243
Misuse of Drugs Act 380
MMR vaccine 12
mobility and safety 251–79
   anatomy and physiology 253–4
   causes of decline in mobility 272*t*
   falls, risk management and moving and
      handling techniques 258–70
   moving and handling children and infants 254–5
   moving and handling equipment to support
      people with impaired mobility 270–8
   moving and handling plans 252
   moving and handling risk assessment 255–6
   moving and handling risk assessment, case study 256
   patient categorisation on level of assistance
      needed 271
   Positive Eight 252
   safety techniques and devices 256–8
moisture lesions 153*t*, 163–5
   vs. pressure damage 164–5
morphine 355, 356
Morse, A. M. 131
mouth 145*f*
   candida infection 145, 324
   see also oral care
moving and handling *see* mobility and safety
muscle power 95–6, 99, 100
   MRC scale 95*f*, 96

muscle tone 95, 99, 100
muscles 253
musculoskeletal system 253
Muslims 141, 217, 334, 368, 407
mycosis 324

nail care 151
naloxone 381
narcolepsy 128
nasal cannula 293, 293f, 296t
nasal sprays/drops 395–6
nasal suctioning 308–9
nasogastric (NG) feeding tubes 181–8, 393
    factors to consider 187–8
    feeding/medication via 187–8
    feeding methods 182–3
    insertion and removal - adult 183–4
    insertion and removal - infant/child 185–6
    medication via 187–8, 193
    and pressure damage 162
    risks associated with insertion 187
    tubes in situ 186f
nasojejunal (NJ) tube 182, 393
    feeding methods 182–3
nasopharyngeal (NP) airways 304, 403f
National Council for Palliative Care 364
National Infection Prevention and Control Manual 342
National Institute for Health Research (NIHR)
    report 58
National Institute of Health and Care Excellence
        (NICE) 17, 106–7, 162, 192, 243, 301, 352
    Chronic Pain Guidelines 123
    5 Rs of fluid therapy 191
National Patient Safety Agency (NPSA) 181
National standards of healthcare cleanliness 340
nausea and vomiting 200–5
    assessing 203
    case study 204–55
    common causes 200–1t
    control and treatment 202
    end of life care 356
    medications that can cause 202
    non-pharmaceutical management 205
    pharmaceutical management 205
    post-operative 202
    vomiting in babies and children 201
nebulisers 302, 405, 405f
    vs. inhalers for children with asthma 302
needle fear 407
negative fluid balance 196
negative predictive value 14–15
negative pressure therapy 154–6
Neisseria meningitis 320f
neonates, infection risk 330
neurological examination 95–101, 95f, 97f, 98f
neurotransmitters 204
NEWS2 107, 108f, 112, 291
    calculating 114–15, 115f
    escalation of care 115–16, 116f
NEWT guidelines 392, 393

NHS 36, 301, 366
nitrates in urine 219
Noblit G. W. 10
nocturia 211
non-randomised controlled trials 7
non-verbal communication 55–6, 139, 140, 141
    and end of life care 363
Nordenfelt, L. 120
Normal Saline 192, 195
NREM (Non-Rapid Eye Movement) sleep 125
Nurse Prescribers 382–3, 382t
Nursing and Midwifery Council (NMC) 121
    'Care and respect every time' 122–3
    The Code 23, 122, 254, 359, 360, 361, 368, 420–1
    standards of proficiency 4, 24, 29, 382
    standards of proficiency covered in present
        volume 71, 119, 135, 171, 209, 251, 283,
        313, 315, 349, 375
nursing formula 386
nursing in action 24–5
Nursing Process 30, 30f, 41
    clinical reasoning in 32f
nutrition 172, 177, 205
    anatomy and physiology 173–4, 173f
    assisting patients with eating 179–81
    assisting patients with eating, case study 181
    nasogastric feeding tubes 181–8
    nausea and vomiting 200–5
    needs across lifespans/cultures 175–7
    nutritional assessment 177–8
    patient not eating, nursing in action 24–5
    total parenteral nutrition (TPN) 192

obesity, and risk of falls 259
observational study design 8, 9
occupational safety, prevention and exposure
        management 343
odds ratio 7, 8
    formula for calculating 8f
oedema see fluid retention
older adults
    aspiration pneumonia 200
    constipation risks 216
    COPD 292
    death in care settings 352
    dehydration risk 189–91
    falls 258, 260, 261
    incontinence 210
    malnutrition risk 260
    nutritional needs 176
    past medical history 74
    remote consultations 39, 40
    UTI detection 222–3
ondansetron 356
open and closed questions 57, 57t
opioids 356
optic drops 397–8
    case study 398
oral administration of medication 391–2
    enteral tube 187–8, 393

release 392–3
oral care 144–7
  deceased persons 370
oral suctioning 306–8
  Yankauer suction catheter 306f
organ donation 361
Organ Donation (Deemed Consent) Act (2019) 361
organic brain disorders, and risk of falls 258–9
Orlando, I. J. 30
oropharyngeal (OP) airways 302f, 303, 303f
osmotic pressure 175
Ostaszkiewicz, J. 242
osteoporosis 18, 21, 23, 421
ottic drops 396–7
ovarian cancer 355
oxycodone 356
oxygen 284, 285, 286–7
oxygen saturations 112–13, 291
oxygen therapy 290–8
  case study 291–2
  children and patients with complex needs 296
  commencing, managing, and discontinuing
    297–8
  devices and equipment 292–6, 296t
  and pressure damage 161

pain 123–4
  case study 124
  as communication barrier 29–30, 52, 66
  end of life care 355–6
  and non-verbal communication 139
  physical and emotional 119
  and soft tissue injury 262
pain assessment 75–7
  children 76, 76f
  patients with communication difficulties 76–7
  SOCRATES 75
pain management 123, 132
  following falls 266
pain sensation 96, 100, 101
palliative care 352
  definition 352
  vs. end of life care 352
  law applied to 359–62
  planning 357–9, 359t
  specialist roles and organizations in the
    community 364–7
palliative care/end of life care (EoLC), definition 352
pancreas 212
pancreatic cancer 6
paracetamol overdoses 77
passive hoists and slings 275–8, 275f, 277f
  use to mobilise person from bed to chair 276–7
past medical history (PMHx) 74
patches (medication) 394
  irritant/allergic reactions 395, 395t
pathophysiology 365
patient advocates 44
patient-centred/person-centred care 17, 29, 30,
  172, 364

patient group direction (PGD) 295, 379,
  380, 383, 391
patient information for assessment 33–5
patient specific direction (PSD) 383
patients' and carers' knowledge 16–17
peak expiratory flow measurement 298–302
  case study 300–1
  peak flow meter 299f
PEO (Population-Exposure-Outcome)
  format 19
Percutaneous Endoscope Gastronomy (PEG) tube
  182, 393
  feeding methods 182–3
percutaneous exposure 328
peristalsis 174, 211
peristomal 211
peristomal skin conditions 237–8
person-to-person transmission 328
personal knowledge 16
personal protective equipment (PPE) 140,
  211, 335–7, 342
  tips 337
personalised care and support plan 352
PH, urine 219
pharmacokinetics 240, 392
pharmacovigilance 380, 421
phenomenology 11
PICO (Population-Intervention-Comparison-
  Outcome) format 5, 18–19
placebo effect 6
plaster casts, and pressure damage 161
pleural rub 84
polyuria 211, 216
POM (prescription only medication) 379t, 391
populations 8, 9
positive fluid balance 196
positive predictive value 14–15
post-surgery eating and drinking assistance 179
PPE see personal protective equipment
PR (per rectum) 211, 240
precordial 102
prescriptions 383
presenting complaint (PC) 73
pressure damage/pressure ulcers 153t, 156–63
  adjunct equipment 160–1
  body map with pressure points 158f
  device related 161–3
  initial skin assessment 157
  vs. moisture lesions 164–5
  patient experience 139
  pressure ulcer definition 156
  pressure ulcer grades 159t
  pressure ulcer treatment 163
  risk assessment 159–60
pressurised metered dose inhalers 403–4, 403f
prevalence 7
prions 315, 316f
privacy
  and after death care 368, 369
  and handovers 61

and personal care 140
and skin assessment for pressure damage 157
procedure pads 164
pronation 254
propagate 324
prospective studies 9
proteins in urine 219
protozoa 315, 316f, 322
PU (passed urine) 211
pulse oximetry 112, 291
pulse rate 110
PVR (post void residual) 211
pyloric stenosis 201

qualitative data 10
    analysis 10
qualitative studies 11, 21
    PEO format 19
quantitative data 10
quasi-experimental design 7

Ramipril 204, 334
randomised controlled trials (RCTs) 5–6
    double-blind 6
recreational drugs 75
    see also controlled drugs; illegal drugs
rectal administration of medication 399–401, 399f
reflex arc 98f
reflex testing 98–9, 100, 101
regurgitation (heart valves) 86
relationships
    developing nurse-patient 53–4
    forging, and critical practice 17
relative risk 8
    calculating 9f
religion 364 see also cultural and religious
        differences
REM (Rapid Eye Movement) sleep 125
remote consultations 36–40
    confidentiality 37
    limitations of 39–40
    medical records and documentation 37–8
    new experiences 38
    patient assessment 33, 38
    physical assessment/examination 38–9
    safety-netting and aftercare plan 39, 39t
renal system 213f
repositioning 162
    end of life 357
research evidence 16
resistance (airways) 285, 288
respiration 288
    external 285–7, 287f
    internal 287, 287f
respiratory and cough hygiene 334–5
    use of masks 335
respiratory care 283–311
    airway devices 302–4
    airway suctioning 305–9, 306f
    anatomy and physiology 284–8

breathlessness assessment 288–90, 289t, 290t
fractional exhaled nitric oxide (FENO) 302
humidification 298
oxygen therapy 290–8
peak expiratory flow measurement 298–302, 299f
sputum sample 309–10, 309t
respiratory rate 83, 109
respiratory system 285f
    overview and function 284
respiratory tract infections 309, 314
respiratory tract secretion, at end of life 356–7
rest 119, 124, 125, 132
Restless Leg Syndrome (RSL) 128
Resuscitation Council 423
retching 200
retraction and protraction 254
retrospective studies 8, 9
Rhynas, S. 72
RICE (Rest-Ice-Compression-Elevation) 216–2, 266
rigours 322, 323
ringworm 325
Risk of Death and Severe Harm from Ingesting
        Superabsorbent Polymer Gel Granules 342
routine investigations 101–6
    electrocardiogram (ECG) 101–4
    venipuncture 104–6
Royal College of General Practitioners 39
Royal College of Nursing (RCN) 336, 419
    principles 121, 122f
Royal Pharmaceutical Society (RPS) 419
Roycroft-Malone, J. 16, 25

SADPERSONS scale 78–9, 78f
SBAR format 61, 62, 62t
search strategies 18–21, 18f
    research question 18–19
    keywords 19
    refining search 19–20
    sources 20
    output 20
sedation
    risk assessment 45
    terminal agitation 357
self-awareness 57
self-harm 77
    types 77
sensation testing 96–8, 99–100, 100–1
sensible fluid loss 175, 197
sensitivity (of tests) 13, 14–15
serum osmolality 190
service user zone 332
sharps, safe disposal 342–3
shaving 147–8
    deceased persons 370
Sherratt, R. 191
side effects 422
sign language 59
silver surfers 40
skin
    anatomy and physiology 136–9, 394

changes in dying process 354
functions 139
layers 137, 138f, 393f, 410f
reactions in allergy 422f
structure 137f
SKIN bundle 160
skin integrity 136, 153–67
moisture lesions 163–5
peristomal skin conditions 237–8
pressure damage 156–65, 158f, 159t
wound treatment 154–6, 165–7
wound types 153, 153–4t
skin tone
and allergic reactions 422
and cyanosis 289
and erythema 157, 159
sleep 124–32
amount needed 126
bedtime routine 126–7
and depression, case study 124
'a good night's sleep' 125
quality in hospitals 130–1
quality in hospitals, case study 130
what it is 125
sleep apnoea 128
case study 128–9
Continuous Positive Airway Pressure (CPAP)
machine 129, 129f
sleep deprivation/insomnia 127–8
sleep disturbances/disorders 128–30
sleep hygiene 131–2
slide sheets 271f, 273–5, 369
small intestine 211
SMART plans 420
smoking 7, 9, 75, 292, 309
SOCRATES 75
social history (SH, SHx) 75
sodium (Na) balance 215
soft mist inhalers 404f, 405
soft tissue damage 261–2
soft touch 96, 99–100
somatisation 123
specificity (of tests) 13–14, 14–15
SPICE 19
SPIDER 19
SPIKES 63–4
spinal cord injuries (SCI) 260
spinal examination, post trauma 267
spine assessment 81
spiritual care, at end of life 363–4
sprains, classification 262
sputum sample 309–10
sputum types and causes 309t
standard infection control precautions
(SICP) 328, 331
staphylococcus aureus 319, 320f, 333
stenosis 86
sterilisation 339
stoma care 234–8
after death 370

case study 237
changing/emptying colostomy bag 235–6
faecal diversion 234–5
peristomal skin conditions 237–8
stomas 211, 213, 234
sizing 235
stomach 211, 212f
Strauss, A. L. 11
streptococcus 320f
stress, and gastrointestinal disorders 242–3
stridor 84
structural racism 17
study design 5–12
Level 1: systematic review and meta-analysis 5
Level 2: randomised controlled trials (RCTs) 5–6
Level 3: well-deigned controlled trials without
randomisation 7
Level 4: case control and cohort studies 7–8
Level 5: meta-synthesis 10–11
Level 6: case study or qualitative study 11
Level 7: opinions of authorities or expert
committees 12
subcutaneous 324
subcutaneous injections 410–12, 410f
subcutaneous mycosis 324
subjects (experimental) 5
subjective-objective data 33–4, 33t
suicidal ideation/suicidality 78
and IBD 244
suicide risk assessment 78–9, 78f
superficial mycosis 324
supinations 254
supplementary prescribers 383
suppositories 238, 400
administering 239–40
surgical scrub 333
surgical wounds 154t
after death care 370
swallowing difficulties 179
sympathy vs. empathy 54
syringe drivers 355
systematic reviews 5
PICO model 5
systems reviews 73–4
systemic mycosis 324
systole 86

tablets 391, 391f
spitting and crushing 391–2
teeth brushing 146–7
temperature taking 113
tendons 253–4
terminal agitation 357
Thalidomide 378
thematic analysis 10
thyroid pathology, and heart rate 110
time constraints, as communication barrier 66
TIME principle 165
topical medication 391
Topical Negative Pressure (TNP) therapy 154–6

total parenteral nutrition (TPN) 192
transgender patients 11, 148, 259
transmission based precautions (TBPs) 343
Traumatic Brain Injury (TBI) 261
trigeminal nerve divisions 93f
true negatives 13, 13f
true positives 13, 13f
TWOC (trial without catheter) 211, 233
tympanic thermometers 113

unconscious patients
    hair care 152
    oral care 145–6
    oropharyngeal (OP) airways 303
UNICEF 175
United Nations Convention on the Rights of the
    Child (1989) 175
upper limb neurological examination 99–100
urinalysis ('dip stick' test) 219–23
    reagent strip/result 222, 222f
    taking a midstream specimen of urine (MSU)
        and 221–2
urinary retention 223, 357
    nursing in action 24
urinary tract infection (UTI) detection in older
        adults and catheter users 222–3
urine
    clarity 219
    colour 217–18, 218–19t
    odour 219
    osmolarity 219
urine output 197, 215
urobilin 217
urostomy 211, 234
    case study 234

vagina 401–2, 401f
vaginal administration of medication 402–3
    self-administration 403
validity 4
valve pathologies 86
venepuncture 104–6

venous leg ulcers 153t
ventilation (breathing) 284–5, 288
ventilators
    care bundle 45t
    importance of monitoring 41
verbal communication 55, 55t, 59
    at end of life 363
verbal orders (for medication) 384
violent patients 266–7
virtual assessment 33, 38–9
virtual private network system (VPN) 37
virulence 325–6, 326f
viruses 315, 316f, 321–2
visual impairment 40, 60, 149, 245
voiding 211
vomiting see nausea and vomiting

wafer preparations 391, 391f
Wakefield, A. 12
washing
    deceased persons 370
    see also bathing; hand washing
weaning 176
Wed Nos project 382
wheeze 83–4
Wong-Baker Pain Rating Scale 76, 76f
World Health Organisation (WHO) 61, 120, 131,
        175, 176, 190, 191, 323, 352, 356, 408
    5 Moments for Hand Hygiene 332
    Guidelines on Hand Hygiene 332
wounds
    assessing need for cleaning 166
    clean vs. sterile technique 165–6
    dressing 167
    nursing in action 24, 25
    simple dressing and suture removal 167
    sterile gloves debate 166
    treatment 165–7
    types 153, 153–4t

yeast 324
Yellow Card Scheme 421